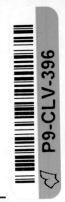

Nutrition Facts Manual

A Quick Reference

Nutrition Facts Manual

A Quick Reference

Abby Stolper Bloch, MS, RD
Maurice E. Shils, MD, ScD

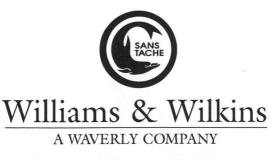

Williams & Wilkins

A WAVERLY COMPANY

BALTIMORE • PHILADELPHIA • LONDON • PARIS • BANGKOK
HONG KONG • MUNICH • SYDNEY • TOKYO • WROCLAW

1996

Executive Editor: Donna Balado
Development Editor: Victoria Vaughn
Production Coordinator: Marette D. Magargle
Book Project Editor: Susan Rockwell
Typesetting: Clarinda
Printing: Victor Graphics
Binding: Victor Graphics

Copyright © 1996
Williams & Wilkins
Rose Tree Corporate Center
1400 North Providence Road
Building II, Suite 5025
Media, PA 19063-2043 USA

Accurate indications, adverse reactions, and dosage schedules for drugs are provided in this book, but it is possible they may change. The reader is urged to review the package information data of the manufacturers of the medications mentioned.

Nutrition facts manual : a quick reference / editors, Maurice E.
  Shils, James A. Olson, Moshe Shike.
      p.   cm.
    Compilation of the appendices for Modern nutrition in health and
  disease. 8th ed. 1994.
    1. Nutrition--Tables.   I. Shils, Maurice E. (Maurice Edward),
  1914-   . II. Olson, James A.   III. Shike, Moshe.   IV. Modern
  nutrition in health and disease.
    [DNLM: 1. Nutritional Requirements--tables.   2. Nutritive Value-
  -tables.   QU 16 N9755 1995]
  QP141.N779   1995
  613.2--dc20
  DNLM/DLC
  for Library of Congress   95-36795
                                                            CIP

Printed in the United States of America

The Publishers have made every effort to trace the copyright holders for borrowed material. If they have inadvertently overlooked any, they will be pleased to make the necessary arrangements at the first opportunity.

                                        96 97 98 99
                    1   2   3   4   5   6   7   8   9   10

Reprints of chapters may be purchased from Williams & Wilkins in quantities of 100 or more. Call Isabella Wise, Special Sales Department, (800) 358-3583.

PREFACE

Nutrition Facts Manual: A Quick Reference is a derivative publication of the Appendices of the 8th edition of Modern Nutrition in Health and Disease.

Surveys conducted by the Publisher have indicated support for a paper-backed separate publication of the material in the Appendices and we, the Editors of the 8th edition, have supported this concept. Donna Balado, Acquisitions Editor of Williams and Wilkins, made the suggestion which has led to this publication in a smaller format for easier transport and use.

Winston-Salem, North Carolina   Maurice E. Shils, MD, ScD
Ames, Iowa   James Allen Olson, PhD
New York, New York   Moshe Shike, MD

INTRODUCTION

The Nutrition Facts Manual-A Quick Reference offers some 150 tables, graphs, menus and guidelines designed to serve as ready references for the dietitian/nutritionist, physician, other health professionals, students, and science writers who need factual answers.

Each major topic with its subtopics is listed by title and page in the detailed table of contents.

The conversion tables between traditional units and those of the International System and other physical data are followed by recommended dietary intakes of the United States, World Health Organization and four other countries. Dietary guidelines from a number of industrialized or developed countries are presented as are growth standards and other anthropometric data by age and sex in five major tables and sub-tables. The nutrient contents of various beverages and foods are covered in seven tables and sub-tables. Major attention is also given to food exchanges by ethnic and racial backgrounds. A variety of therapeutic diets are presented in terms of their objectives and recommendations with sample menus and food values. Finally, there is miscellaneous material with metabolic data, effects of foods on drug absorptions and sources of enteral formulas.

Detailed nutrient composition data on individual oral and tube feeding formulations are not included because their frequent changes make printed formulas quickly obsolete: instead, Table A-37 lists types and names of various formulas with the addresses and phone numbers of sources that provide current detailed information.

The sources of information in the tables are indicated either by a source reference in the literature and/or to the appropriate chapter in the 8th edition of Modern Nutrition in Health and Disease.

New York, New York   Abby Stolper Bloch
Winston Salem, North Carolina   Maurice E. Shils

CONTENTS

A–12 ● PHYSICAL GROWTH STANDARDS

A–13 ● ADULT WEIGHTS AND HEIGHTS BY RACE, SEX, AGE, AND PERCENTILES

A—14 ● WEIGHT AND SKINFOLD ● THICKNESS DATA

A—15 ● BODY FAT ESTIMATIONS FROM SKINFOLD DATA

*Table added to Appendices since publication of the 8th edition of *Modern Nutrition in Health and Disease.*

*Table added to Appendices since publication of the 8th edition of *Modern Nutrition in Health and Disease.*

TABLE A—1A. CONVERSION FACTORS BETWEEN TRADITIONAL AND SI UNITS

Factors for converting nutrients expressed in metric or millequivalent units into International System (SI) units.

1. Definitions

   a. Equivalent weight (EW) = atomic weight of element/valence of ionic form. Example with magnesium: atomic wt = 24, valence = 2+; therefore EW = 12

   b. Quantity of an electrolyte in milliequivalents per liter (mEq/1) = mg of electrolyte/L/EW. Example: 48 mg of magnesium/L/12 = 4 mEq/L

   c. Quantity of an electrolyte in mg/dl = (mEq/L ×EW)/10

   d. To convert mg/dl (= mg%) of an electrolyte to mEq/L mg/dl ×10/EW = mEq/L

   e. 1 mol = 1 molecular or atomic weight of element or compound in grams (GMWt). In solutions this is usually expressed as moles per liter; i.e., 1 mol/L = 1 M; 1 mM (mmol) = 1 mol $\times 10^{-3}$; 1 μM (μmol) = 1 mol $\times 10^{-6}$; 1 nM (nmol) = 1 mol $\times 10^{-9}$

   f.
      (1) To convert mEq/L of an electrolyte or other ions in solution to mmol/L: mEq/L divided by valence = mmol/L; e.g., (a) 2 mEq/L of magnesium (Mg^{2+}) = 2/2 = 1 mmol/L; e.g., (b) 140 mEq Na^+/L = 140/L = 140 mmol/L

      (2) To convert mg/dl to mmol/L: (mg/dl ×10/EW) divided by valence = mmol/L; e.g.,
      2 mg/dl of magnesium = (2 ×10/12) divided by 2 = 0.83 mmol/L

      (3) For organic substances: mmol/L = wt in mg/L/MW (in mg)

2. SI units for expressing clinical laboratory data

   These units are now widely used and are increasingly required for publication of scientific data in physical, biologic, and biomedical publications. Extensive SI conversion tables have been published together with an explanation of the rationale for their use and technical aspects of usage.[1-3]

   a. The base units of interest in physical quantities used in clinical chemistry are:

Quantity	Base Unit
mass	kilogram
time	second
amount	mole
length	meter

   A derived unit for energy is the kjoule(kJ) 4.18 kJ = 1 kcal
   1 MJ = 239 kcal

   b. Prefixes and symbols for decimal multiples and submultiples include:

Factor	Prefix	Symbol	Factor	Prefix	Symbol
10^9	giga	G	10^{-3}	milli	m
10^6	mega	M	10^{-6}	micro	u
10^3	kilo	k	10^{-9}	nano	n
10^2	hecto	h	10^{-12}	pico	p
10^1	deka	da	10^{-15}	femto	f
10^{-1}	deci	d	10^{-18}	atto	a
10^{-2}	centi	c			

3. Conversion factors for selected compounds of nutrition interest*

Component	(1) Present Unit	(2) Conversion Factor	(3) SI Unit Symbol	(4) Mass Conversion Factor
Albumin (s)	g/dl	10	g/L	—
Aluminum (s)	μg/L	37.04	nmol/L	μg/27 = mol
Amino acids	(see ref. 3, p. 119 for individual amino acids)			
Amino acid nitrogen (p)	mg/dl	0.714	mmol/L	mg/14 = mmol
Ascorbic acid (p)	mg/dl	56.78	μmol/L	mg/176 = mmol
Calcium (s)	mg/dl	0.250	mmol/L	mg/40 = mmol
Calcium (s)	mEq/dl	0.500	mmol/L	mEq/2 = mmol
β-Carotene† (s)	μ/dl	0.0186	μmol/L	ug/536.85 umol
Chloride (s)	mEq/L	1.00	mmol/L	mEq = mmol
Cholesterol (p)	mg/dl	0.0259	mmol/L	mg/386.6 = mmol
Copper (s)	μg/dl	0.157	μmol/L	μg/63.5 = umol
Cyanocobalamin (B$_{12}$)	pg/ml	0.738	pmol/L	pg/1355 = pmol
Ethanol (p)	mg/dl	0.217	mmol/L	mg/46 = mmol
Folic acid	ng/ml	2.265	nmol/L	ng/441.4 = nmol
Glucose (p)	mg/dl	0.0555	mmol/L	mg/180.2 = mmol
Iron (s)	μg/dl	0.179	μmol/L	μg/55.9 = umol
Phosphate (p) (as phosphorus)	mg/dl	0.323	mmol/L	mg/31 = mmol
Potassium (s)	mEq/L	1.000	mmol/L	mEq = mmol
Potassium	mg/dl	0.256	mmol/L	mg/39.1 = mmol
Magnesium (s)	mg/dl	0.411	mmol/L	mg/24.3 = mmol
Pyridoxal (B)	ng/ml	5.981	nmol/L	ng/167 = nmol
Retinol† (p,s)	μg/dl	0.0349	μmol/L	μg/286 = umol
Riboflavin (s)	μg/dl	26.57	nmol/L	μg/376 = nmol
Sodium (s)	mEq/L	1.00	mmol/L	mEq = mmol
Thiamin HCl (U)	μg/24 hr	0.00298	μmol/d	μg/337 = umol
α-Tocopherol (p)	mg/dl	23.22	μmol/L	μg/431 = umol
Vitamin D$_3$	μg/dl	26.01	nmol/L	μg/384 = umol
Calcidiol	ng/ml	2.498	nmol/L	ng/400 = nmol
Zinc (s)	μg/dl	0.153	μmol/L	μg/65.4 = umol

*To convert metric or equivalent unit per unit volume (column 1) to S.I. units per liter (column 3), multiply by the conversion factor in column 2. p = plasma; s = serum; B = blood; U = urine.

†See Appendix table A—1b for detailed conversion figures for retinol and carotene

REFERENCES

1. Young, D.S.: Ann. Intern. Med., *106*:114, 1987.
2. Lundberg, G.D., Iberson, C., Radulescu, G.: JAMA, *255*: 2329, 1986.
3. Monsen, E.R.: J. Am. Diet. Assoc., *87*:356, 1987.

TABLE A—1B. FACTORS AND FORMULAS USED IN INTERCONVERTING UNITS OF VITAMIN A AND CAROTENOIDS

Factors
- 1 nmol retinol = 286.42 ng
- 1 nmol retinoic acid = 300.42 ng
- 1 nmol β-carotene = 536.85 ng

1 μg retinol equivalent (μg RE)
- = 1 μg all-*trans* retinol
- = 3.49 nmol all-*trans* retinol
- = 6 μg all-*trans* β-carotene
- = 11.18 nmol all-*trans* β-carotene
- = 12 μg other all-*trans* provitamin A carotenoids
- = 3.33 IU_a (the international unit of all-*trans* retinol)
- = 10 IU_c (the international unit of all-*trans* β-carotene)

1 IU_a
- = 0.3 μg all-*trans* retinol
- = 0.3 μg RE
- = 1.05 nmol all-*trans* retinol
- = 1.8 μg all-*trans* β-carotene
- = 3.35 nmol all-*trans* β-carotene
- = 3 IU_c
- = 3.6 μg other all-*trans* provitamin A carotenoids

1 IU_c
- = 0.6 μg all-*trans* β-carotene
- = 1.12 nmol all-*trans* β-carotene
- = 0.1 μg RE
- = 0.33 IU_a
- = 1.2 μg other all-*trans* provitamin A carotenoids

Formulas and Examples: All-*trans* configurations of retinol and carotenoids are assumed

1. μg RE = μg retinol + μg β-carotene/6
   A diet contains 500 μg retinol and 1800 μg β-carotene. Then,

$$\mu g\ RE = 500 + 1800/6 = 800\ \mu g\ RE$$

2. μg RE = IU_a/3.33 + IU_c/10
   A diet contains 1667 IU_a of retinol and 3000 IU_c of β-carotene. Then,

$$\mu g\ RE = 1667/3.33 + 3000/10 = 800\ \mu g\ RE$$

3. μg RE = μg β-carotene/6 + μg other provitamin A carotenoids/12
   A serving of sweet potato contains 2400 μg of β-carotene and 480 μg of other provitamin A carotenoids. Then,

$$\mu g\ RE = 2400/6 + 480/12 = 440\ \mu g\ RE$$

(continued)

4.
$$\% \ \mu g \ RE \ as \ retinol = \left[1.5 - \frac{0.15 \ total \ IU}{total \ RE} \right] \times 100$$

$$\% \ \mu g \ RE \ as \ carotenoids = \left[\frac{0.15 \ total \ IU}{total \ RE} - 0.5 \right] \times 100$$

A 100-g portion of cheese contains a total of 300 μg RE and a total of 1200 IU, in which 1 IU_a has been *assumed* to equal 1 IU_c. Then,

$$\% \ RE \ as \ retinol = \left[1.5 - \frac{0.15 \times 1200}{300} \right] \times 100 = 90\%$$

$$\% \ RE \ as \ carotenoids = \left[\frac{0.15 \times 1200}{300} - 0.5 \right] \times 100 = 10\%$$

In this sample of cheese, therefore, 270 μg (270 μg RE) is present as retinol and 180 μg, or 30 μg RE, is present as β-carotene or its equivalent of other provitamin A carotenoids.

5.
$$IU_a = \frac{10 \ \mu g \ RE - total \ IU}{2}$$

$$IU_c = \frac{3 \ total \ IU - 10 \ \mu g \ RE}{2}$$

In a cheese sample containing a total of 300 μg RE and a total of 1200 IU, in which 1 IU_a is *assumed* to equal 1 IU_c,

$$IU_a = \frac{10 \times 300 - 1200}{2} = 900$$

$$IU_c = \frac{3 \times 1200 - 10 \times 300}{2} = 300$$

Note: Assumptions used from revised sections of the United States Department of Agriculture's *Handbook 8* (i.e., 8.1–8.10) are (a) that 1 IU_a = 1 IU_c and (b) that 1 RE = 1 μg of retinol = 6 μg of β-carotene = 12 μg of other provitamin A carotenoids.

In some cases, small negative values for IU_c are obtained when the values for total IU and total RE are given for foods containing only preformed vitamin A_1 particularly in fortified foods like margarine. This aberrant calculation results from the rounding of analytic values. Similarly, small negative values for IU_a may result for foods containing only carotenoids. In both cases, the negative values should be taken as zero.

Prepared by J.A. Olson. For further discussion of these interconversions, see Chapter 16.

TABLE A-1C. ATOMIC WEIGHTS (ALPHABETIC ORDER)

ELEMENT	SYMBOL	ATOMIC NUMBER	ATOMIC WEIGHT	ELEMENT	SYMBOL	ATOMIC NUMBER	ATOMIC WEIGHT
Actinium	Ac	89	227.0278*	Neodymium	Nd	60	144.24
Aluminum	Al	13	26.981539	Neon	Ne	10	20.1797
Americium	Am	95	243.0614*	Neptunium	Np	93	237.0482*
Antimony	Sb	51	121.75	Nickel	Ni	28	58.69
Argon	Ar	18	39.948	Niobium	Nb	41	92.90638
Arsenic	As	33	74.92159	Nitrogen	N	7	14.00674
Astatine	At	85	209.9871*	Nobelium	No	102	259.1009*
Barium	Ba	56	137.327	Osmium	Os	76	190.2
Berkelium	Bk	97	247.0703*	Oxygen	O	8	15.9994
Beryllium	Be	4	9.012182	Palladium	Pd	46	106.42
Bismuth	Bi	83	208.98037	Phosphorus	P	15	30.973762
Boron	B	5	10.811	Platinum	Pt	78	195.08
Bromine	Br	35	79.904	Plutonium	Pu	94	244.0642*
Cadmium	Cd	48	112.411	Polonium	Po	84	208.9824*
Calcium	Ca	20	40.078	Potassium	K	19	39.0983
Californium	Cf	98	251.0796*	Praseodymium	Pr	59	140.90765
Carbon	C	6	12.011	Promethium	Pm	61	144.9127*
Cerium	Ce	58	140.115	Protactinium	Pa	91	231.0359*
Cesium	Cs	55	132.90543	Radium	Ra	88	226.0254*
Chlorine	Cl	17	35.4527	Radon	Rn	86	222.0176*
Chromium	Cr	24	51.9961	Rhenium	Re	75	186.207
Cobalt	Co	27	58.93320	Rhodium	Rh	45	102.90550
Copper	Cu	29	63.546	Rubidium	Rb	37	85.4678
Curium	Cm	96	247.0703*	Ruthenium	Ru	44	101.07
Dysprosium	Dy	66	162.50	Samarium	Sm	62	150.36
Einsteinium	Es	99	252.083*	Scandium	Sc	21	44.955910
Erbium	Er	68	167.26	Selenium	Se	34	78.96
Europium	Eu	63	151.965	Silicon	Si	14	28.0855

(Continued)

TABLE A–1C. (CONTINUED)

ELEMENT	SYMBOL	ATOMIC NUMBER	ATOMIC WEIGHT	ELEMENT	SYMBOL	ATOMIC NUMBER	ATOMIC WEIGHT
Fermium	Fm	100	257.0951*	Silver	Ag	47	107.8682
Fluorine	F	9	18.9984032	Sodium	Na	11	22.989768
Francium	Fr	87	223.0197*	Strontium	Sr	38	87.62
Gadolinium	Gd	64	157.25	Sulfur	S	16	32.066
Gallium	Ga	31	69.723	Tantalum	Ta	73	180.9479
Germanium	Ge	32	72.61	Technetium	Tc	43	97.9072*
Gold	Au	79	196.96654	Tellurium	Te	52	127.60
Hafnium	Hf	72	178.49	Terbium	Tb	65	158.92534
Helium	He	2	4.002602	Thallium	Tl	81	204.3833
Holmium	Ho	67	164.93032	Thorium	Th	90	232.0381
Hydrogen	H	1	1.00794	Thulium	Tm	69	168.93421
Indium	In	49	114.82	Tin	Sn	50	118.710
Iodine	I	53	126.90447	Titanium	Ti	22	47.88
Iridium	Ir	77	192.22	Tungsten	W	74	183.85
Iron	Fe	26	55.847	Unnilquadium	Unq	104	261.11*
Krypton	Kr	36	83.80	Unnilpentium	Unp	105	262.114*
Lanthanum	La	57	138.9055	Unnilhexium	Unh	106	263.118*
Lawrencium	Lr	103	262.11*	Unnilseptium	Uns	107	262.12*
Lead	Pb	82	207.2	Uranium	U	92	238.0289
Lithium	Li	3	6.941	Vanadium	V	23	50.9415
Lutetium	Lu	71	174.967	Xenon	Xe	54	131.29
Magnesium	Mg	12	24.3050	Ytterbium	Yb	70	173.04
Manganese	Mn	25	54.93805	Yttrium	Y	39	88.90585
Mendelevium	Md	101	258.10*	Zinc	Zn	30	65.39
Mercury	Hg	80	200.59	Zirconium	Zr	40	91.224
Molybdenum	Mo	42	95.94				

*Relative atomic mass of the isotope of that element with the longest known half-life.
(Based on 1987 IUPAC Table of Standard Atomic Weights of the Elements. *In* The Merck Index. 11th Ed. Rahway, NJ, Merck & Co., 1989.)

TABLE A—1D. WEIGHTS AND MEASURES

VOLUMES:

Apothecaries' Measure	Metric	Household
1 fluid dram (fl dr)	4 milliliter (ml)	1 teaspoon (tsp)
2 fl dr	8 ml	1 dessert spoonful
½ fluid ounce (fl oz)	15 ml	1 tablespoon (Tbsp) (3 tsp)
1 fl oz.	30 ml	2 Tbsp (⅛ cup)
1-½ fl oz	45 ml	1 jigger
2 fl oz	59 ml	4 Tbsp (¼ cup)
2-⅔ fl oz	80 ml	5-⅓ Tbsp (⅓ cup)
4 fl oz	118 ml	8 Tbsp (½ cup)
8 fl oz	237 ml	1 cup
16 fl oz	473 ml	1 pint (pt)
32 fl oz	947 ml	1 quart (qt)
128 fl oz	3,785 ml	1 gallon (gal)
3.38 fl oz	1 deciliter (dl) (100 ml)	
2.11 pt	1 liter (L) (1,000 ml)	

WEIGHTS:

Avoirdupois	Metric
	1 femtogram (fg) (10^{-15} g)
	1 picogram (pg) (10^{-12} g)
	1 nanogram (ng) (10^{-9} g)
	1 microgram (μg) (10^{-6} g)
1 grain (gr)	0.065 g (65 mg)
1 gram (0.035 oz)	15.432 gr
1 scruple (20 gr)	1.296 g
1 dram (dr) (= drachm) (27.3 gr)	1.77 g
1 oz (16 dr)	28.35 g
1 lb (16 oz)	453.59 g
1 ton (2,000 lb)	0.91 metric tons
1.015 gr	1 milligram (mg) (10^{-3} g)
	1 centigram (cg) (10^{-2} g)
	1 decigram (dg) (10^{-1} g)
15.4 gr (0.035 oz)	1 gram (g)
2.2 lb	1 kilogram (kg) (10^{3} g)

LENGTH/AREA:

	Metric
1 angstrom (A)	10 millimeter (mm)
1/2500 inch (in)	1 micron (μ) (10^{-3} mm) = micrometer (μm)
0.039 in	1 mm
0.39 in	1 centimeter (cm)
1 in	2.54 cm
1 foot (ft) (12 in)	30.5 cm
39.4 in	1 meter (m)
1 yard (yd) (3 ft)	0.9 m
1 rod (5.5 yd)	4.95 m
1093.6 yd (0.62 mile)	1 kilometer (km)
1 mile (mi) (5280 ft)	1.61 km
1 acre (160 square rods)	0.4 hectare

TABLE A–1D. (CONTINUED)

TEMPERATURE CONVERSIONS:

F to C: 5/9 (F − 32)
C to F: (9/5 × C) + 32

ELECTROLYTE DATA:

Ion		Weight (1)	Valence (2)	Equivalent Wt* 1 ÷ 2
Bicarbonate	HCO_3^-	61.0	1	61.0
Calcium	Ca^{2+}	40.1	2	20.0
Chloride	Cl^-	35.5	1	35.5
Magnesium	Mg^{2+}	24.3	2	12.2
Phosphate[†]	HPO_4^{2-}	96.0	2	48.0[†]
Potassium	K^+	39.1	1	39.1
Sodium	Na^+	23.0	1	23.0
Sulfate	SO_4^{2-}	96.1	2	48.0

*Milliequivalent (mEq) = equivalent weight in milligrams (mg). To convert mg quantities of all electrolytes to mEq:

$$\frac{mg\ of\ electrolyte}{equivalent\ weight\ in\ mg} = mEq$$

To convert mEq quantities of all electrolytes to mg:

$$mEq \times equivalent\ wt = mg$$

To convert mg/dl to mEq/L:

$$\frac{mg/dl \times 10}{equivalent\ wt\ in\ mg} = mEq/L$$

To convert mEq/L to mg/dl: mEq/L × equivalent wt in mg × 0.1

†At the normal pH of plasma, 20% of the total inorganic phosphate radical is combined with one equivalent of base as BH_2PO_4, and 80% with two equivalents of base as B_2HPO_4. Under these conditions, base equivalence is therefore 0.2 + (0.8 × 2) = 1.8, and the equivalent weight of 53.3 is obtained by dividing the ionic weight by 1.8 instead of by 2. For phosphorus content of phosphate solutions, 1 mEq provides approximately 15 mg, and 1 mmol provides approximately 31 mg.

TABLE A-2A. MEDIAN HEIGHTS AND WEIGHTS AND RECOMMENDED ENERGY INTAKE IN THE UNITED STATES[a]

CATEGORY	AGE (YEARS) OR CONDITION	WEIGHT (kg)	WEIGHT (lb)	HEIGHT (cm)	HEIGHT (in)	REE[b] (kcal/day)	AVERAGE ENERGY ALLOWANCE (kcal)[c] Multiples of REE	Per kg	Per day[d]
Infants	0.0–0.5	6	13	60	24	320		108	650
	0.5–1.0	9	20	71	28	500		98	850
Children	1–3	13	29	90	35	740		102	1,300
	4–6	20	44	112	44	950		90	1,800
	7–10	28	62	132	52	1,130		70	2,000
Males	11–14	45	99	157	62	1,440	1.70	55	2,500
	15–18	66	145	176	69	1,760	1.67	45	3,000
	19–24	72	160	177	70	1,780	1.67	40	2,900
	25–50	79	174	176	70	1,800	1.60	37	2,900
	51+	77	170	173	68	1,530	1.50	30	2,300
Females	11–14	46	101	157	62	1,310	1.67	47	2,200
	15–18	55	120	163	64	1,370	1.60	40	2,200
	19–24	58	128	164	65	1,350	1.60	38	2,200
	25–50	63	138	163	64	1,380	1.55	36	2,200
	51+	65	143	160	63	1,280	1.50	30	1,900
Pregnant	1st trimester					—			+0
	2nd trimester								+300
	3rd trimester								+300
Lactating	1st 6 months								+500
	2nd 6 months								+500

[a]Median Height/Weight used by the RDA are those which are the medians for the U.S. population of designated age as reported in NHANES II.
[b]Calculations based on WHO equation derived from BMR data (Table A–7a), then rounded.
[c]In the range of light to moderate activity, the coefficient of variation is ±20%.
[d]Figure is rounded.
(From Food and Nutrition Board, National Research Council: Recommended Dietary Allowances. 10th Ed. Washington, D.C., National Academy Press, 1989, p. 33.)

TABLE A–2B. RECOMMENDED DIETARY ALLOWANCES[a], REVISED 1989 (DESIGNED FOR THE MAINTENANCE OF GOOD NUTRITION OF PRACTICALLY ALL HEALTHY PEOPLE IN THE UNITED STATES)

CATEGORY	AGE (YEARS) OR CONDITION	WEIGHT[b] (kg)	WEIGHT[b] (lb)	HEIGHT[b] (cm)	HEIGHT[b] (in)	PROTEIN (G)	FAT-SOLUBLE VITAMINS Vita-min A (µg RE)[c]	Vita-min D (µg)[d]	Vita-min E (mg α-TE)[e]	Vita-min K (µg)
Infants	0.0–0.5	6	13	60	24	13	375	7.5	3	5
	0.5–1.0	9	20	71	28	14	375	10	4	10
Children	1–3	13	29	90	35	16	400	10	6	15
	4–6	20	44	112	44	24	500	10	7	20
	7–10	28	62	132	52	28	700	10	7	30
Males	11–14	45	99	157	62	45	1,000	10	10	45
	15–18	66	145	176	69	59	1,000	10	10	65
	19–24	72	160	177	70	58	1,000	10	10	70
	25–50	79	174	176	70	63	1,000	5	10	80
	51+	77	170	173	68	63	1,000	5	10	80
Females	11–14	46	101	157	62	46	800	10	8	45
	15–18	55	120	163	64	44	800	10	8	55
	19–24	58	128	164	65	46	800	10	8	60
	25–50	63	138	163	64	50	800	5	8	65
	51+	65	143	160	63	50	800	5	8	65
Pregnant						60	800	10	10	65
Lactating	1st 6 months					65	1,300	10	12	65
	2nd 6 months					62	1,200	10	11	65

[a]The allowances, expressed as average daily intakes over time, are intended to provide for individual variations among most normal persons as they live in the United States under usual environmental stresses. Diets should be based on a variety of common foods in order to provide other nutrients for which human requirements have been less well defined. See text for detailed discussion of allowances and of nutrients not tabulated.

[b]Weights and heights of reference adults are actual medians for the U.S. population of the designated age, as reported by NHANES II. The median weights and heights of those under 19 years of age were taken from Hamill et al. (1979). The use of these figures does not imply that the height-to-weight ratios are ideal.

[c]Retinol equivalents. 1 retinol equivalent = 1 µg retinol or 6 µg β-carotene. See text for calculation of vitamin A activity of diets as retinol equivalents.

[d]As cholecalciferol. 10 µg cholecalciferol = 400 IU of vitamin D.

[e]α-Tocopherol equivalents. 1 mg d-α tocopherol = 1 α-TE. See text for variation in allowances and calculation of vitamin E activity of the diet as α-tocopherol equivalents.

[f]1 NE (niacin equivalent) is equal to 1 mg of niacin or 60 mg of dietary tryptophan.

(From Food and Nutrition Board, National Research Council: Recommended Dietary Allowances. 10th Ed. Washington, D.C., National Academy Press, 1989.)

TABLE A–2B. (CONTINUED)

WATER-SOLUBLE VITAMINS | | | | | | | MINERALS

Vitamin C (mg)	Thiamin (mg)	Riboflavin (mg)	Niacin (mg NE)f	Vitamin B$_6$ (mg)	Folate (µg)	Vitamin B$_{12}$ (µg)	Calcium (mg)	Phosphorus (mg)	Magnesium (mg)	Iron (mg)	Zinc (mg)	Iodine (µg)	Selenium (µg)
30	0.3	0.4	5	0.3	25	0.3	400	300	40	6	5	40	10
35	0.4	0.5	6	0.6	35	0.5	600	500	60	10	5	50	15
40	0.7	0.8	9	1.0	50	0.7	800	800	80	10	10	70	20
45	0.9	1.1	12	1.1	75	1.0	800	800	120	10	10	90	20
45	1.0	1.2	13	1.4	100	1.4	800	800	170	10	10	120	30
50	1.3	1.5	17	1.7	150	2.0	1,200	1,200	270	12	15	150	40
60	1.5	1.8	20	2.0	200	2.0	1,200	1,200	400	12	15	150	50
60	1.5	1.7	19	2.0	200	2.0	1,200	1,200	350	10	15	150	70
60	1.5	1.7	19	2.0	200	2.0	800	800	350	10	15	150	70
60	1.2	1.4	15	2.0	200	2.0	800	800	350	10	15	150	70
50	1.1	1.3	15	1.4	150	2.0	1,200	1,200	280	15	12	150	45
60	1.1	1.3	15	1.5	180	2.0	1,200	1,200	300	15	12	150	50
60	1.1	1.3	15	1.6	180	2.0	1,200	1,200	280	15	12	150	55
60	1.1	1.3	15	1.6	180	2.0	800	800	280	15	12	150	55
60	1.0	1.2	13	1.6	180	2.0	800	800	280	10	12	150	55
70	1.5	1.6	17	2.2	400	2.2	1,200	1,200	320	30	15	175	65
95	1.6	1.8	20	2.1	280	2.6	1,200	1,200	355	15	19	200	75
90	1.6	1.7	20	2.1	260	2.6	1,200	1,200	340	15	16	200	75

TABLE A–2C. ESTIMATED SAFE AND ADEQUATE DAILY DIETARY INTAKES OF SELECTED VITAMINS AND MINERALS*

CATEGORY	AGE (years)	VITAMINS	
		BIOTIN (µg)	PANTOTHENIC ACID (mg)
Infants	0–0.5	10	2
	0.5–1	15	3
Children and adolescents	1–3	20	3
	4–6	25	3–4
	7–10	30	4–5
	11+	30–100	4–7
Adults		30–100	4–7

TRACE ELEMENTS†

CATEGORY	AGE (years)	COPPER (mg)	MANGANESE (mg)	FLUORIDE (mg)	CHROMIUM (µg)	MOLYBDENUM (µg)
Infants	0–0.5	0.4–0.6	0.3–0.6	0.1–0.5	10–40	15–30
	0.5–1	0.6–0.7	0.6–1.0	0.2–1.0	20–60	20–40
Children and adolescents	1–3	0.7–1.0	1.0–1.5	0.5–1.5	20–80	25–50
	4–6	1.0–1.5	1.5–2.0	1.0–2.5	30–120	30–75
	7–10	1.0–2.0	2.0–3.0	1.5–2.5	50–200	50–150
	11+	1.5–2.5	2.0–5.0	1.5–2.5	50–200	75–250
Adults		1.5–3.0	2.0–5.0	1.5–4.0	50–200	75–250

*Because there is less information on which to base allowances, these figures are not given in the main table of RDA and are provided here in the form of ranges of recommended intakes.

†Because the toxic levels for many trace elements may be only several times usual intakes, the upper levels for the trace elements given in this table should not be habitually exceeded.

(From Food and Nutrition Board, National Research Council: Recommended Dietary Allowances. 10th Ed. Washington, D.C., National Academy Press, 1989, p. 284.)

TABLE A–3A. SUMMARY OF EXAMPLES OF RECOMMENDED NUTRIENTS BASED ON ENERGY EXPRESSED AS DAILY RATES, CANADA

AGE	SEX	ENERGY (kcal)	THIAMIN (mg)	RIBOFLAVIN (mg)	NIACIN (ne[b])	n-3 PUFA[a] (g)	n-6 PUFA (g)
Months							
0–4	Both	600	0.3	0.3	4	0.5	3
5–12	Both	900	0.4	0.5	7	0.5	3
Years							
1	Both	1100	0.5	0.6	8	0.6	4
2–3	Both	1300	0.6	0.7	9	0.7	4
4–6	Both	1800	0.7	0.9	13	1.0	6
7–9	M	2200	0.9	1.1	16	1.2	7
	F	1900	0.8	1.0	14	1.0	6
10–12	M	2500	1.0	1.3	18	1.4	8
	F	2200	0.9	1.1	16	1.2	7
13–15	M	2800	1.1	1.4	20	1.5	9
	F	2200	0.9	1.1	16	1.2	7
16–18	M	3200	1.3	1.6	23	1.8	11
	F	2100	0.8	1.1	15	1.2	7
19–24	M	3000	1.2	1.5	22	1.6	10
	F	2100	0.8	1.1	15	1.2	7
25–49	M	2700	1.1	1.4	19	1.5	9
	F	1900	0.8[c]	1.0[c]	14[c]	1.1[c]	7[c]
50–74	M	2300	0.9	1.2	16	1.3	8
	F	1800	0.8[c]	1.0[c]	14[c]	1.1[c]	7[c]
75+	M	2000	0.8	1.0	14	1.1	7
	F[d]	1700	0.8[c]	1.0[c]	14[c]	1.1[c]	7[c]
Pregnancy (additional)							
1st trimester		100	0.1	0.1	1	0.05	0.3
2nd trimester		300	0.1	0.3	2	0.16	0.9
3rd trimester		300	0.1	0.3	2	0.16	0.9
Lactation (additional)		450	0.2	0.4	3	0.25	1.5

[a]PUFA, Polyunsaturated fatty acids.
[b]NE, Niacin equivalents.
[c]Level below which intake should not fall.
[d]Assumes moderate (more than average) physical activity.
(From Health and Welfare Canada: Nutrition Recommendations. The Report of the Scientific Review Committee. Ottawa: Supply and Services Canada, 1990. Reproduced with permission of the Minister of Supply and Services Canada 1992.)

TABLE A–3B. SUMMARY OF EXAMPLES OF RECOMMENDED NUTRIENT INTAKE BASED ON AGE AND BODY WEIGHT EXPRESSED AS DAILY RATES, CANADA

AGE	SEX	WEIGHT (kg)	PRO-TEIN (g)	VIT. A (RE)[a]	VIT. D (µg)	VIT. E (mg)	VIT. C (mg)	FO-LATE (µg)	VIT. B$_{12}$ (µg)	CAL-CIUM (mg)	PHOS-PHO-RUS (mg)	MAG-NE-SIUM (mg)	IRON (mg)	IODINE (µg)	ZINC (mg)
Months															
0–4	Both	6.0	12[b]	400	10	3	20	25	0.3	250[c]	150	20	0.3[d]	30	2[d]
5–12	Both	9.0	12	400	10	3	20	40	0.4	400	200	32	7	40	3
Years															
1	Both	11	13	400	10	3	20	40	0.5	500	300	40	6	55	4
2–3	Both	14	16	400	5	4	20	50	0.6	550	350	50	6	65	4
4–6	Both	18	19	500	5	5	25	70	0.8	600	400	65	8	85	5
7–9	M	25	26	700	2.5	7	25	90	1.0	700	500	100	8	110	7
	F	25	26	700	2.5	6	25	90	1.0	700	500	100	8	95	7
10–12	M	34	34	800	2.5	8	25	120	1.0	900	700	130	8	125	9
	F	36	36	800	2.5	7	25	130	1.0	1100	800	135	8	110	9
13–15	M	50	49	900	2.5	9	30[e]	175	1.0	1100	900	185	10	160	12
	F	48	46	800	2.5	7	30[e]	170	1.0	1000	850	180	13	160	9

16–18 M	62	58	1000	2.5	10	40[e]	220	1.0	900	1000	230	10	160	12
F	53	47	800	2.5	7	30[e]	190	1.0	700	850	200	12	160	9
19–24 M	71	61	1000	2.5	10	40[e]	220	1.0	800	1000	240	9	160	12
F	58	50	800	2.5	7	30[e]	180	1.0	700	850	200	13	160	9
25–49 M	74	64	1000	2.5	9	40[e]	230	1.0	800	1000	250	9	160	12
F	59	51	800	2.5	6	30[e]	185	1.0	700	850	200	13	160	9
50–74 M	73	63	1000	5	7	40[e]	230	1.0	800	1000	250	9	160	12
F	63	54	800	5	6	30[e]	195	1.0	800	850	210	8	160	9
75+ M	69	59	1000	5	6	40[e]	215	1.0	800	1000	230	9	160	12
F	64	55	800	5	5	30[e]	200	1.0	800	850	210	8	160	9
Pregnancy (additional)													
1st trimester		5	0	2.5	2	0	200	0.2	500	200	15	0	25	6
2nd trimester		20	0	2.5	2	10	200	0.2	500	200	45	5	25	6
3rd trimester		24	0	2.5	2	10	200	0.2	500	200	45	10	25	6
Lactation (additional)		20	400	2.5	3	25	100	0.2	500	200	65	0	50	6

[a] Retinol Equivalents.

[b] Protein is assumed to be from breast milk and must be adjusted for infant formula.

[c] Infant formula with high phosphorus should contain 375 mg calcium.

[d] Breast milk is assumed to be the source of the mineral.

[e] Smokers should increase vitamin C by 50%.

(From Health and Welfare Canada: Nutrition Recommendations. The Report of the Scientific Review Committee. Ottawa, Supply and Services Canada, 1990. Reproduced with permission of the Minister of Supply and Services Canada 1992.)

TABLE A—4A. ESTIMATED AVERAGE REQUIREMENTS (EAR) FOR ENERGY, UNITED KINGDOM

AGE	EAR MJ/D (KCAL/D) Males	Females
0—3 months	2.28 (545)	2.16 (515)
4—6 months	2.89 (690)	2.69 (645)
7—9 months	3.44 (825)	3.20 (765)
10—12 months	3.85 (920)	3.61 (865)
1—3 years	5.15 (1,230)	4.86 (1,165)
4—6 years	7.16 (1,715)	6.46 (1,545)
7—10 years	8.24 (1,970)	7.28 (1,740)
11—14 years	9.27 (2,220)	7.92 (1,845)
15—18 years	11.51 (2,755)	8.83 (2,110)
19—50 years	10.60 (2,550)	8.10 (1,940)
51—59 years	10.60 (2,550)	8.00 (1,900)
60—64 years	9.93 (2,380)	7.99 (1,900)
65—74 years	9.71 (2,330)	7.96 (1,900)
75+ years	8.77 (2,100)	7.61 (1,810)
Pregnancy		+0.80*(200)
Lactation:		
1 month		+1.90 (450)
2 months		+2.20 (530)
3 months		+2.40 (570)
4—6 months (Group 1)		+2.00 (480)
4—6 months (Group 2)		+2.40 (570)
>6 months (Group 1)		+1.00 (240)
>6 months (Group 2)		+2.30 (550)

*last trimester only

(From Report on Health and Social Subjects: Dietary Reference Values for Food and Energy and Nutrients for the United Kingdom. London, Her Majesty's Stationery Office, 1991.)

TABLE A—4B. REFERENCE NUTRIENT INTAKES FOR PROTEIN, UNITED KINGDOM

AGE	REFERENCE NUTRIENT INTAKE[a] (g/d)	
0—3 months	12.5[b]	
4—6 months	12.7	
7—9 months	13.7	
10—12 months	14.9	
1—3 years	14.5	
4—6 years	19.7	
7—10 years	28.3	
Males		
11—14 years	42.1	
15—18 years	55.2	
19—50 years	55.5	
50+ years	53.3	
Females		
11—14 years	41.2	
15—18 years	45.0	
19—50 years	45.0	
50+ years	46.5	
Pregnancy[c]		+ 6
Lactation[c]		
0—4 months		+11
4+ months		+ 8

[a]These figures, based on egg and milk protein, assume complete digestibility.

[b]No values for infants 0 to 3 months are given by WHO. The reference nutrient intake is calculated from the recommendations of Committee on Medical Aspects of Food Policy (COMA).

[c]To be added to adult requirement through all stages of pregnancy and lactation.

(From Report on Health and Social Subjects: No. 41, Dietary Reference Values for Food Energy and Nutrients for the United Kingdom, Report of the Panel on Dietary Reference Values of the Committee on Medical Aspects of Food Policy. London, Her Majesty's Stationery Office, 1991.)

TABLE A–4C. REFERENCE NUTRIENT INTAKES FOR VITAMINS, UNITED KINGDOM

AGE	THIAMIN (mg/d)	RIBOFLAVIN (mg/d)	NIACIN (NICOTINIC ACID EQUIVALENT) (mg/d)	VITAMIN B$_6$ (mg/d[a])	VITAMIN B$_{12}$ (µg/d)	FOLATE (µg/d)	VITAMIN C (mg/d)	VITAMIN A (µg/d)	VITAMIN D (µg/d)
0–3 months	0.2	0.4	3	0.2	0.3	50	25	350	8.5
4–6 months	0.2	0.4	3	0.2	0.3	50	25	350	8.5
7–9 months	0.2	0.4	4	0.3	0.4	50	25	350	7
10–12 months	0.3	0.4	5	0.4	0.4	50	25	350	7
1–3 years	0.5	0.6	8	0.7	0.5	70	30	400	7
4–6 years	0.7	0.8	11	0.9	0.8	100	30	500	—
7–10 years	0.7	1.0	12	1.0	1.0	150	30	500	—
Males									
11–14 years	0.9	1.2	15	1.2	1.2	200	35	600	—
15–18 years	1.1	1.3	18	1.5	1.5	200	40	700	—
19–50 years	1.0	1.3	17	1.4	1.5	200	40	700	—
50+ years	0.9	1.3	16	1.4	1.5	200	40	700	**
Females									
11–14 years	0.7	1.1	12	1.0	1.2	200	35	600	—
15–18 years	0.8	1.1	14	1.2	1.5	200	40	600	—
19–50 years	0.8	1.1	13	1.2	1.5	200	40	600	—
50+ years	0.8	1.1	12	1.2	1.5	200	40	600	**
Pregnancy	+0.1[b]	+0.3	*	*	*	+100	+10	+100	10
Lactation									
0–4 months	+0.2	+0.5	+2	*	+0.5	+60	+30	+350	10
4+ months	+0.2	+0.5	+2	*	+0.5	+60	+30	+350	10

*No increment
**After age 65 the RNI is 10 µg/d for men and women
[a]Based on protein providing 14.7% of EAR for energy
[b]For last trimester only

(From Report on Health and Social Subjects: No. 41, Dietary Reference Values for Food Energy and Nutrients for the United Kingdom. Report of the Panel on Dietary Reference Values of the Committee on Medical Aspects of Food Policy. London, Her Majesty's Stationery Office, 1991.)

AGE	CALCIUM (mmol/d)	PHOSPHORUS[1] (mmol/d)	MAGNESIUM (mmol/d)	SODIUM[2] (mmol/d)	POTASSIUM[3] (mmol/d)	CHLORIDE[4] (mmol/d)	IRON (μmol/d)	ZINC (μmol/d)	COPPER (μmol/d)	SELENIUM (μmol/d)	IODINE (μmol/d)
0–3 months	13.1	13.1	2.2	9	20	9	30	60	5	0.1	0.4
4–6 months	13.1	13.1	2.5	12	22	12	80	60	5	0.2	0.5
7–9 months	13.1	13.1	3.2	14	18	14	140	75	5	0.1	0.5
10–12 months	13.1	13.1	3.3	15	18	15	140	75	5	0.1	0.5
1–3 years	8.8	8.8	3.5	22	20	22	120	75	6	0.2	0.6
4–6 years	11.3	11.3	4.8	30	28	30	110	100	9	0.3	0.8
7–10 years	13.8	13.8	8.0	50	50	50	160	110	11	0.4	0.9
Males											
11–14 years	25.0	25.0	11.5	70	80	70	200	140	13	0.6	1.0
15–18 years	25.0	25.0	12.3	70	90	70	200	145	16	0.9	1.0
19–50 years	17.5	17.5	12.3	70	90	70	160	145	19	0.9	1.0
50+ years	17.5	17.5	12.3	70	90	70	160	145	19	0.9	1.0
Females											
11–14 years	20.0	10.0	11.5	70	80	70	260[5]	140	13	0.6	1.0
15–18 years	20.0	20.0	12.3	70	90	70	260[5]	110	16	0.8	1.1
19–50 years	17.5	17.5	10.9	70	90	70	260[5]	110	19	0.8	1.1
50+ years	17.5	17.5	10.9	70	90	70	160	110	19	0.8	1.1
Pregnancy	*	*	*	*	*	*	*	*	*	*	*
Lactation											
0–4 months	+14.3	+14.3	+2.1	*	*	*	*	+90	+5	+0.2	*
4+ months	+14.3	+14.3	+2.1	*	*	*	*	+40	+5	+0.2	*
0–3 months	525	400	55	210	800	320	1.7	4.0	0.2	10	50
4–6 months	525	400	60	280	850	400	4.3	4.0	0.3	13	60
7–9 months	525	400	75	320	700	500	7.8	5.0	0.3	10	60
10–12 months	525	400	80	350	700	500	7.8	5.0	0.3	10	60

(Continued)

TABLE A–4D. (CONTINUED)

AGE	CAL-CIUM (mmol/d)	PHOS-PHO-RUS[1] (mmol/d)	MAGNE-SIUM (mmol/d)	SODI-UM[2] (mmol/d)	POTAS-SIUM[3] (mmol/d)	CHLOR-IDE[4] (mmol/d)	IRON (μmol/d)	ZINC (μmol/d)	COP-PER (μmol/d)	SELE-NIUM (μmol/d)	IODINE (μmol/d)
1–3 years	350	270	85	500	800	800	6.9	5.0	0.4	15	70
4–6 years	450	350	120	700	1,100	1,100	6.1	6.5	0.6	20	100
7–10 years	550	450	200	1,200	2,000	1,800	8.7	7.0	0.7	30	110
Males											
11–14 years	1,000	775	280	1,600	3,100	2,500	11.3	9.0	0.8	45	130
15–18 years	1,000	775	300	1,600	3,500	2,500	11.3	9.5	1.0	70	140
19–50 years	700	550	300	1,600	3,500	2,500	8.7	9.5	1.2	75	140
50+ years	700	550	300	1,600	3,500	2,500	8.7	9.5	1.2	75	140
Females											
11–14 years	800	625	280	1,600	3,100	2,500	14.8[5]	9.0	0.8	45	130
15–18 years	800	625	300	1,600	3,500	2,500	14.8[5]	7.0	1.0	60	140
19–50 years	700	550	270	1,600	3,500	2,500	14.8[5]	7.0	1.2	60	140
50+ years	700	550	270	1,600	3,500	2,500	8.7	7.0	1.2	60	140
Pregnancy	*	*	*	*	*	*	*	*	*	*	*
Lactation											
0–4 months	+550	+440	+50	*	*	*	*	+6.0	+0.3	+15	*
4+ months	+550	+440	+50	*	*	*	*	+2.5	+0.3	+15	*

*No increment
[1]Phosphorus RNI is set equal to calcium in molar terms
[2]1 mmol sodium = 23 mg
[3]1 mmol potassium = 39 mg
[4]1 mmol = 35.5 mg
[5]Insufficient for women with high menstrual losses where the most practical way of meeting iron requirements is to take iron supplements

(From Report on Health and Social Subjects: No. 41, Dietary Reference Values for Food Energy and Nutrients for the United Kingdom, Report of the Panel on Dietary Reference Values of the Committee on Medical Aspects of Food Policy. London, Her Majesty's Stationery Office, 1991.)

TABLE A—4E. SAFE INTAKES, UNITED KINGDOM

NUTRIENT	SAFE INTAKE
Vitamins	
Pantothenic acid	
adults	3—7 mg/d
infants	1.7 mg/d
Biotin	10—200 μg/d
Vitamin E	
men	above 4 mg/d
women	above 3 mg/d
infants	0.4 mg/g polyunsaturated fatty acids
Vitamin K	
adults	1 μg/kg/d
infants	10 μg/d
Minerals	
Manganese	
adults	1.4 mg (26 μmol)/d
infants and children	16 μg (0.3 μmol)/d
Molybdenum	
adults	50—400 μg/d
infants, children, and adolescents	0.5—1.5 μg/kg/d
Chromium	
adults	25 μg (0.5 μmol)/d
children and adolescents	0.1—1.0 μg (2—20 μmol)/kg/d
Fluoride (for infants only)	0.05 mg (3 μmol)/kg/d

For some nutrients, which are known to have important functions in humans, the Panel found insufficient reliable data on human requirements and were unable to set any dietary reference values for these. However, they decided on grounds of prudence to set a safe intake, particularly for infants and children. The safe intake was judged to be a level or range of intake at which there is no risk of deficiency and below a level where there is risk of undesirable effects. They are not therefore intended as a "toxic level," and although exceeding these safe intakes would not necessaily result in undesirable effects, equally there is no evidence for any benefits. The Panel agreed that the safe range of intakes set for the nutrients need not be exceeded.

(From Report on Health and Social Subjects: No. 41, Dietary Reference Values for Food Energy and Nutrients for the United Kingdom, Report of the Panel on Dietary Reference Values of the Committee on Medical Aspects of Food Policy. London, Her Majesty's Stationery Office, 1991.)

TABLE A–5A. RECOMMENDED DIETARY ALLOWANCES FOR PERSONS WITH LOW ACTIVITY, JAPAN

AGE (YR)	ENERGY (kcal) M	ENERGY (kcal) F	PROTEIN (g) M	PROTEIN (g) F	FAT (%)	CALCIUM (g) M	CALCIUM (g) F	IRON (mg) M	IRON (mg) F	VITAMIN A (IU) M	VITAMIN A (IU) F	VITAMIN B₁ (mg) M	VITAMIN B₁ (mg) F	VITAMIN B₂ (mg) M	VITAMIN B₂ (mg) F	NIACIN (mg) M	NIACIN (mg) F	ASCORBIC ACID (mg)	VITAMIN D (IU)
15~	2,350	2,000	85	70	25~30	0.8			12			0.9	0.8	1.3	1.1	16	13		
16~	2,400	1,950	80	70		0.8		12				1.0	0.8	1.3	1.1	16	13		
17~	2,400	1,900	80	70		0.8						1.0	0.8	1.3	1.0	16	13		
18~	2,350	1,850	75	65		0.7						0.9	0.7	1.3	1.0	16	12		
19~	2,300	1,850	75	60		0.7						0.9	0.7	1.3	1.0	15	12		
20~29	2,250	1,800	70	60		0.6	0.6		12	2,000	1,800	0.9	0.7	1.2	1.0	15	12	50	100
30~39	2,200	1,750	70	60								0.9	0.7	1.2	1.0	15	12		
40~49	2,150	1,700	70	60								0.9	0.7	1.2	0.9	14	11		
50~59	2,000	1,650	70	60								0.8	0.7	1.1	0.9	13	11		
60~64	1,850	1,550	70	60	20~25	0.6		10				0.7	0.6	1.0	0.9	12	10		
65~69	1,800	1,500	70	60								0.7	0.6	1.0	0.9	12	10		
70~74	1,650	1,450	65	55								0.7	0.6	1.0	0.9	12	10		
75~79	1,600	1,400	65	55					†10			0.7	0.6	1.0	0.9	12	10		
80~	1,500	1,250	65	55								0.7	0.6	1.0	0.9	12	10		
1st Half Pregnancy*	+150		+10			+0.4	+0.4		+3		+0		+0.1		+0.1		+1	+10	+300
Last Half Pregnancy	+350		+20		25~30		+0.4		+8		+200		+0.2		+0.2		+2	+10	+300
Lactation	+700		+20				+0.5		+8		+1,400		+0.3		+0.4		+5	+40	+300

*Pregnancy increases are shown for convenience; however, values apply to each activity level.
†Decrease to 10 mg after menopause.
(From the Health Promotion and Nutrition Division, Health Policy Bureau, Ministry of Health and Welfare, Tokyo, Japan, 1991.)

TABLE A–5B. RECOMMENDED DIETARY ALLOWANCES FOR PERSONS WITH MEDIUM ACTIVITY OR GROWTH STAGES, JAPAN

AGE	AVERAGE HEIGHT (CM) M	F	AVERAGE WEIGHT (kg) M	F	ENERGY (kcal) M	F	PROTEIN (g) M	F	FAT (%)	CALCIUM (g) M	F	IRON (mg) M	F	VITAMIN A (IU) M	F	VITAMIN B₁ (mg) M	F	VITAMIN B₂ (mg) M	F	NIACIN (mg) M	F	ASCORBIC ACID (mg)	VITAMIN D (IU)
0~mo					120/kg	120/kg	3.3/kg		45	0.4	0.4	6	6	1,300	1,300	0.4	0.4	0.5	0.5	6	4	40	400
2~mo					110/kg	110/kg	2.5/kg		45	0.4	0.4	6	6	1,300	1,300	0.5	0.5	0.7	0.6	6	6	40	400
6~mo					100/kg	100/kg	3.0/kg		30~40	0.4	0.4	6	6	1,000	1,000	0.7	0.7	0.8	0.7	6	6	40	400
1~yr	80.7	79.6	10.95	10.35	960	910	30	30	25~30	0.4	0.4	7	7	1,000	1,000	0.6	0.6	0.9	0.8	8	8	40	100
2~	90.0	89.1	13.24	12.74	1,200	1,150	35	35	25~30	0.4	0.4	7	7	1,000	1,000	0.6	0.6	0.9	0.8	8	8	40	100
3~	97.3	96.6	15.04	14.70	1,400	1,350	40	40	25~30	0.4	0.4	8	8	1,000	1,000	0.7	0.7	1.0	0.9	10	9	40	100
4~	104.3	103.7	16.97	16.69	1,550	1,450	45	45	25~30	0.4	0.4	8	8	1,000	1,000	0.7	0.7	1.0	0.9	10	10	40	100
5~	110.8	110.3	19.04	18.78	1,600	1,500	50	50	25~30	0.4	0.4	8	8	1,000	1,000	0.8	0.8	1.0	0.9	11	10	40	100
6~	117.0	116.5	21.35	21.04	1,700	1,600	55	50	25~30	0.5	0.5	9	9	1,000	1,000	0.8	0.8	1.1	1.0	11	11	40	100
7~	122.7	122.2	23.85	23.44	1,800	1,650	60	55	25~30	0.5	0.5	9	9	1,200	1,200	0.9	0.8	1.1	1.0	12	11	40	100
8~	128.3	127.9	26.70	26.24	1,900	1,750	65	60	25~30	0.6	0.6	9	9	1,200	1,200	0.9	0.8	1.2	1.1	12	12	40	100
9~	133.5	133.6	29.76	29.50	1,950	1,850	65	65	25~30	0.6	0.6	9	9	1,200	1,200	1.0	0.8	1.2	1.1	13	12	40	100
10~	138.8	139.8	33.21	33.54	2,050	1,950	70	70	25~30	0.6	0.6	10	10	1,200	1,200	1.0	0.8	1.3	1.1	13	13	40	100
11~	144.6	146.5	37.26	38.46	2,150	2,100	75	75	25~30	0.7	0.7	10	10	1,200	1,200	1.0	0.8	1.3	1.2	14	14	40	100
12~	151.4	151.9	42.29	43.31	2,350	2,250	80	80	25~30	0.8	0.7	10	10	1,200	1,200	1.1	0.9	1.4	1.3	15	15	40	100
13~	159.0	155.4	48.34	47.43	2,500	2,300	85	80	25~30	0.9	0.7	10	12	1,500	1,500	1.1	0.9	1.5	1.3	16	15	40	100
14~	164.9	157.1	53.87	50.32	2,600	2,300	85	75	25~30	0.8	0.7	10	12	1,500	1,500	1.1	0.9	1.5	1.3	17	15	40	100
15~	168.5	157.6	57.98	51.99	2,700	2,250	85	70	25~30	0.8	0.7	10	12	1,500	1,500	1.1	0.9	1.5	1.3	17	15	40	100
16~	169.9	158.0	60.21	52.87	2,700	2,200	80	70	25~30	0.8	0.7	12	12	1,500	1,500	1.0	0.8	1.4	1.2	18	14	50	100
17~	170.8	158.1	61.55	52.92	2,700	2,150	80	70	25~30	0.8	0.7	12	12	1,500	1,500	1.0	0.8	1.4	1.2	18	14	50	100
18~	171.3	158.1	62.18	52.52	2,650	2,100	75	65	25~30	0.7	0.7	12	12	1,500	1,500	1.0	0.8	1.4	1.2	17	14	50	100
19~	171.5	158.1	62.41	52.02	2,600	2,050	75	60	25~30	0.7	0.7	12	12	1,500	1,500	1.0	0.8	1.4	1.2	17	14	50	100
20~29	171.1	157.7	64.00	51.83	2,550	2,000	70	60	20~25	0.6	0.6	10	12*	2,000	1,800	1.0	0.8	1.4	1.2	17	14	50	100
30~39	169.8	156.7	65.48	54.09	2,500	2,000	70	60	20~25	0.6	0.6	10	12*	2,000	1,800	1.0	0.8	1.4	1.2	17	14	50	100
40~49	167.8	154.6	65.10	55.14	2,400	1,950	70	60	20~25	0.6	0.6	10	12*	2,000	1,800	1.0	0.8	1.4	1.2	16	13	50	100
50~59	164.2	151.9	61.93	54.13	2,250	1,850	70	60	20~25	0.6	0.6	10	12*	2,000	1,800	0.9	0.7	1.3	1.0	15	13	50	100
60~64	162.1	149.8	59.41	52.49	2,100	1,750	70	60	20~25	0.6	0.6	10	10	2,000	1,800	0.9	0.7	1.3	1.0	15	12	50	100
65~69	160.8	148.3	57.61	51.02	2,000	1,700	70	60	20~25	0.6	0.6	10	10	2,000	1,800	0.9	0.7	1.3	1.0	15	12	50	100
70~74	159.7	145.7	55.83	49.26	1,850	1,600	65	55	20~25	0.6	0.6	10	10	2,000	1,800	0.8	0.7	1.2	1.0	14	12	50	100
75~79	158.7	145.0	54.07	47.22	1,750	1,550	65	55	20~25	0.6	0.6	10	10	2,000	1,800	0.8	0.7	1.2	1.0	14	12	50	100
80~	157.6	142.4	52.38	44.53	1,650	1,400	65	55	20~25	0.6	0.6	10	10	2,000	1,800	0.8	0.7	1.2	1.0	14	12	50	100

*Decrease to 10 mg after menopause.

(From the Health Promotion and Nutrition Division, Health Policy Bureau, Ministry of Health and Welfare, Tokyo, Japan, 1991.)

TABLE A–5C. RECOMMENDED DIETARY ALLOWANCES FOR PERSONS WITH MEDIUM-HIGH ACTIVITY, JAPAN

AGE	ENERGY (kcal) M	F	PROTEIN (g) M	F	FAT (%)	CALCIUM (g) M	F	IRON (mg) M	F	VITAMIN A (IU) M	F	VITAMIN B₁ (mg) M	F	VITAMIN B₂ (mg) M	F	NIACIN (mg) M	F	ASCORBIC ACID (mg)	VITAMIN D (IU)
15~	3,200	2,650	100	85	25~30	0.8	0.6	12	12	2,000	1,800	1.3	1.1	1.8	1.5	21	17	50	100
16~	3,200	2,600	95	80								1.3	1.0	1.8	1.4	21	17		
17~	3,200	2,550	95	80		0.7						1.3	1.0	1.8	1.4	21	17		
18~	3,150	2,500	90	75								1.3	1.0	1.7	1.4	21	17		
19~	3,100	2,450	90	70								1.2	1.0	1.7	1.3	20	16		
20~29	3,050	2,400	85	70		0.6			12			1.2	1.0	1.7	1.3	20	16		
30~39	2,950	2,350	85	70								1.2	0.9	1.6	1.3	19	16		
40~49	2,850	2,300	85	70				10				1.1	0.9	1.6	1.3	19	15		
50~59	2,700	2,200	85	70					*			1.1	0.9	1.5	1.2	18	15		
60~64	2,450	2,050	80	70					10			1.0	0.8	1.3	1.1	16	14		
65~69	2,350	2,000	80	70								1.0	0.8	1.3	1.1	16	14		

*Decrease to 10 mg after menopause.
(From the Health Promotion and Nutrition Division, Health Policy Bureau, Ministry of Health and Welfare, Tokyo, Japan, 1991.)

TABLE A—5D. RECOMMENDED DIETARY ALLOWANCES FOR PERSONS WITH HIGH ACTIVITY, JAPAN

AGE	ENERGY (kcal) M	F	PRO-TEIN (g) M	F	FAT (%)	CALCIUM (g) M	F	IRON (mg) M	F	VITAMIN A (IU) M	F	VITA-MIN B₁ (mg) M	F	VITA-MIN B₂ (mg) M	F	NIACIN (mg) M	F	AS-COR-BIC ACID (mg)	VITA-MIN D (IU)
15~	3,750	3,100	115	95		0.8		12	12			1.5	1.2	2.1	1.7	25	20		
16~	3,750	3,050	110	95		0.8						1.5	1.2	2.1	1.7	25	20		
17~	3,750	2,950	110	95		0.7						1.5	1.2	2.1	1.6	25	19		
18~	3,700	2,900	105	90		0.7						1.5	1.2	2.0	1.6	24	19		
19~	3,700	2,850	105	85		0.7						1.5	1.1	2.0	1.6	24	19		
20~29	3,550	2,800	100	85	25~30	0.6	0.6	10	12	2,000	1,800	1.4	1.1	2.0	1.5	23	18	50	100
30~39	3,450	2,750	100	85		0.6			12			1.4	1.1	1.9	1.5	23	18		
40~49	3,350	2,700	100	85		0.6			*			1.3	1.0	1.8	1.5	22	18		
50~59	3,150	2,600	100	85		0.6						1.3	1.0	1.7	1.4	21	17		
60~64	2,850	2,400	95	80		0.6			10			1.1	1.0	1.6	1.3	19	16		
65~69	2,750	2,300	95	80								1.1	1.0	1.6	1.3	19	16		

*Decrease to 10 mg after menopause.

(From the Health Promotion and Nutrition Division, Health Policy Bureau, Ministry of Health and Welfare, Tokyo, Japan, 1991.)

Comments
1. These general guidelines are not for individual daily values. For individual nutrient requirements, other tables must be used.
2. An individual should take no more than 10 mg sodium daily.
3. Vitamin E: Males should have at least 8 mg, females should have at least 7 mg.
4. For those in the low activity category, more exercise is recommended. The values in Table A—5c represent the ideal intake for adults. These values are reflective of individuals who exercise accordingly.

TABLE A–6. RECOMMENDED DAILY DIETARY ALLOWANCES, KOREA*

CATEGORY	AGE (years)	WEIGHT (kg)	HEIGHT (cm)	ENERGY (kcal)	PRO-TEIN (g)	VITA-MIN A (re)†	Vita-min B₁ (mg)	VITA-MIN B₂ (mg)	NIA-CIN (mg)	VITA-MIN C (mg)	VITA-MIN D (µg)‡	CAL-CIUM (mg)	IRON (mg)§
Infants													
	0–3 mo	5.5	58.5	800	25	350	0.40	0.48	6.4	35	10	400	10
	4–6 mo	8.4	67.5	900	25	350	0.45	0.54	7.2	35	10	400	10
	7–9 mo	9.5	76.0	1,000	30	350	0.50	0.60	8.0	35	10	400	15
	10–12 mo	10.4	79.0	1,100	30	350	0.55	0.66	8.0	35	10	400	15
Children													
	1–3	12.6	87.0	1,200	35	350	0.60	0.72	8.0	40	10	500	15
	4–6	19.0	110.0	1,300	40	400	0.75	0.90	10.0	40	10	600	10
	7–9	26.0	130.0	1,800	50	500	0.90	1.08	12.0	40	10	700	10
Males													
	10–12	36.0	144.0	2,100	60	600	1.05	1.26	14.0	50	10	800	15
	13–15	51.0	161.0	2,600	80	700	1.30	1.36	17.0	50	10	800	18
	16–19	59.0	169.0	2,500	75	700	1.25	1.50	16.5	55	10	800	18
	20–29	64.0	170.5	2,500	70	700	1.25	1.50	16.5	55	5	600	10
	30–49	65.0	168.5	2,500	70	700	1.25	1.50	16.5	55	5	600	10
	50–64	63.0	168.0	2,200	70	700	1.10	1.32	14.5	55	5	600	10
	65 or older	61.0	167.0	1,900	70	700	1.00	1.20	13.0	55	5	600	10

		Weight	Height	Energy	Protein	Vit A					Vit D	Ca	Fe
Females	10–12	37.0	145.0	2,000	60	600	1.00	1.20	13.0	50	10	800	18
	13–15	48.0	155.0	2,300	65	700	1.15	1.38	15.0	50	10	800	18
	16–19	52.0	158.0	2,200	60	700	1.10	1.32	14.5	55	10	700	18
	20–29	52.5	159.5	2,000	60	700	1.00	1.20	13.0	55	5	600	18
	30–49	55.0	158.0	2,000	60	700	1.00	1.20	13.0	55	5	600	18
	50–64	54.0	156.0	1,900	60	700	1.00	1.20	13.0	55	5	600	10
	65 or older	53.0	156.0	1,600	60	700	1.00	1.20	13.0	55	5	600	10
Pregnancy	First half			+150	+30	+0	+0.40	+0.30	+2.0	+15	+5	+400	+2
	Second half			+350	+30	+100	+0.40	+0.30	+2.0	+15	+5	+400	+2
Lactation				+700	+30	+300	+0.60	+0.50	+6.0	+35	+5	+500	+2

*The allowances for energy are based on individuals of moderate activity. Data in this table are intended to provide only a standard figure under usual environment and given conditions.

†Retinol equivalent: 1 RE = 1 μg retinol = 6 μg β-carotene

‡Vitamin D : 10 μg = 400 IU.

§Supplemental iron should be taken to meet the increased requirement during pregnancy and lactation.

(From the Ministry of Health and Social Affairs, Kyonggi, Korea, 1989.)

TABLE A—7A. EQUATIONS FOR PREDICTING BASAL METABOLIC RATE FROM BODY WEIGHT (W)*

AGE RANGE (years)	KCAL$_{th}$/DAY	CORRELATION COEFFICIENT	SD†	MJ/DAY	CORRELATION COEFFICIENT	SD
Males						
0–3	60.9 W − 54	0.97	53	0.255 W − 0.226	0.97	0.222
3–10	22.7 W + 495	0.86	62	0.0949 W + 2.07	0.86	0.259
10–18	17.5 W + 651	0.90	100	0.0732 W + 2.72	0.90	0.418
18–30	15.3 W + 679	0.65	151	0.0640 W + 2.84	0.65	0.632
30–60	11.6 W + 879	0.60	164	0.0485 W + 3.67	0.60	0.686
> 60	13.5 W + 487	0.79	148	0.0565 W + 2.04	0.79	0.619
Females						
0–3	61.0 W − 51	0.97	61	0.255 W − 0.214	0.97	0.255
3–10	22.5 W + 499	0.85	63	0.0941 W + 2.09	0.85	0.264
10–18	12.2 W + 746	0.75	117	0.0510 W + 3.12	0.75	0.489
18–30	14.7 W + 496	0.72	121	0.0615 W + 2.08	0.72	0.506
30–60	8.7 W + 829	0.70	108	0.0364 W + 3.47	0.70	0.452
> 60	10.5 W + 596	0.74	108	0.0439 W + 2.49	0.74	0.452

*Since the present report was compiled, the data base for the equations contained in Schofield, W. N., et al.: Hum. Nutr. Clin. Nutr. *39(Suppl.)*, 1985 has been slightly expanded. They therefore differ from the equations shown in this table, but the differences are negligible.

†Standard deviation of differences between actual BMR and predicted estimates.

(From Energy and Protein Requirements: Report of a Joint FAO/WHO/UNU Expert Consultation. Technical Report Series No. 724. Geneva, World Health Organization, 1985, p. 71.)

TABLE A—7B. EXAMPLES OF PREDICTED BASAL METABOLIC RATE (BMR) IN SUBJECTS OF THE SAME HEIGHT BUT DIFFERENT WEIGHTS, PREDICTED FROM ACTUAL WEIGHT AND FROM MEDIAN ACCEPTABLE WEIGHT FOR HEIGHT

	MAN, AGE 40, HEIGHT 1.8 M			WOMAN, AGE 25, HEIGHT 1.5 M		
	Position in range*			Position in range*		
	Upper	Median	Lower	Upper	Median	Lower
BMI†	25	22	20	24	21	19
Wt(kg)	81.0	71.3	64.8	54.0	47.2	42.7
BMR‡ from actual wt						
kcal$_{th}$/day	1,820	1,710	1,630	1,290	1,190	1,120
MJ/day	7.61	7.15	6.82	5.39	4.98	4.68
BMR from median wt						
kcal$_{th}$/day	1,710	1,710	1,710	1,190	1,190	1,190
MJ/day	7.15	7.15	7.15	4.97	4.97	4.97

*Acceptable range of BMI (see Annex 2A in original reference).
†Body mass index = wt(kg)/ht²(m).
‡Predicted from equations in Table A—7a.
(From Energy and Protein Requirements: Report of a Joint FAO/WHO/UNU Expert Consultation. Technical Report Series No. 724, Geneva, World Health Organization, 1985, p. 72.)

TABLE A–7C. BASAL METABOLIC RATES OF ADOLESCENT BOYS AND GIRLS

AGE (years)	HEIGHT* (cm)	WEIGHT† (kg)	BMR‡ Total (kcal_th/day)	(MJ/day)	per kg (kcal_th/day)	(MJ/day)
Boys						
10–11	140	32.2	1215	5.08	37.7	0.16
11–12	147	37.0	1300	5.43	35.1	0.15
12–13	153	40.9	1370	5.73	33.4	0.14
13–14	160	47.0	1465	6.12	31.4	0.13
14–15	166	52.6	1570	6.57	29.9	0.12
15–16	171	58.0	1665	6.96	28.7	0.12
16–17	175	62.7	1750	7.32	27.9	0.12
17–18	177	65.0	1790	7.48	27.5	0.12
Girls						
10–11	142	33.7	1160	4.85	34.3	0.14
11–12	148	38.7	1220	5.10	31.5	0.13
12–13	155	44.0	1280	5.38	29.1	0.12
13–14	159	48.8	1340	5.60	27.5	0.12
14–15	161	51.4	1375	5.75	26.7	0.11
15–16	162	53.0	1395	5.83	26.3	0.11
16–17	163	54.0	1405	5.87	26.0	0.11
17–18	164	54.4	1410	5.89	25.9	0.11

*Median height for age from NCHS standards.
†Median weight for height and age from Baldwin's standards (Annex 2(B) of original reference.
‡Boys: BMR = 17.5 W + 651 kcal_th/day (2.72 MJ/day). Girls: 12.2 W + 746 kcal_th/day (3.12 MJ/day).
(From Energy and Protein Requirements: Report of a joint FAO/WHO/UNU Expert Consultation. Technical Report Series No. 724. Geneva, World Health Organization, 1985, p. 72.)

TABLE A-7D. BASAL METABOLIC RATE IN ADULT MEN AND WOMEN IN RELATION TO HEIGHT AND MEDIAN ACCEPTABLE WEIGHT FOR HEIGHT* (VALUES GIVEN IN KCAL$_{TH}$ WITH MJ IN PARENTHESES)

HEIGHT (m)	WEIGHT† (kg)	18–30 YEARS		30–60 YEARS		>60 YEARS	
		Per kg per day	Per day	Per kg per day	Per day	Per kg per day	Per day
Men							
1.5	49.5	29.0 (121)	1440 (6.03)	29.4 (123)	1450 (6.07)	23.3 (98)	1150 (4.81)
1.6	56.5	27.4 (115)	1540 (6.44)	27.2 (114)	1530 (6.40)	22.2 (93)	1250 (5.23)
1.7	63.5	26.0 (109)	1650 (6.90)	25.4 (106)	1620 (6.78)	21.2 (89)	1350 (5.65)
1.8	71.5	24.8 (104)	1770 (7.41)	23.9 (99)	1710 (7.15)	20.3 (85)	1450 (6.07)
1.9	79.5	23.9 (100)	1890 (7.91)	22.7 (95)	1800 (7.53)	19.6 (82)	1560 (6.53)
2.0	88	23.0 (96)	2030 (8.49)	21.6 (90)	1900 (7.95)	19.0 (80)	1670 (6.99)
Women							
1.4	41	26.7 (112)	1100 (4.60)	28.8 (120)	1190 (4.98)	25.0 (105)	1030 (4.31)
1.5	47	25.2 (105)	1190 (4.98)	26.3 (110)	1240 (5.19)	23.1 (97)	1090 (4.56)
1.6	54	23.9 (100)	1290 (5.40)	24.1 (101)	1300 (5.44)	21.6 (90)	1160 (4.85)
1.7	61	22.9 (96)	1390 (5.82)	22.4 (94)	1360 (5.69)	20.3 (85)	1230 (5.15)
1.8	68	22.0 (92)	1500 (6.28)	20.9 (87)	1420 (5.94)	19.3 (81)	1310 (5.48)

*BMR from equations in Table A–7a rounded to 10 kcal$_{th}$.

†Weight taken as median acceptable weight for height: body mass index (wt/ht^2) = 22 in men, 21 in women.

(From Energy and Protein Requirements: Report of a joint FAO/WHO/UNU Expert Consultation. Technical Report Series No. 724. Geneva, World Health Organization, 1985, p. 72.)

TABLE A–8A. CALCULATED ENERGY REQUIREMENTS OF INFANTS FROM BIRTH TO 1 YEAR

AGE (months)	INTAKE*		CALCULATED ENERGY REQUIREMENT†		MEDIAN BODY WEIGHT‡		TOTAL REQUIREMENT			
							Boys		Girls	
	(kcal$_{th}$/kg per day)	(kJ/kg per day)	(kcal$_{th}$/kg per day)	(kJ/kg per day)	Boys (kg)	Girls (kg)	(kcal$_{th}$/day)	(kJ/day)	(kcal$_{th}$/day)	(kJ/day)
0.5	118	494	124	519	3.8	3.6	470	1,965	445	1,860
1–2	114	477	116	485	4.75	4.35	550	2,300	505	2,115
2–3	107	448	109	456	5.6	5.05	610	2,550	545	2,280
3–4	101	423	103	431	6.35	5.7	655	2,740	590	2,470
4–5	96	402	99	414	7.0	6.35	695	2,910	630	2,635
5–6	93	389	96.5	404	7.55	6.95	730	3,055	670	2,800
6–7	91	381	95	397	8.05	7.55	765	3,220	720	3,010
7–8	90	377	94.5	395	8.55	7.95	810	3,390	750	3,140
8–9	90	377	95	397	9.0	8.4	855	3,580	800	3,350
9–10	91	381	99	414	9.35	8.75	925	3,870	865	3,620
10–11	93	389	100	418	9.7	9.05	970	4,060	905	3,790
11–12	97	406	104.5	437	10.05	9.35	1,050	4,395	975	4,080
12	102	427								

*Observed intakes at ages indicated, from data of sources given in original publication. Average intake predicted from equation (age in months): 1 (kcal$_{th}$/kg) = 123 − 8.9 age + 0.59 age. See original reference.

†Requirement over interval indicated, calculated as predicted intake + 5‰. See original reference.

‡NCHS median weights at midpoint of month.

(From Energy and Protein Requirements: Report of a Joint FAO/WHO/UNU Expert Consultation. Technical Report Series No. 724. Geneva, World Health Organization, 1985, p. 91.)

TABLE A–8B. ESTIMATED AVERAGE DAILY ENERGY INTAKES AND REQUIREMENTS, AGES 1 TO 10 YEARS

BOYS

Age (years)	Intake* (kcal_th/day)	(MJ/day)	Requirement† (kcal_th/day)	(MJ/day)
1–2	1,140	4.76	1,200	5.02
2–3	1,340	5.60	1,410	5.89
3–4	1,490	6.23	1,560	6.52
4–5	1,610	6.73	1,690	7.07
5–6	1,720	7.19	1,810	7.57
6–7	1,810	7.57	1,900	7.94
7–8	1,895	7.92	1,990	8.32
8–9	1,970	8.24	2,070	8.66
9–10	2,045	8.55	2,150	8.99

GIRLS

Age (years)	Intake* (kcal_th/day)	(MJ/day)	Requirement† (kcal_th/day)	(MJ/day)
1–2	1,090	4.56	1,140	4.76
2–3	1,250	5.23	1,310	5.48
3–4	1,370	5.73	1,440	6.02
4–5	1,465	6.12	1,540	6.44
5–6	1,550	6.48	1,630	6.81
6–7	1,620	6.77	1,700	7.11
7–8	1,685	7.05	1,770	7.40
8–9	1,740	7.28	1,830	7.65
9–10	1,795	7.51	1,880	7.86

REQUIREMENT BY WEIGHT‡

	Boys		Girls	
	(kcal_th/kg per day)	(kJ/kg per day)	(kcal_th/kg per day)	(kJ/kg per day)
	104	435	108	452
	104	410	102	427
	99	414	95	397
	95	397	92	385
	92	385	88	368
	88	368	83	347
	83	347	76	318
	77	322	69	268
	72	301	62	259

*From data of Ferro-Luzzi and Durnin. Rome, FAO, 1981 (Document ESN: FAO/WHO/UNU/EPR/81/9).
†Intakes +5%. See original reference.
‡From NCHS median weights at midyear.
(From Energy and Protein Requirements: Report of a Joint FAO/WHO/UNU Expert consultation. Technical Report Series No. 724. Geneva, World Health Organization, 1985, pp. 94 and 95.)

TABLE A–8C. CALCULATED AVERAGE ENERGY EXPENDITURE AND OBSERVED INTAKES AND COMPARISON WITH RECOMMENDATIONS OF 1971 COMMITTEE FOR ADOLESCENTS AGED 10 TO 18 YEARS

AGE (years)	EXPENDITURE (× BMR)*	EXPENDITURE (kcal_th/day)	(MJ/day)	INTAKE† (kcal_th/day)	(MJ/day)	1971 COMMITTEE‡ RECOMMENDED REQUIREMENT (kcal_th/day)	(MJ/day)
Boys							
10–11	1.76	2,140	8.95	2,110	8.82	2,500	10.46
11–12	1.73	2,240	9.37	2,170	9.07	2,600	10.87
12–13	1.69	2,310	9.66	2,200	9.20	2,700	11.29
13–14	1.67	2,440	10.20	2,280	9.53	2,800	11.71
14–15	1.65	2,590	10.83	2,340	9.79	2,900	12.13
15–16	1.62	2,700	11.29	2,390	9.99	3,000	12.55
16–17	1.60	2,800	11.71	2,440	10.20	3,050	12.76
17–18	1.60	2,870	12.0	2,490	10.41	3,100	12.97
Girls							
10–11	1.65	1,910	7.99	1,850	7.74	2,300	9.62
11–12	1.63	1,980	8.28	1,890	7.90	2,350	9.83
12–13	1.60	2,050	8.57	1,930	8.07	2,400	10.04
13–14	1.58	2,120	8.87	1,970	8.24	2,450	10.25
14–15	1.57	2,160	9.03	2,010	8.40	2,500	10.46
15–16	1.54	2,140	8.95	2,050	8.57	2,500	10.46
16–17	1.53	2,130	8.91	2,080	8.70	2,420	10.12
17–18	1.52	2,140	8.95	2,120	8.87	2,340	9.79

*Expenditure calculated as in original publication.
†Intakes from reference in original publication.
‡Reference in original 1971 publication. (cf ref. d)
(From Energy and Protein Requirements: Report of a Joint FAO/WHO/UNU Expert consultation. Technical Report Series No. 724. Geneva, World Health Organization, 1985, p. 98.)

TABLE A–8D. DERIVATION OF AVERAGE VALUES OF THE ENERGY COST OF THREE GRADES OF PHYSICAL ACTIVITY AT WORK FOR WOMEN AND MEN*

	WOMEN†				MEN‡			
	Cost/min (kcal$_{th}$)	(kJ)	Average cost × BMR (gross)	(net)	Cost/min (kcal$_{th}$)	(kJ)	Average cost × BMR (gross)	(net)
Light work								
75% of time sitting or standing	1.51	6.3			1.79	7.5		
25% of time standing and moving	1.70	7.1			2.51	10.5		
Average	1.56	6.5	1.7	0.7	1.99	8.3	1.7	0.7
Moderate work								
25% of time sitting or standing	1.51	6.3			1.79	7.5		
75% of time spent on specific occupational activity	2.20	9.2			3.61	15.1		
Average	2.03	8.5	2.2	1.2	3.16	13.2	2.7	1.7
Heavy work								
40% of time sitting or standing	1.51	6.3			1.79	7.5		
60% of time spent on specific occupational activity	3.21	13.4			6.22	26.0		
Average	2.54	10.6	2.8	1.8	4.45	18.6	3.8	2.8

*Times and energy costs of sitting, standing, moving around, and work tasks are composite values derived from published and unpublished data (Annex 5) in original reference.
†Based on young adult females (18–30 years). Wt 55 kg, BMR 0.90 kcal$_{th}$(3.8 kJ)/min (Table A–7a.)
‡Based on young adult males (18–30 years). Wt 65 kg, BMR 1.16 kcal$_{th}$(4.9 kJ)/min (Table A–7a.)
(From Energy and Protein Requirements: Report of a Joint FAO/WHO/UNU Expert Consultation. Technical Report Series No. 724. Geneva, World Health Organization, 1985, p. 76.)

TABLE A—8E. AVERAGE DAILY ENERGY REQUIREMENT OF ADULTS WHOSE OCCUPATIONAL WORK IS CLASSIFIED AS LIGHT, MODERATE, OR HEAVY, EXPRESSED AS A MULTIPLE OF BASAL METABOLIC RATE

	LIGHT	MODERATE	HEAVY
Men	1.55	1.78	2.10
Women	1.56	1.64	1.82

(From Energy and Protein Requirements: Report of a Joint FAO/WHO/UNU Expert Consultation. Technical Report Series No. 724. Geneva, World Health Organization, 1985, p. 78.)

TABLE A—8F. ESTIMATES OF ENERGY COST OF WEIGHT GAIN*

SUBJECTS		ENERGY COST	
		($kcal_{th}$/g)	(kJ/g)
Premature infants		4.9	20.5
Premature infants		5.7	23.8
Normal infants		5.6	23.4
Infants recovering from malnutrition		5.55	23.2
		4.6	19.2
		3.5	14.6
		4.4	18.4
		7.1	29.7
Adults, recovering from anorexia nervosa		6.4	26.7
Adults, intentional overfeeding		8.2	34.3
Pregnancy	Theoretic estimate[†]	6.4	26.7

*See original references for data sources.
[†]Calculated as 80,000 $kcal_{th}$ (335 mJ) stored for 12.5 kg of weight gain.
(From Energy and Protein Requirements: Report of a Joint FAO/WHO/UNU Expert Consultation. Technical Report Series No. 724. Geneva, World Health Organization, 1985, p. 185.)

TABLE A-8G. NOMOGRAM FOR ESTIMATION OF CALORIC REQUIREMENTS

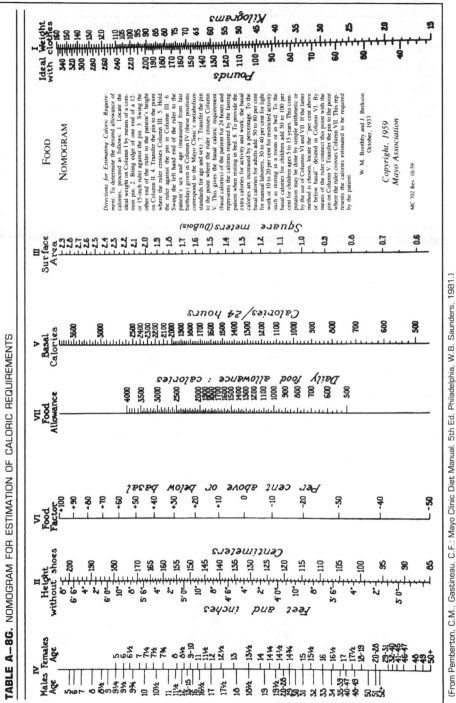

FOOD NOMOGRAM

Directions for Estimating Caloric Requirement. To determine the desired allowance of calories, proceed as follows: 1. Locate the ideal weight on Column I by means of a common pin. 2. Bring edge of one end of a 12- or 15-inch ruler against the pin. 3. Swing the other end of the ruler to the patient's height on Column II. 4. Transfer the pin to the point where the ruler crosses Column III. 5. Hold the ruler against the pin in Column III. 6. Swing the left hand end of the ruler to the patient's sex and age (measured from last birthday) given in Column IV (these positions correspond to the Mayo Clinic's metabolism standards for age and sex). 7. Transfer the pin to the point where the ruler crosses Column V. This gives the basal caloric requirement (basal calories) of the patient for 24 hours and represents the calories required by the fasting patient when resting in bed. 8. To provide the extra calories for activity and work, the basal calories are increased by a percentage. To the basal calories for adults add: 50 to 80 per cent for manual laborers, 30 to 40 per cent for light work or 10 to 20 per cent for restricted activity such as resting in a room or in bed. To the basal calories for children add 50 to 100 per cent for children ages 5 to 15 years. This computation may be done by simple arithmetic or by the use of Columns VI and VII. If the latter method is chosen, locate the "per cent above or below basal" desired in Column VI. By means of the ruler connect this point with the pin on Column V. Transfer the pin to the point where the ruler crosses Column VII. This represents the calories estimated to be required by the patient.

Copyright, 1959
Mayo Association

W. M. Boothby and J. Berkson
October, 1933

MC 702 Rev. 10-59

(From Pemberton, C.M., Gastineau, C.F.: Mayo Clinic Diet Manual. 5th Ed. Philadelphia, W.B. Saunders, 1981.)

TABLE A—9A. VALUES FOR THE DIGESTIBILITY OF PROTEIN IN MAN*

PROTEIN SOURCE	TRUE DIGESTIBILITY (mean ±SD)	DIGESTIBILITY RELATIVE TO REFERENCE PROTEINS
Egg	97 ± 3	
Milk, cheese	95 ± 3 95	100
Meat, fish	94 ± 3	
Maize	85 ± 6	89
Rice, polished	88 ± 4	93
Wheat, whole	86 ± 5	90
Wheat, refined	96 ± 4	101
Oatmeal	86 ± 7	90
Millet	79	83
Peas, mature	88	93
Peanut butter	95	100
Soyflour	86 ± 7	90
Beans	78	82
Maize + beans	78	82
Maize + beans + milk	84	88
Indian rice diet	77	81
Indian rice diet + milk	87	92
Chinese mixed diet	96	98[†]
Brazilian mixed diet	78	82
Filipino mixed diet	88[‡]	93
American mixed diet	96[‡]	101
Indian rice + bean diet	78[‡]	82

*See original reference for data sources.
[†]Relative to egg measured in the same study.
[‡]Recalculated from apparent digestibility, using F_K = 12 mg N/kg (see original text).
(From Energy and Protein Requirements: Report of a Joint FAO/WHO/UNU Expert Consultation. Technical Report Series No. 724. Geneva, World Health Organization, 1985, p. 119.)

TABLE A–9B-1. DAILY AVERAGE (PER KG) ENERGY REQUIREMENTS AND SAFE LEVEL OF PROTEIN INTAKE FOR INFANTS AND CHILDREN AGED 3 MONTHS TO 10 YEARS (SEXES COMBINED UP TO 5 YEARS)

AGE	MEDIAN WEIGHT (kg)	ENERGY REQUIREMENT				SAFE LEVEL OF PROTEIN INTAKE (g/kg)*
		(kcal$_{th}$/kg)		(kJ/kg)		
Months						
3–6	7.0	100		418		1.85
6–9	8.5	95		397		1.65
9–12	9.5	100		418		1.50
Years						
1–2	11.0	105		439		1.20
2–3	13.5	100		418		1.15
3–5	16.5	95		397		1.10
		Boys	Girls	Boys	Girls	
5–7	20.5	90	85	377	356	1.00
7–10	27.0	78	67	326	280	1.00

*Minimum level considered safe.
(From Diet, Nutrition and the Prevention of Chronic Diseases: Report of a WHO Study Group. Technical Report Series No. 797. Geneva, World Health Organization, 1990, pp. 167–168.

TABLE A–9B-2. DAILY AVERAGE ENERGY REQUIREMENTS AND SAFE LEVEL OF PROTEIN INTAKE FOR ADOLESCENTS AGED 10 TO 18 YEARS

AGE (years)	MEDIAN WEIGHT (kg)	ENERGY REQUIREMENT		SAFE LEVEL OF PROTEIN INTAKE (g/kg)*
		(kcal$_{th}$)	(kJ)	
Boys				
10–12	34.5	2,200	9,200	1.00
12–14	44.0	2,400	10,000	1.00
14–16	55.5	2,650	11,100	0.95
16–18	64.0	2,850	11,900	0.90
Girls				
10–12	36.0	1,950	8,200	1.00
12–14	46.5	2,100	8,800	0.95
14–16	52.0	2,150	9,000	0.90
16–18	54.0	2,150	9,000	0.80

*Minimum level considered safe.
(From Diet, Nutrition and the Prevention of Chronic Diseases: Report of a WHO Study Group. Technical Report Series No. 797. Geneva, World Health Organization, 1990, pp. 167–168.)

TABLE A–9B-3. DAILY AVERAGE ENERGY REQUIREMENTS AND SAFE LEVEL OF PROTEIN INTAKE FOR ADULTS*

WEIGHT (kg)	ENERGY REQUIREMENT						SAFE LEVEL OF PROTEIN INTAKE (g/day)†
	18–30 years		30–60 years		Over 60 years		
	(kcal$_{th}$)	(kJ)	(kcal$_{th}$)	(kJ)	(kcal$_{th}$)	(kJ)	
Men							
50	2,300	9,700	2,350	9,700	1,850	7,700	37.5
55	2,400	10,100	2,450	10,100	1,950	8,300	41.0
60	2,550	10,600	2,500	10,400	2,100	8,600	45.0
65	2,700	11,300	2,600	10,900	2,200	9,100	49.0
70	2,800	11,700	2,700	11,200	2,300	9,600	52.5
75	2,900	12,300	2,800	11,800	2,400	10,000	56.0
80	3,050	12,900	2,900	12,000	2,500	10,400	60.0
Women							
40	1,700	7,200	1,900	7,900	1,650	6,800	30.0
45	1,850	7,700	1,950	8,300	1,700	7,100	34.0
50	1,950	8,200	2,050	8,500	1,800	7,500	37.5
55	2,100	8,600	2,100	8,800	1,900	7,900	41.0
60	2,200	9,200	2,200	9,000	1,950	8,200	45.0
65	2,300	9,800	2,250	9,400	2,050	8,500	49.0
70	2,450	10,300	2,300	9,600	2,150	8,900	52.5
75	2,550	10,800	2,400	10,000	2,200	9,300	56.0

*For a basal metabolic rate factor of 1.6.
†Minimum level considered safe.
(From Diet, Nutrition and the Prevention of Chronic Diseases: Report of a WHO Study Group. Technical Report Series No. 797. Geneva, World Health Organization, 1990, pp. 167–168.)

TABLE A–10. RECOMMENDED DIETARY ALLOWANCES OF VITAMINS AND MINERALS

AGE	VITAMIN A[a,b] SAFE LEVEL (µg retinol/day) M	F	FOLATE[a] (µg/day) M	F	VITAMIN B$_{12}$[a] (µg/day) M	F	VITAMIN C[c] (mg/day) M	F	VITAMIN D[c] (µg/day) M	F	IRON[a,d] ABSORBED (µg/kg per day) M	F	ZINC[e] (mg/day) M	F
Infants (months)														
0–3	350	350		16	0.1	0.1	20	20	10	10		120		3.1
4–6	350	350		24	0.1	0.1	20	20	10	10		120		3.1
7–9	350	350		32	0.1	0.1	20	20	10	10		120		2.8
10–12	350	350		32	0.1	0.1	20	20	10	10		120		2.8
Children and adults (years)														
1–2	400	400		50	1.0	1.0	20	20	10	10		56	4.0	3.9
3–4	400	400		50	1.0	1.0	20	20	10	10		44	4.0	3.9
5–6	400	400		102	1.0	1.0	20	20	10	10		40	4.0	3.9
7–10	400	400		102	1.0	1.0	20	20	2.5	2.5		40	4.0	3.9
11–12	500	500		102	1.0	1.0	20	20	2.5	2.5		40	7.0	6.6
13–14	600	600		170	1.0	1.0	30	30	2.5	2.5	34	40	7.0	6.6
15–16	600	500	200	170	1.0	1.0	30	30	2.5	2.5	34	40	7.0	5.5
17–18	600	500	200	170	1.0	1.0	30	30	2.5	2.5	34	40	7.0	5.5
19+	600	500	200	170	1.0	1.0	30	30	2.5	2.5	18	43	5.5	5.5
Pregnant women		600		370 to 470		1.4		50		10		f		6.4 to 7.5
Lactating women		850		270		1.3		50		10		24		13.7
Postmenopausal women		500		170		1.0		30		2.5		18		5.5

[a]Adapted from reference 1.
[b]Minimum level considered safe.
[c]Adapted from reference 2; 2.5 µg of cholecalciferol are equivalent to 100 IU of vitamin D.
[d]The amount of absorbed iron is a variable proportion of the intake, depending on the type of diet.
[e]Adapted from reference 3.
[f]Requirements during pregnancy depend on the woman's iron status before pregnancy.

REFERENCES

1. FAO Food and Nutrition Series No. 23. Rome, Food and Agriculture Organization, 1988.
2. WHO Technical Report Series No. 452. Geneva, World Health Organization, 1970.
3. WHO Technical Report Series No. 532. Geneva, World Health Organization, 1973.
   (From Diet, Nutrition and the Prevention of Chronic Diseases; Report of a WHO Study Group. Technical Report Series No. 797. Geneva, World Health Organization, 1990, p. 169.)

TABLE A-11A. HEIGHT-WEIGHT TABLES: THEIR SOURCES AND DEVELOPMENT (SIDNEY ABRAHAM)

The Metropolitan Life Insurance Company presented their height and weight tables derived from data of the Build Study, 1979.[1] Metropolitan Life had previously utilized data from life insurance mortality studies compiled in the early 1900s and late 1950s to develop desirable weight tables in 1942,[2] 1943,[3] and 1959.[4] These studies reported the prevalence of mortality among insured persons according to variations in body build (height and weight) and also presented the average weight for height of persons by age. Such studies were designed to determine which groups (those underweight or overweight) showed a proportionately higher prevalence of mortality to yield information for underwriting purposes and for warranting changes in insurance policy premiums.

AVERAGE WEIGHT BY HEIGHT TABLES AND AGE-GROUP

Mortality Studies. In the American life insurance industry, interest in build (height and weight) as factors that influence mortality dates back to 1885. In that year, the Union Mutual Life Insurance Company published a pamphlet containing the results of a study of the company's records on mortality in relation to build.[5] The first indepth study on the subject was presented in 1901 by a representative of the New York Life Insurance Company at the twelfth annual meeting of the Association of Life Insurance Medical Directors of America.[6] In this presentation it was pointed out that a certain amount of overweight had previously been looked on favorably. Nonetheless, the summary of this report noted that: "First among life insurance risks [is that] the [health] hazard increases in proportion to the degree of over- or underweight, second, whereas among overweights the mortality to be expected increases with [the] increased age of [the] applicant, among underweights the mortality decreases with advancing years."

Height-Weight Tables. The first height-weight table based on a considerable volume of statistics and taking age into account was the "Shepherd Table." This table was prepared in 1897 and was based on 74,162 male applicants accepted for life insurance in the United States and Canada.[7]

The basic study of height and weight based on life insurance statistics, however, was made as part of the Medico-Actuarial Mortality Investigation of 1912.[8] This study and the tables derived therefrom were the basis of the

(From Clinical Consultations in Nutrition Support, 3:5–8, 1983. Reprinted with permission of Sidney Abraham and Clinical Consultants in Nutrition Support.)

height-weight tables prepared for the general population. In addition to the study of the prevalence of mortality of certain groups of the insured population, the 1912 investigation included a study of the height and weight of a sample of persons insured from 1885 to 1900. The height and weight were recorded with the subjects wearing shoes and street clothes. A total of 221,819 men residing in the United States and Canada were included in this sample. At least 40% of the weights were estimated by the medical examiners. The data as tabulated were then smoothed to provide the figures for the height-weight age tables, and the adjusted tables became the basis for height-weight tables for males in the United States at this time.

Substantially the same procedure was employed to develop height-weight tables for women, but to secure enough cases for the preparation of tables it was necessary to add 126,504 policies issued after 1900 to the 10,000 included in the 1885 to 1900 sample.

In the Medical Impairment Study of 1929,[9] height-weight data were again collected on 667,000 men and 85,000 women. The average weights of both men and women in the 1929 study were not significantly different from those observed in the Medico-Actuarial Mortality Investigation. In fact, differences were so small that it was decided not to revise the standard height-weight tables except for those individuals younger than age 15.

TABLES OF "IDEAL" OR "DESIRABLE" WEIGHTS

An article presented in 1920, "Is the 'Average' the Same as the 'Normal' for Weight and Blood Pressure?"[10] illustrates an important development in the preparation of height-weight tables. In this paper the "normal" weight group is defined as that having the lowest mortality rate. The article presented a table of "normal" weights, so defined, for medium-sized men averaging 68 inches in height, and several discussants added their tables of similarly defined normal weights for men of small, medium, and tall height. In 1922, complete height-weight tables were presented that showed this normal weight for each inch of height and for each age group.[11] In general, all such tables of normal weight indicated that the ideal weight in terms of mortality was the average weight for height at age 30.

METROPOLITAN LIFE DEVELOPS "IDEAL" HEIGHT-WEIGHT TABLES

Desirable Weight Tables, 1942 and 1943. The concept of a "normal" weight, represented by the average weight of men at age 30, plus an awareness of the shortcomings of height and weight alone as complete indications of obesity, led to the development of "ideal" weight tables by the Metropolitan Life Insurance company.[2,3] Although employed for many purposes, these tables were originally intended for use in health education. The basic data were derived from the standard height-weight tables of the Medico-Actuarial Study of 1912, using the average weight for each inch of height at age 30 for men and at age 25 for women. Arbitrary ranges were then developed, using the base figures as reference points. These ranges are approximately the standard deviation of average weights for a given height and include the lightest weight for persons with small frames to the heaviest weight for persons with large frames. The total was then arbitrarily divided into three overlapping ranges, and the resulting figures represented ideal weights for individuals of small, medium, and large frames. However, no definition of frame size was presented.

These tables were intended to aid people in achieving a weight below the average for their height. Before these tables were developed, only average weights for each inch of height by age and sex were available. The new approach represented a change in concept between average weight (assuming that the average value is optimal for health) and desirable weight (weight based on the criterion of longevity). The concept underlying these tables deemphasized the use of a single average at each height and refuted the popular notion that weight increments attendant with advancing age were normal and therefore not harmful.

Desirable Weight Tables, 1959. The next study of build in relation to mortality was made in conjunction with the Build and Blood Pressure Study of 1959.[4] This investigation was based on the combined experience of 26 life insurance companies in the United States and Canada from 1935 to 1954 and involved observation of nearly 5 million insured persons for periods up to 20 years. Only those insured persons ages 15 through 69 were included. The height and weight data were recorded with the subjects wearing street shoes and indoor clothing. More than 90% of the insured persons were reported to have been actually weighed and measured at the time of examination for life insurance. The study presented average weights for men and women for each inch of height, ranging from 62 to 76 inches for men and from 58 to 72 inches for women. To provide some indication of the sole effect of weight on mortality, persons with heart disease, cancer, or diabetes were excluded.

When the Build and Blood Pressure Study was completed, the "ideal weight" table, originally developed by the Metropolitan Life Insurance company in 1942 and 1943, was revised to conform to the latest data. The new table, called the "desirable weight" table (Table A–11b) was derived directly from weights associated with lowest mortality. Ranges of "desirable weight" for individuals 25 years and older with small, medium, and large frames were given, but again, no definition of frame size was included.

1983 Metropolitan Height-Weight Tables. Data published by the Society of Actuaries and the Association of Life Insurance Medical Directors of America in the Build Study, 1979,[1] are the source for the 1983 Metropolitan Life Insurance Height-Weight Tables (Table A–11c). The data are from 25 life insurance companies in the United States and Canada and show the prevalence of mortality from 1954 to 1972 of approximately 4.2 million insured men and women. Almost 90% of the recorded weights submitted for the study was obtained by actually weighing the applicants. As in the 1959 Build and Blood Pressure Study, applicants with major disease conditions at the time of policy issuance were excluded from the study. The terms "ideal body weight" and "desirable body weight," used in the earlier tables were not applied to the new height and weight tables because of the various misinterpretations of their meaning.

The findings from the Build Study, 1979, showed that the gap between the weights based on lowest mortality and average weights has narrowed considerably since the 1959 Build and Blood Pressure Study. Metropolitan Life considered this factor in developing the 1983 height-weight tables. Weight for height has increased in contrast to the 1959 tables, but the increased weights are still less than the average weights (see Table A–11f). Additionally, the increases in weight are not uniformly distributed throughout the 1983 height-weight tables. For each frame size, the weight increases for tall men or women were not as large as those for short men or women or for those of medium height.

In conjunction with investigations based on the life insurance data previously enumerated, long-term studies such as the Framingham Heart Study[12] and the Manitoba Study[13] all indicate that the weight associated with the greatest longevity tends to be below the average weight of the population under consideration and that "slimmer is better," provided that the underweight is not associated with a medical history of significant impairment.

FRAME SIZE

The 1983 Metropolitan height-weight tables relate weight to body frame size. A distinction is made among persons with small, medium, and large frames. The previous Metropolitan height-weight tables also related weight to body frame size, but although the body frame sizes were statistically defined, no generally accepted method of measuring frame size was provided. Body frame size is an integral factor in considering variation in weight, assuming that persons with larger frames have larger lean body mass and therefore weigh more. In the 1983 tables, elbow breadth is now used to determine frame size in men and women (Table A–11d). The frame sizes were developed from elbow breadth measurements taken from the first National Health and Nutrition Examination Survey, 1971 to 1975,[14] and were distributed so that 50% of the population falls within the medium frame and 25% each falls within the small and large frames.

SUMMARY

Major insurance mortality studies on insured populations in the United States and Canada conducted in 1912 by the Actuarial Society of America[8] and in 1959 and 1979 by the Society of Actuaries and the Association of Life Insurance Medical Directors of America[1,4] analyzed the mortality experience among insured persons according to variations of weight by height. The studies also presented data on the distribution of weight and height. The earliest study showed that the lowest mortality by build (weight for height) was found for those somewhat overweight at younger ages and among those underweight at older ages. In later mortality studies, it was generally found that insured persons whose weight was below the average lived longer than those whose weights were above average.

Since 1942, the Metropolitan Life Insurance Company has developed weight tables from data derived from each of the three major studies. The weights in each of the tables at given heights for men and women are classified according to frame size and refer to the weights associated with lowest mortality of policyholders. The weights were those obtained when the individual was originally insured. Because it is recognized that height and weight alone are incomplete indicators of excess weight, the weight tables also considered measurements of body build. In the tables issued in the 1940s,[2,3] 1959,[4] and 1983, three groups of frame size were identified. In each frame size, weight was given as a range rather than as a single value. However, no objective method was presented to estimate frame size in the earlier two tables. In the 1983 Metropolitan Height-Weight Tables, elbow breadth, unaffcted by degree of adiposity and closely representative of bony dimension, was suggested to estimate frame size in the three categories of body build.

The views herein are solely those of the author and do not necessarily represent those of the National Center for Health Statistics.

REFERENCES

1. Build Study, 1979: Society of Actuaries and Association of Life Insurance Medical Directors of America. Philadelphia, Recording and Statistical Corporation, 1980.
2. Ideal Weight for Men: Stat. Bull. Metropol. Life Insur. Co., *23*:6, 1942.
3. Ideal weights for Woman: Stat. Bull. Metropol. Life Insur. Co., *24*:6, 1943.
4. New Weight Standards for Men and Women: Stat. Bull. Metropol. Life Insur. Co., *40*:1, 1959.
5. Grant, F. S.: Proc. Assoc. Life Insur. Med. Dir. Am., *2*:323−327, 1902.
6. Rogers, O. H.: Proc. Assoc. Life Insur. Med. Dir. Am., *1*:280−288, 1901.
7. Shepherd, G. R.: Proc. Assoc. Life Insur. Med. Dir. Am., *6*:46−58, 1912.
8. Medico-Actuarial Mortality Investigation. New York, Actuarial Society of America, 1912.
9. Medical Impairment Study, 1929. New York, The Association of Life Insurance Medical Directors of America and the Actuarial Society of America, 1931.
10. Hunter, A.: Trans. Actuar. Soc. Am., *21*:365−370, 1920.
11. Knight, A. S.: Proc. Assoc. Life Insur. Med. Dir. Am., *9*:193−199, 1922.
12. Hubert, H. B., Feinleib, M., McNamara, P. M., et al.: Circulation, *5*:968−977, 1983.
13. Rabkin, S. W., Mathewson, F. A. L., Hsu, P. H.: Am. J. Cardiol., *39*:452−458, 1977.
14. Public Use Data Tape, NHANES I—Anthropometry, goniometry, skeletal age, bone density, and cortical thickness, ages 1−74. Tape No. 4111, National Health and Nutrition Examination Survey, 1971−1975. Hyattsville, MD, National Center for Health Statistics.

TABLE A–11B. DESIRABLE WEIGHTS FOR MEN AND WOMEN AGED 25 AND OVER (IN POUNDS) BY HEIGHT AND FRAME, IN INDOOR CLOTHING), 1959

MEN (IN SHOES, ONE-INCH HEELS)

HEIGHT FEET	INCHES	SMALL FRAME	MEDIUM FRAME	LARGE FRAME
5	2	112–120	118–129	126–141
5	3	115–123	121–133	129–144
5	4	118–126	124–136	132–148
5	5	121–129	127–139	135–152
5	6	124–133	130–143	138–156
5	7	128–137	134–147	142–161
5	8	132–141	138–152	147–166
5	9	136–145	142–156	151–170
5	10	140–150	146–160	155–174
5	11	144–154	150–165	159–179
6	0	148–158	154–170	164–184
6	1	152–162	158–175	168–189
6	2	156–167	162–180	173–194
6	3	160–171	167–185	178–199
6	4	164–175	172–190	182–204

WOMEN (IN SHOES, TWO-INCH HEELS)

HEIGHT FEET	INCHES	SMALL FRAME	MEDIUM FRAME	LARGE FRAME
4	10	92–98	96–107	104–119
4	11	94–101	98–110	106–122
5	0	96–104	101–113	109–125
5	1	99–107	104–116	112–128
5	2	102–110	107–119	115–131
5	3	105–113	110–122	118–134
5	4	108–116	113–126	121–138
5	5	111–119	116–130	125–142
5	6	114–123	120–135	129–146
5	7	118–127	124–139	133–150
5	8	122–131	128–143	137–154
5	9	126–135	132–147	141–158
5	10	130–140	136–151	145–163
5	11	134–144	140–155	149–168
6	0	138–148	144–159	153–173

(Data adapted from new weight standards for men and women. Stat. Bull. Metropol. Life Insur. Co., *40:*1, 1959.)

TABLE A–11C. HEIGHT-WEIGHT TABLES, 1983

MEN

HEIGHT FEET	INCHES	SMALL FRAME	MEDIUM FRAME	LARGE FRAME
5	2	128–134	131–141	138–150
5	3	130–136	133–143	140–153
5	4	132–138	135–145	142–156
5	5	134–140	137–148	144–160
5	6	136–142	139–151	146–164
5	7	138–145	142–154	149–168
5	8	140–148	145–157	152–172
5	9	142–151	148–160	155–176
5	10	144–154	151–163	158–180
5	11	146–157	154–166	161–184
6	0	149–160	157–170	164–188
6	1	152–164	160–174	168–192
6	2	155–168	164–178	172–197
6	3	158–172	167–182	176–202
6	4	162–176	171–187	181–207

WOMEN

HEIGHT FEET	INCHES	SMALL FRAME	MEDIUM FRAME	LARGE FRAME
4	10	102–111	109–121	118–131
4	11	103–113	111–123	120–134
5	0	104–115	113–126	122–137
5	1	106–118	115–129	125–140
5	2	108–121	118–132	128–143
5	3	111–124	121–135	131–147
5	4	114–127	124–138	134–151
5	5	117–130	127–141	137–155
5	6	120–133	130–144	140–159
5	7	123–136	133–147	143–163
5	8	126–139	136–150	146–167
5	9	129–142	139–153	149–170
5	10	132–145	142–156	152–173
5	11	135–148	145–159	155–176
6	0	138–151	148–162	158–179

Weight according to frame (ages 25 to 59) for men wearing indoor clothing weighing 5 lb, shoes with one-inch heels; for women, indoor clothing weighing 3 lb, shoes with one-inch heels.

Reprinted with permission from the Metropolitan Life Insurance Company, New York.)

TABLE A—11D. HEIGHT AND ELBOW BREADTH FOR MEN AND WOMEN*

HEIGHT IN ONE-INCH HEELS	ELBOW BREADTH
Men	
5'2"–5'3"	2½"–2⅞"
5'4"–5'7"	2⅝"–2⅞"
5'8"–5'11"	2¾"–3"
6'0"–6'3"	2¾"–3⅛"
6'4"	2⅞"–3¼"
Women	
4'10"–4'11"	2¼"–2½"
5'0"–5'3"	2¼"–2½"
5'4"–5'7"	2⅜"–2⅝"
5'8"–5'11"	2⅜"–2⅝"
6'0"	2½"–2¾"

*See Table A—11f; see Table A—11g for data on frame size by elbow breadth from NHANES I and II.

Extend your arm and bend the forearm upward at a 90° angle. Keep fingers straight and turn the inside of your wrist toward your body. If you have a caliper, use it to measure the space between the two prominent bones on either side of your elbow. Without a caliper, place thumb and index finger of your other hand on these two bones. Measure the space between your fingers against a ruler or tape measure. Compare it with these tables that list elbow measurements for medium-frame men and women. Measurements lower than those listed indicate you have a small frame. Higher measurements indicate a larger frame.

(Reprinted with permission from Metropolitan Life Insurance Company, New York.)

TABLE A–11E. HEIGHT-WEIGHT TABLES (METRIC UNITS), 1983*

MEN

HEIGHT (cm)	SMALL FRAME (kg)	MEDIUM FRAME (kg)	LARGE FRAME (kg)
157.5	58.2–60.9	59.4–64.1	62.7–68.2
160	59.1–61.8	60.5–65.0	63.6–69.5
162.5	60.0–62.7	61.4–65.9	64.5–70.9
165	60.9–63.7	62.3–67.3	65.5–72.7
167.5	61.8–64.5	63.2–68.6	66.4–74.5
170	62.7–65.9	64.5–70.0	67.7–76.4
173	63.6–67.3	65.9–71.4	69.1–78.2
175	64.5–68.6	67.3–72.7	70.5–80.0
178	65.4–70.0	68.6–74.1	71.8–81.8
180	66.4–71.4	70.0–75.5	73.2–83.6
183	67.7–72.7	71.4–77.3	74.5–85.6
185.5	69.1–74.5	72.7–79.1	76.4–87.3
188	70.5–76.4	74.5–80.9	78.2–89.5
190.5	71.8–78.2	75.9–82.7	80.0–91.8
193	73.6–80.0	77.7–85.0	82.3–94.1

WOMEN

HEIGHT (cm)	SMALL FRAME (kg)	MEDIUM FRAME (kg)	LARGE FRAME (kg)
147.5	46.4–50.5	49.5–55.0	53.6–59.5
150	46.8–51.4	50.5–55.9	54.5–60.9
152.5	47.3–52.3	51.4–57.3	55.5–62.3
155	48.2–53.6	52.3–58.6	56.8–63.6
157.5	49.1–55.0	53.6–60.0	58.2–65.0
160	50.5–56.4	55.0–61.4	59.5–66.8
162.5	51.8–57.7	56.4–62.7	60.9–68.6
165	53.2–59.1	57.7–64.1	62.3–70.5
167.5	54.5–60.5	59.1–65.5	63.6–72.3
170	55.9–61.8	60.5–66.8	65.0–74.1
173	57.3–63.2	61.8–68.2	66.4–75.9
175	58.6–64.5	63.2–69.5	67.7–77.3
178	60.0–65.9	64.5–70.9	69.1–78.6
180	61.4–67.3	65.9–72.3	70.5–80.0
183	62.3–68.6	67.3–73.6	71.8–81.4

*The 1983 Metropolitan Height-Weight Tables are based on the 1979 Build Study.
The values are statistical computations from individuals ranging from 25 to 59 years of weights by height and body frame at which mortality has been found to be lowest or longevity the highest. Metropolitan Life does not advocate the use of the term "ideal," which has different meanings to various individuals, because the term was used originally in their 1942 to 1943 tables. If one wishes to use these tables in the sense that they are "ideal" in terms of lowest mortality, they are "appropriate" in that context. These tables do not provide weights related to minimizing illness, optimizing job performance, or creating the best appearance.
(Reprinted with permission from the Metropolitan Life Insurance Company, New York.)

TABLE A–11F. AVERAGE WEIGHTS BY HEIGHT AND AGE GROUP: 1959 AND 1979 BUILD AND BLOOD PRESSURE STUDIES

MEN	HEIGHT														
	5'2"	5'3"	5'4"	5'5"	5'6"	5'7"	5'8"	5'9"	5'10"	5'11"	6'0"	6'1"	6'2"	6'3"	6'4"
15–16 Years*															
1959 Study	107	112	117	122	127	132	137	142	146	150	154	159	164	169	†
1979 Study	112	116	121	127	133	137	143	148	153	159	162	168	173	178	184
Weight Change	+5	+4	+4	+5	+6	+5	+6	+6	+7	+9	+8	+9	+9	+9	—
17–19 Years															
1959 Study	119	123	127	131	135	139	143	147	151	155	160	164	168	172	176
1979 Study	124	129	132	137	141	145	150	155	159	164	168	174	179	185	190
Weight Change	+5	+6	+5	+6	+6	+6	+7	+8	+8	+9	+8	+10	+11	+13	+14
20–24 Years															
1959 Study	128	132	136	139	142	145	149	153	157	161	166	170	174	178	181
1979 Study	130	136	139	143	148	153	157	163	167	171	176	182	187	193	198
Weight Change	+2	+4	+3	+4	+6	+8	+8	+10	+10	+10	+10	+12	+13	+15	+17
25–29 Years															
1959 Study	134	138	141	144	148	151	155	159	163	167	172	177	182	186	190
1979 Study	134	140	143	147	152	156	161	166	171	175	181	186	191	197	202
Weight Change	+0	+2	+2	+3	+4	+5	+6	+7	+8	+8	+9	+9	+9	+11	+12
30–39 Years															
1959 Study	137	141	145	149	153	157	161	165	170	174	179	183	188	193	199
1979 Study	138	143	147	151	156	160	165	170	174	179	184	190	195	201	206
Weight Change	+1	+2	+2	+2	+3	+3	+4	+5	+4	+5	+5	+7	+7	+8	+7
40–49 Years															
1959 Study	140	144	148	152	156	161	165	169	174	178	183	187	192	197	203
1979 Study	140	144	149	154	158	163	167	172	176	181	186	192	197	203	208
Weight Change	+0	+0	+1	+2	+2	+2	+2	+3	+2	+3	+3	+5	+5	+6	+5
50–59 Years															
1959 Study	142	145	149	153	157	162	166	170	175	180	185	189	194	199	205
1979 Study	141	145	150	155	159	164	168	173	177	182	187	193	198	204	209
Weight Change	−1	+0	+1	+2	+2	+2	+2	+3	+2	+2	+2	+4	+4	+5	+4
60–69 Years															
1959 Study	139	142	146	150	154	159	163	168	173	178	183	188	193	198	204
1979 Study	140	144	149	153	158	163	167	172	176	181	186	191	196	200	207
Weight Change	+1	+2	+3	+3	+4	+4	+4	+4	+3	+3	+3	+3	+3	+2	+3

(Continued)

TABLE A—11F. (continued)

WOMEN	HEIGHT														
	4'10"	4'11"	5'0"	5'1"	5'2"	5'3"	5'4"	5'5"	5'6"	5'7"	5'8"	5'9"	5'10"	5'11"	6'0"
15—16 Years*															
1959 Study	97	100	103	107	111	114	117	121	125	128	132	136	†	†	†
1979 Study	101	105	109	112	117	121	123	128	131	135	138	142	146	149	152
Weight Change	+4	+5	+6	+5	+6	+7	+6	+7	+6	+7	+6	+6	—	—	—
17—19 Years															
1959 Study	99	102	105	109	113	116	120	124	127	130	134	138	142	147	152
1979 Study	103	108	111	115	119	123	126	129	132	136	140	145	148	150	154
Weight Change	+4	+6	+6	+6	+6	+7	+6	+5	+5	+6	+6	+7	+6	+3	+2
20—24 Years															
1959 Study	102	105	108	112	115	118	121	125	129	132	136	140	144	149	154
1979 Study	105	110	112	116	120	124	127	130	133	137	141	146	149	155	157
Weight Change	+3	+5	+4	+4	+5	+6	+6	+5	+4	+5	+5	+6	+5	+6	+3
25—29 Years															
1959 Study	107	110	113	116	119	122	125	129	133	136	140	144	148	153	158
1979 Study	110	112	114	119	121	125	128	132	134	138	142	148	150	156	159
Weight Change	+3	+2	+1	+3	+2	+3	+3	+3	+1	+2	+2	+4	+2	+3	+1
30—39 Years															
1959 Study	115	117	120	123	126	129	132	135	139	142	146	150	154	159	164
1979 Study	113	115	118	121	124	128	131	134	137	141	145	150	153	159	164
Weight Change	-2	-2	-2	-2	-2	-1	-1	-1	-2	-1	-1	0	-1	0	0
40—49 Years															
1959 Study	122	124	127	130	133	136	140	143	147	151	155	159	164	169	174
1979 Study	118	121	123	127	129	133	136	139	143	147	150	155	158	162	168
Weight Change	-4	-3	-4	-3	-4	-3	-4	-4	-4	-4	-5	-4	-6	-7	-6
50—59 Years															
1959 Study	125	127	130	133	136	140	144	148	152	156	160	164	169	174	180
1979 Study	121	125	127	131	133	137	141	144	147	152	156	159	162	166	171
Weight Change	-4	-2	-3	-2	-3	-3	-3	-4	-5	-4	-4	-5	-7	-8	-9
60—69 Years															
1959 Study	127	129	131	134	137	141	145	149	153	157	161	165	†	†	†
1979 Study	123	127	130	133	136	140	143	147	150	155	158	161	163	167	172
Weight Change	-4	-2	-1	-1	-1	-1	-2	-2	-3	-2	-3	-4	—	—	—

*Height in shoes (feet and inches) and weight in indoor clothing (pounds).

†Average weights omitted in classes with too few cases for analysis.

(Data from Association of Life Insurance Medical Directors of America and Society of Actuaries. Compiled by Seltzer, F.: Dietetic Currents, 10:17—22, 1983. Reprinted with permission of Ross Laboratories, Columbus, Ohio.)

TABLE A−11G. FRAME SIZE BY ELBOW BREADTH (cm) OF UNITED STATES MALE AND FEMALE ADULTS DERIVED FROM THE COMBINED NHANES I AND II DATA SETS*

AGE (YEARS)	FRAME SIZE		
	SMALL	MEDIUM	LARGE
MEN			
18−24	≤6.6	>6.6 AND <7.7	≥7.7
25−34	≤6.7	>6.7 AND <7.9	≥7.9
35−44	≤6.7	>6.7 AND <8.0	≥8.0
45−54	≤6.7	>6.7 AND <8.1	≥8.1
55−64	≤6.7	>6.7 AND <8.1	≥8.1
65−74	≤6.7	>6.7 AND <8.1	≥8.1
WOMEN			
18−24	≤5.6	>5.6 AND <6.5	≥6.5
25−34	≤5.7	>5.7 AND <6.8	≥6.8
35−44	≤5.7	>5.7 AND <7.1	≥7.1
45−54	≤5.7	>5.7 AND <7.2	≥7.2
55−64	≤5.8	>5.8 AND <7.2	≥7.2
65−74	≤5.8	>5.8 AND <7.2	≥7.2

*The tenth and ninetieth percentiles, respectively, represent the predicted mean ±1.282 times the SE. Similarly, the fifteenth and eighty-fifth percentiles are the predicted mean minus and plus, respectively, 1.036 times the SE of the regression equation. There were significant black-white population differences in weight and body composition when age and height were considered. However, when the comparisons were made with reference to age, height, and frame size, there were only minor interpopulation differences. For this reason, all races (white, black, and other) included in the NHANES I and II surveys were merged together for the purpose of calculating percentiles of anthropometric measurements.

(Combined NHANES I and II data sets from Frisancho, A.R.: Am, J. Clin. Nutr., *40*:808−819, 1984, with permission.)

TABLE A-11H. COMPARISON OF THE WEIGHT-FOR-HEIGHT TABLES FROM ACTUARIAL DATA (BUILD STUDY): NON-AGE-CORRECTED METROPOLITAN LIFE INSURANCE COMPANY AND AGE-SPECIFIC GERONTOLOGY RESEARCH CENTER RECOMMENDATIONS*

HEIGHT	METROPOLITAN 1983 WEIGHTS FOR AGES 25-59†		GERONTOLOGY RESEARCH CENTER WEIGHT RANGE FOR MEN AND WOMEN BY AGE (YEARS)				
	MEN	WOMEN	25	35	45	55	65
ft-in			lb				
4-10	—	100-131	84-111	92-119	99-127	107-135	115-142
4-11	—	101-134	87-115	95-123	103-131	111-139	119-147
5-0	—	103-137	90-119	98-127	106-135	114-143	123-152
5-1	123-145	105-140	93-123	101-131	110-140	118-148	127-157
5-2	125-148	108-144	96-127	105-136	113-144	122-153	131-163
5-3	127-151	111-148	99-131	108-140	117-149	126-158	135-168
5-4	129-155	114-152	102-135	112-145	121-154	130-163	140-173
5-5	131-159	117-156	106-140	115-149	125-159	134-168	144-179
5-6	133-163	120-160	109-144	119-154	129-164	138-174	148-184
5-7	135-167	123-164	112-148	122-159	133-169	143-179	153-190
5-8	137-171	126-167	116-153	126-163	137-174	147-184	158-196
5-9	139-175	129-170	119-157	130-168	141-179	151-190	162-201
5-10	141-179	132-173	122-162	134-173	145-184	156-195	167-207
5-11	144-183	135-176	126-167	137-178	149-190	160-201	172-213
6-0	147-187	—	129-171	141-183	153-195	165-207	177-219
6-1	150-192	—	133-176	145-188	157-200	169-213	182-225
6-2	153-197	—	137-181	149-194	162-206	174-219	187-232
6-3	157-202	—	141-186	153-199	166-212	179-225	192-238
6-4	—	—	144-191	157-205	171-218	184-231	197-244

*Values in this table are for height without shoes and weight without clothes. To convert inches to centimeters, multiply by 2.54; to convert pounds to kilograms, multiply by 0.455.

†The weight range is the lower weight for small frame and the upper weight for large frame.

(Gerontology Research Center data from Andres, R.: Mortality and obesity: the rationale for age-specific height-weight tables. *In* Principles of Geriatric Medicine. Edited by R. Andres, E. Bierman, and W. R. Hazzard. New York, McGraw-Hill, 1985, pp. 311–318.)

TABLE A—11I. NOMOGRAPH FOR ESTIMATING BODY MASS INDEX (kg/m^2)*

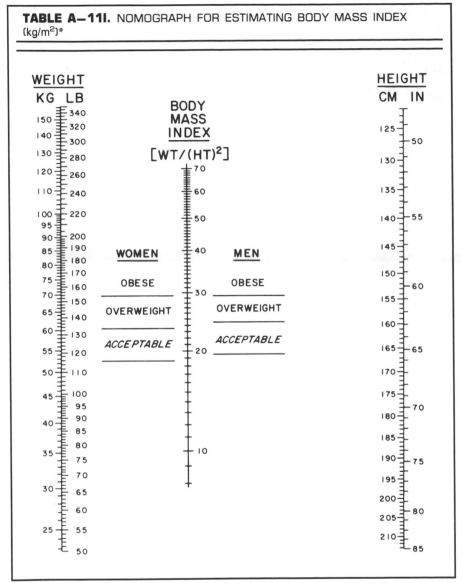

WEIGHT
KG LB

BODY
MASS
INDEX
$[WT/(HT)^2]$

WOMEN

OBESE

OVERWEIGHT

ACCEPTABLE

MEN

OBESE

OVERWEIGHT

ACCEPTABLE

HEIGHT
CM IN

*The ratio of weight/height^2 emerges from varied epidemiologic studies as the most generally useful index of relative body mass in adults. This nomograph facilitates use of this relationship in clinical situations. While showing the range of weight given as desirable in life insurance studies, the scale expresses relative weight as a continuous variable. This method encourages use of clinical judgment in interpreting "overweight" and "underweight" and in accounting for muscular and skeletal contributions to measured mass.

From Bray GA; Definitions, measurements, and classifications of the syndromes of obesity. Int J Obesity 2(2):99—112, 1978.

TABLE A–11J. DESIRABLE BODY MASS INDEX (BMI) IN RELATION TO AGE

Age (years)	BMI (kg/m^2)
19–24	19–24
25–34	20–25
35–44	21–26
45–54	22–27
55–65	23–28
>65	24–29

(From Committee on Diet and Health, Food and Nutrition Board, National Research Council. Diet and Health: Implications for Reducing Chronic Disease Risk. Washington, D.C., National Academy Press, 1989, p. 564.)

TABLE A–12A. FETAL GROWTH STANDARDS: INTRAUTERINE WEIGHT* AND LENGTH† CHARTS

INTRAUTERINE WEIGHT CHART
BOTH SEXES

INTRAUTERINE LENGTH CHART
BOTH SEXES

*Fetal body weight percentiles from 28 to 43 weeks of gestation.
†Fetal body length percentiles from 28 to 43 weeks of gestation.
(From Naeye, R.L., Dixon J.B.: Pediatr. Res., 12:989, 1978.)

TABLE A–12B-1. PHYSICAL GROWTH NCHS PERCENTILES: GIRLS FROM BIRTH TO 36 MONTHS

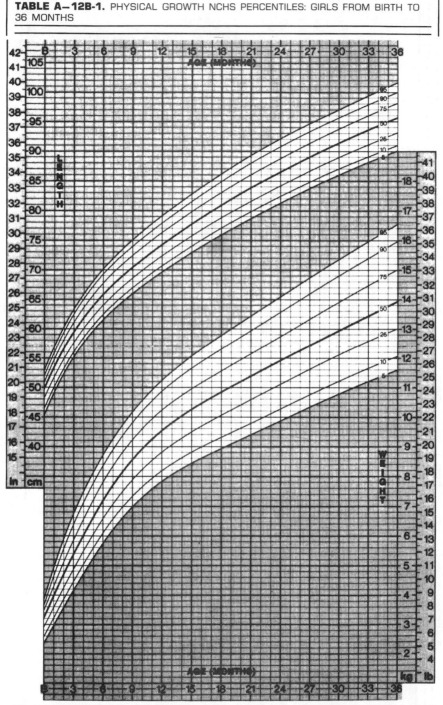

(Courtesy of Ross Laboratories, who adapted the growth curves from the original data: National Center for Health Statistics, NCHS Growth Charts, 1976. Monthly Vital Statistics Report, Vol. 25, No. 3, Suppl. (HRA) 76–1120. Rockville, MD, Health Resources Administration, June, 1976. Data from The Fels Research Institute, Yellow Springs, Ohio.)

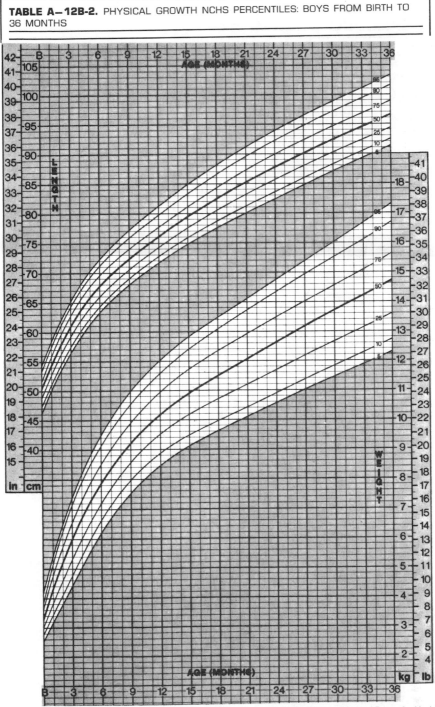

(Courtesy of Ross Laboratories, who adapted the growth curves from the original data: National Center for Health Statistics, NCHS Growth Charts, 1976. Monthly Vital Statistics Report, Vol. 25, No. 3, Suppl. (HRA) 76—1120. Rockville, MD, Health Resources Administration, June, 1976. Data from The Fels Research Institute, Yellow Springs, Ohio.)

TABLE A—12C-1. PHYSICAL GROWTH NCHS PERCENTILES: GIRLS FROM 2 TO 18 YEARS

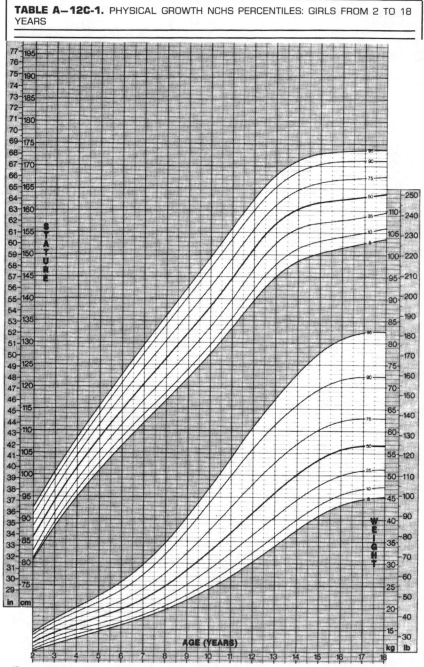

(Courtesy of Ross Laboratories, who adapted the growth curves from the original data: National Center for Health Statistics, NCHS Growth Charts, 1976. Monthly Vital Statistics Report, Vol. 25, No. 3, Suppl. (HRA) 76—1120. Rockville, MD, Health Resources Administration, June, 1976. Data from The Fels Research Institute, Yellow Springs, Ohio.)

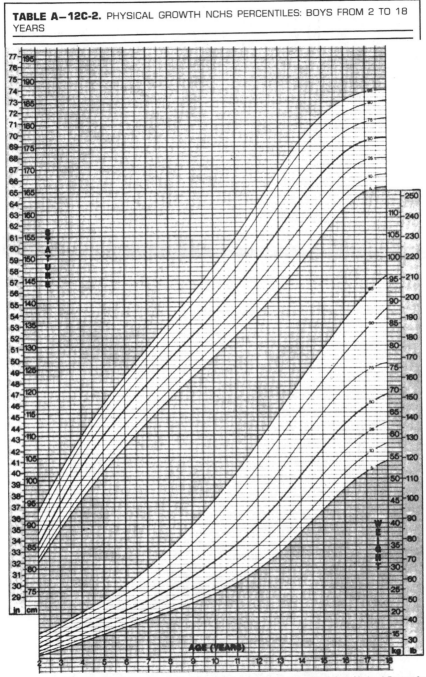

(Courtesy of Ross Laboratories, who adapted the growth curves from the original data: National Center for Health Statistics, NCHS Growth Charts, 1976. Monthly Vital Statistics Report, Vol. 25, No. 3, Suppl. (HRA) 76—1120. Rockville, MD, Health Resources Administration, June, 1976. Data from The Fels Research Institute, Yellow Springs, Ohio.)

TABLE A–12D. HEIGHT IN CENTIMETERS FOR PERSONS 2 TO 19 YEARS OF AGE: NUMBER EXAMINED, MEAN, STANDARD DEVIATION, AND SELECTED PERCENTILES BY SEX AND AGE, UNITED STATES, 1976 TO 1980*

SEX AND AGE (years)	NUMBER OF EXAMINED PERSONS	MEAN	STANDARD DEVIATION	PERCENTILE								
				5th	10th	15th	25th	50th	75th	85th	90th	95th
Male												
2	375	91.2	4.3	84.5	85.8	85.5	88.2	91.3	94.2	95.8	96.6	97.6
3	418	99.2	4.5	92.0	94.3	94.9	96.5	98.8	102.0	103.9	105.0	107.0
4	404	106.0	5.2	97.8	99.5	100.5	102.5	106.4	109.2	111.0	112.4	115.0
5	397	112.6	5.4	104.0	105.8	107.2	109.4	112.6	115.6	118.1	119.6	121.2
6	133	119.5	5.1	111.2	112.6	114.5	115.9	120.1	122.6	124.7	125.5	126.8
7	148	125.1	5.9	115.4	117.6	119.1	121.8	125.9	128.1	130.2	131.5	133.6
8	147	129.9	7.0	118.6	122.0	123.5	125.3	130.6	134.1	136.5	138.0	142.0
9	145	135.5	5.8	125.9	126.4	129.4	131.2	136.1	139.6	141.2	143.1	144.7
10	157	141.6	7.3	130.3	132.8	134.0	137.0	141.5	146.4	149.6	150.6	153.0
11	155	146.0	7.8	133.1	135.9	138.0	141.1	145.6	151.2	153.9	155.2	160.2
12	145	152.5	7.9	139.0	142.6	144.9	147.5	152.0	158.0	160.5	162.0	164.4
13	173	158.9	8.3	144.4	147.6	149.7	152.6	159.7	165.0	168.7	169.5	171.6
14	186	167.5	8.3	153.9	156.5	159.1	162.5	167.5	173.1	176.5	178.7	180.6
15	184	170.8	6.7	160.1	162.0	162.6	165.7	171.1	175.5	177.5	178.2	181.9
16	178	173.8	6.4	163.0	164.7	167.4	169.8	173.7	178.1	180.3	182.6	186.1
17	173	175.1	7.1	164.1	167.3	168.4	170.6	174.9	179.7	182.8	184.3	187.5
18	164	176.9	6.7	166.5	168.8	169.9	172.3	176.9	180.9	183.9	185.1	189.6
19	148	176.5	6.7	164.5	168.2	169.4	171.8	176.9	181.1	183.5	184.8	187.2

Female	n	Mean	SD									
2	336	89.7	4.2	83.1	84.4	85.5	86.7	89.8	92.2	93.6	94.9	97.2
3	366	97.5	4.8	89.6	91.1	92.5	94.5	97.6	100.8	102.5	103.4	104.5
4	396	104.6	5.0	96.1	98.2	99.5	101.5	104.5	108.2	109.8	110.7	112.4
5	364	111.6	5.3	103.0	105.1	106.4	108.1	111.6	115.2	116.5	118.8	120.3
6	135	118.4	6.1	109.9	111.1	111.5	113.3	118.5	122.2	124.5	126.5	128.7
7	157	123.7	6.7	113.3	116.6	117.4	119.6	124.1	128.1	130.1	132.2	134.7
8	123	130.2	5.7	120.8	123.4	124.4	125.8	130.6	133.2	135.4	137.5	140.5
9	149	134.4	7.6	124.0	126.4	127.8	129.0	134.8	139.0	140.7	142.6	147.1
10	136	141.9	6.5	131.6	133.6	135.1	137.6	141.6	146.3	148.1	150.4	153.8
11	140	147.9	7.8	134.7	139.3	140.6	142.2	147.9	152.2	154.7	156.9	162.7
12	147	154.4	7.2	143.9	145.7	146.7	149.2	154.8	158.6	161.9	164.7	165.9
13	162	158.9	6.6	149.0	150.3	152.7	155.3	159.0	163.0	164.5	166.9	170.3
14	178	160.8	6.4	151.0	152.7	154.5	156.7	160.9	165.1	166.9	168.2	172.3
15	145	163.2	6.2	153.0	155.2	157.1	159.1	163.1	167.1	170.2	172.4	173.5
16	170	162.9	6.1	152.0	154.5	157.2	159.1	163.2	166.4	169.4	171.4	173.3
17	134	163.5	5.7	153.8	156.8	158.5	160.4	163.1	166.7	169.7	170.7	172.2
18	170	162.4	6.8	150.7	154.2	155.6	158.0	162.7	166.2	169.1	171.5	174.0
19	158	163.5	5.6	153.8	156.8	157.7	159.7	163.7	167.2	169.5	170.4	172.1

*Height without shoes.

(From National Center for Health Statistics: Anthropometric Reference Data and Prevalence of Overweight, United States 1976–1980. DHHS Publication No. 87–1688. Hyattsville, MD, U.S. Department of Health and Human Services, Public Health Service, 1987.)

TABLE A–12E. WEIGHT IN KILOGRAMS FOR PERSONS 6 MONTHS TO 19 YEARS OF AGE: NUMBER EXAMINED, MEAN, STANDARD DEVIATION, AND SELECTED PERCENTILES BY SEX AND AGE, UNITED STATES, 1976 TO 1980*

SEX AND AGE	NUMBER OF EXAMINED PERSONS	MEAN	STANDARD DEVIATION	PERCENTILE										
				5th	10th	15th	25th	50th	75th	85th	90th	95th
Male													
6–11 months	179	9.4	1.3	7.5	7.6	8.2	8.6	9.4	10.1	10.7	10.9	11.4
1 year	370	11.8	1.9	9.6	10.0	10.3	10.8	11.7	12.6	13.1	13.6	14.4
2 years	375	13.6	1.7	11.1	11.6	11.8	12.6	13.5	14.5	15.2	15.8	16.5
3 years	418	15.7	2.0	12.9	13.5	13.9	14.4	15.4	16.8	17.4	17.9	19.1
4 years	404	17.8	2.5	14.1	15.0	15.3	16.0	17.6	19.0	19.9	20.9	22.2
5 years	397	19.8	3.0	16.0	16.8	17.1	17.7	19.4	21.3	22.9	23.7	25.4
6 years	133	23.0	4.0	18.6	19.2	19.8	20.3	22.0	24.1	26.4	28.3	30.1
7 years	148	25.1	3.9	19.7	20.8	21.2	22.2	24.8	26.9	28.2	29.6	33.9
8 years	147	28.2	6.2	20.4	22.7	23.6	24.6	27.5	29.9	33.0	35.5	39.1
9 years	145	31.1	6.3	24.0	25.6	26.0	27.1	30.2	33.0	35.4	38.6	43.1
10 years	157	36.4	7.7	27.2	28.2	29.6	31.4	34.8	39.2	43.5	46.3	53.4
11 years	155	40.3	10.1	26.8	28.8	31.8	33.5	37.3	46.4	52.0	57.0	61.0
12 years	145	44.2	10.1	30.7	32.5	35.4	37.8	42.5	48.8	52.6	58.9	67.5
13 years	173	49.9	12.3	35.4	37.0	38.3	40.1	48.4	56.3	59.8	64.2	69.9
14 years	186	57.1	11.0	41.0	44.5	46.4	49.8	56.4	63.3	66.1	68.9	77.0
15 years	184	61.0	11.0	46.2	49.1	50.6	54.2	60.1	64.9	68.7	72.8	81.3
16 years	178	67.1	12.4	51.4	54.3	56.1	58.7	64.4	73.6	78.1	82.2	91.2
17 years	173	66.7	11.5	50.7	53.4	54.8	58.7	65.8	72.0	76.8	82.3	88.9
18 years	164	71.1	12.7	54.1	56.6	60.3	61.9	70.4	76.6	80.0	83.5	95.3
19 years	148	71.7	11.6	55.9	57.9	60.5	63.8	69.5	77.9	84.3	86.8	92.1

Female

	n											
6–11 months	177	8.8	1.2	6.6	7.3	7.5	7.9	8.9	9.4	10.1	10.4	10.9
1 year	336	10.8	1.4	8.8	9.1	9.4	9.9	10.7	11.7	12.4	12.7	13.4
2 years	336	13.0	1.5	10.8	11.2	11.6	12.0	12.7	13.8	14.5	14.9	15.9
3 years	366	14.9	2.1	11.7	12.3	12.9	13.4	14.7	16.1	17.0	17.4	18.4
4 years	396	17.0	2.4	13.7	14.3	14.5	15.2	16.7	18.4	19.3	20.2	21.1
5 years	364	19.6	3.3	15.3	16.1	16.7	17.2	19.0	21.2	22.8	24.7	26.6
6 years	135	22.1	4.0	17.0	17.8	18.6	19.3	21.3	23.8	26.6	28.9	29.6
7 years	157	24.7	5.0	19.2	19.5	19.8	21.4	23.8	27.1	28.7	30.3	34.0
8 years	123	27.9	5.7	21.4	22.3	23.3	24.4	27.5	30.2	31.3	33.2	36.5
9 years	149	31.9	8.4	22.9	25.0	25.8	27.0	29.7	33.6	39.3	43.3	48.4
10 years	136	36.1	8.0	25.7	27.5	29.0	31.0	34.5	39.5	44.2	45.8	49.6
11 years	140	41.8	10.9	29.8	30.3	31.3	33.9	40.3	45.8	51.0	56.6	60.0
12 years	147	46.4	10.1	32.3	35.0	36.7	39.1	45.4	52.6	58.0	60.5	64.3
13 years	162	50.9	11.8	35.4	39.0	40.3	44.1	49.0	55.2	60.9	66.4	76.3
14 years	175	54.8	11.1	40.3	42.8	43.7	47.4	53.1	60.3	65.7	67.6	75.2
15 years	145	55.1	9.8	44.0	45.1	46.5	48.2	53.3	59.6	62.2	65.5	76.6
16 years	170	58.1	10.1	44.1	47.3	48.9	51.3	55.6	62.5	68.9	73.3	76.8
17 years	134	59.6	11.4	44.5	48.9	50.5	52.2	58.4	63.4	68.4	71.6	81.8
18 years	170	59.0	11.1	45.3	49.5	50.8	52.8	56.4	63.0	66.0	70.1	78.0
19 years	158	60.2	11.0	48.5	49.7	51.7	53.9	57.1	64.4	70.7	74.8	78.1

*Includes clothing weight, estimated as ranging from 0.09 to 0.28 kilogram.
(From National Center for Health Statistics: Anthropometric Reference Data and Prevalence of Overweight, United States 1976–1980. DHHS Publication No. 87–1688. Hyattsville, MD, U.S. Department of Health and Human Services, Public Health Service, 1987.)

TABLE A—12F-1. WEIGHT IN KILOGRAMS OF YOUTHS AGED 12 YEARS AT LAST BIRTHDAY BY SEX AND HEIGHT GROUP IN CENTIMETERS: SAMPLE SIZE, ESTIMATED POPULATION SIZE, MEAN, STANDARD DEVIATION, STANDARD ERROR OF THE MEAN, AND SELECTED PERCENTILES, UNITED STATES, 1966 TO 1970

SEX AND HEIGHT	n	N	$\bar{X}$	s	$s_{\bar{x}}$	PERCENTILE							
						5th	10th	25th	50th	75th	90th	95th	
						in kilograms							
Male													
Under 130	5	15	*	*	*	*	*	*	*	*	*	*	
130.0–134.9	4	8	*	*	*	*	*	*	*	*	*	*	
135.0–139.9	34	111	32.50	3.741	0.727	26.6	27.6	30.2	31.6	34.7	37.7	39.4	
140.0–144.9	80	241	34.28	3.635	0.601	28.1	30.0	31.8	34.1	36.5	38.6	40.7	
145.0–149.9	123	386	39.27	6.243	0.615	32.1	33.2	35.7	38.2	40.9	46.1	52.5	
150.0–154.9	156	513	42.90	6.314	0.480	34.9	36.1	38.2	42.1	46.0	51.6	56.3	
155.0–159.9	135	432	47.35	7.551	0.769	38.3	39.4	41.9	46.2	50.5	57.4	61.9	
160.0–164.9	65	201	50.82	8.735	1.388	42.1	42.7	44.9	48.4	56.0	61.1	67.1	
165.0–169.9	29	88	55.75	8.811	2.031	43.3	46.4	49.0	54.4	59.9	68.3	76.6	
170.0–174.9	8	21	62.37	4.503	1.993	54.0	58.1	60.1	61.0	66.0	69.1	69.5	
175.0–179.9	3	10	*	*	*	*	*	*	*	*	*	*	
180.0–184.9	1	2	*	*	*	*	*	*	*	*	*	*	
185.0–189.9	—	—	—	—	—	—	—	—	—	—	—	—	
190.0–194.9	—	—	—	—	—	—	—	—	—	—	—	—	
195.0 and over	—	—	—	—	—	—	—	—	—	—	—	—	

*Sample too small for analysis.

TABLE A—12F-1. (continued)

Sex and Height	n	N	$\bar{X}$	s	$s_{\bar{x}}$	PERCENTILE in kilograms						
						5th	10th	25th	50th	75th	90th	95th
Female												
Under 130	—	—	—	—	—	—	—	—	—	—	—	—
130.0–134.9	3	10	*	*	*	*	*	*	*	*	*	*
135.0–139.9	12	44	29.41	3.372	0.914	25.0	25.0	26.4	28.9	32.1	34.1	34.2
140.0–144.9	32	116	38.30	7.314	1.194	28.8	30.6	33.3	36.8	41.4	49.2	55.1
145.0–149.9	72	258	39.78	6.205	0.975	31.8	32.8	35.5	38.5	42.8	48.3	50.6
150.0–154.9	147	517	44.00	7.421	0.677	34.4	35.8	38.9	42.8	47.4	52.9	57.4
155.0–159.9	144	525	48.74	8.369	0.714	37.9	39.2	43.0	46.8	53.8	60.7	63.5
160.0–164.9	95	336	53.06	8.010	0.658	42.5	43.9	47.2	51.1	57.2	65.6	69.6
165.0–169.9	31	117	54.89	7.022	1.384	43.9	47.1	50.4	53.1	59.7	64.5	71.3
170.0–174.9	11	42	63.66	14.501	6.214	48.7	50.1	50.8	56.7	82.2	86.0	86.1
175.0–179.9	—	—	—	—	—	—	—	—	—	—	—	—
180.0–184.9	—	—	—	—	—	—	—	—	—	—	—	—
185.0–189.9	—	—	—	—	—	—	—	—	—	—	—	—
190.0–194.9	—	—	—	—	—	—	—	—	—	—	—	—
195.0 and over	—	—	—	—	—	—	—	—	—	—	—	—

n, Sample size; N, estimated number of youths in population in thousands; $\bar{X}$, mean; s, standard deviation; $s_{\bar{x}}$, standard error of the mean. (From National Center for Health Statistics: Height and weight of youths 12–17 years, United States. In Vital and Health Statistics, Series 11, No. 124, Health Services and Mental Health Administration. Washington, D.C., U.S. Government Printing Office, 1973, pp. 282–288.)

TABLE A—12F-2. WEIGHT IN KILOGRAMS OF YOUTHS AGED 13 YEARS AT LAST BIRTHDAY BY SEX AND HEIGHT GROUP IN CENTIMETERS: SAMPLE SIZE, ESTIMATED POPULATION SIZE, MEAN, STANDARD DEVIATION, STANDARD ERROR OF THE MEAN, AND SELECTED PERCENTILES, UNITED STATES, 1966 TO 1970

SEX AND HEIGHT	n	N	$\bar{X}$	s	$s_{\bar{x}}$	PERCENTILE						
						5th	10th	25th	50th	75th	90th	95th
						in kilograms						
Male												
Under 130	—	—	*	—	*	*	*	*	*	*	*	*
130.0–134.9	2	5	*	*	*	*	*	*	*	*	*	*
135.0–139.9	6	25	32.62	5.624	7.716	27.2	27.6	28.9	31.0	34.9	43.1	43.2
140.0–144.9	18	56	36.54	5.852	1.607	30.0	30.5	32.1	36.1	39.2	41.7	53.2
145.0–149.9	65	204	39.03	5.270	0.662	32.4	33.9	36.1	37.9	41.2	44.5	46.4
150.0–154.9	99	312	42.58	6.724	0.865	34.8	36.2	37.9	41.0	45.5	49.4	61.0
155.0–159.9	131	421	47.27	7.482	0.717	37.8	39.2	41.7	45.8	51.1	58.7	61.7
160.0–164.9	125	393	53.01	9.324	0.916	41.5	43.7	46.9	50.4	58.2	64.4	72.5
165.0–169.9	91	285	55.92	8.560	0.833	46.3	47.5	49.3	53.6	59.4	69.0	75.0
170.0–174.9	63	215	62.01	10.362	1.033	51.2	51.6	53.7	60.1	67.0	76.0	85.0
175.0–179.9	19	68	67.92	12.085	3.428	56.3	57.9	60.1	63.3	70.3	88.3	89.0
180.0–184.9	5	15	*	*	*	*	*	*	*	*	*	*
185.0–189.9	—	—	—	—	—	—	—	—	—	—	—	—
190.0–194.9	—	—	—	—	—	—	—	—	—	—	—	—
195.0 and over	—	—	—	—	—	—	—	—	—	—	—	—

Female

Height	n	N	$\bar{X}$	s	$s_{\bar{x}}$	Percentile						
						5th	10th	25th	50th	75th	90th	95th
Under 130	—	—	—	—	—	—	—	—	—	—	—	—
130.0–134.9	—	—	—	—	—	—	—	—	—	—	—	—
135.0–139.9	15	51	37.13	7.317	2.259	26.6	27.5	30.5	36.7	40.1	44.5	56.1
140.0–144.9	47	165	42.23	6.880	0.888	34.7	35.6	38.2	40.5	44.2	53.6	57.6
145.0–149.9	98	329	44.32	7.029	0.787	35.6	36.5	39.2	42.9	47.3	53.7	57.9
150.0–154.9	152	499	49.75	8.757	0.699	39.1	39.9	43.8	48.4	53.8	61.0	65.9
155.0–159.9	156	515	53.16	8.399	0.522	41.2	43.9	47.7	52.2	57.0	63.8	68.5
160.0–164.9	86	284	58.17	9.125	0.921	46.2	47.4	52.2	58.1	61.5	69.3	76.2
165.0–169.9	24	87	58.11	13.209	2.343	46.2	47.1	48.4	52.9	65.3	68.6	96.8
170.0–174.9	3	10	*	*	*	*	*	*	*	*	*	*
175.0–179.9	—	—	—	—	—	—	—	—	—	—	—	—
180.0–184.9	—	—	—	—	—	—	—	—	—	—	—	—
185.0–189.9	—	—	—	—	—	—	—	—	—	—	—	—
190.0–194.9	—	—	—	—	—	—	—	—	—	—	—	—
195.0 and over	—	—	—	—	—	—	—	—	—	—	—	—

n, Sample size; N, estimated number of youths in population in thousands; $\bar{X}$, mean; s, standard deviation; $s_{\bar{x}}$, standard error of the mean. (From National Center for Health Statistics: Height and weight of youths 12–17 years, United States. *In* Vital and Health Statistics, Series 11, No. 124, Health Services and Mental Health Administration. Washington, D.C., U.S. Government Printing Office, 1973, pp. 282–288.)

TABLE A—12F-3. WEIGHT IN KILOGRAMS OF YOUTHS AGED 14 YEARS AT LAST BIRTHDAY BY SEX AND HEIGHT GROUP IN CENTIMETERS: SAMPLE SIZE, ESTIMATED POPULATION SIZE, MEAN, STANDARD DEVIATION, STANDARD ERROR OF THE MEAN, AND SELECTED PERCENTILES, UNITED STATES, 1966 TO 1970

SEX AND HEIGHT	n	N	$\bar{X}$	s	$s_{\bar{x}}$	PERCENTILE (in kilograms)						
						5th	10th	25th	50th	75th	90th	95th
Male												
Under 130	—	—	—	—	—	—	—	—	—	—	—	—
130.0–134.9	—	—	—	—	—	—	—	—	—	—	—	—
135.0–139.9	2	7	*	*	*	*	*	*	*	*	*	*
140.0–144.9	3	13	*	*	*	*	*	*	*	*	*	*
145.0–149.9	11	42	40.51	1.829	0.644	36.9	38.6	39.6	40.6	42.0	42.5	42.7
150.0–154.9	45	135	43.63	6.277	1.182	36.2	37.0	39.0	41.4	48.0	51.7	55.3
155.0–159.9	83	261	47.42	7.822	0.872	37.7	38.7	41.8	46.1	51.2	58.0	62.7
160.0–164.9	96	299	52.28	6.785	0.584	42.5	44.0	47.5	52.1	56.3	61.5	65.1
165.0–169.9	134	432	58.07	9.416	1.054	47.7	49.3	51.6	55.4	62.3	70.6	75.7
170.0–174.9	144	435	62.37	11.516	1.095	49.7	51.0	55.0	59.4	65.6	79.2	86.3
175.0–179.9	71	228	65.54	9.704	1.306	50.9	55.1	58.5	64.7	69.9	74.5	84.0
180.0–184.9	25	81	72.44	13.014	2.298	59.6	60.0	65.1	69.4	77.0	83.0	94.3
185.0–189.9	3	9	*	*	*	*	*	*	*	*	*	*
190.0–194.9	1	3	*	*	*	*	*	*	*	*	*	*
195.0 and over	—	—	—	—	—	—	—	—	—	—	—	—

	n	N	$\bar{X}$	s	$s_{\bar{x}}$							
Female												
Under 130	—	—	—	—	—	—	—	—	—	—	—	—
130.0–134.9	—	—	—	—	—	—	—	—	—	—	—	—
135.0–139.9	1	2	*	*	*	*	*	*	*	*	*	*
140.0–144.9	2	6	*	*	*	*	*	*	*	*	*	*
145.0–149.9	17	52	42.00	5.879	1.683	32.0	35.3	36.3	42.3	47.5	49.5	51.1
150.0–154.9	64	196	48.26	6.797	0.926	37.7	39.2	42.5	47.9	53.3	55.9	58.8
155.0–159.9	157	508	51.35	7.705	0.520	41.2	43.4	46.3	49.6	55.6	62.2	64.3
160.0–164.9	186	603	54.59	8.810	0.707	43.0	45.0	48.4	53.0	59.7	66.7	70.7
165.0–169.9	114	372	58.46	10.185	0.955	45.9	47.5	52.1	56.8	61.8	70.5	76.4
170.0–174.9	36	121	64.37	15.821	2.814	49.2	52.1	56.2	59.8	70.5	72.9	99.4
175.0–179.9	7	28	61.33	5.496	2.620	51.7	52.0	57.7	59.8	64.6	70.2	70.6
180.0–184.9	2	7	*	*	*	*	*	*	*	*	*	*
185.0–189.9	—	—	—	—	—	—	—	—	—	—	—	—
190.0–194.9	—	—	—	—	—	—	—	—	—	—	—	—
195.0 and over	—	—	—	—	—	—	—	—	—	—	—	—

n, Sample size; N, estimated number of youths in population in thousands; $\bar{X}$, mean; s, standard deviation; $s_{\bar{x}}$, standard error of the mean. (From National Center for Health Statistics: Height and weight of youths 12–17 years, United States. In Vital and Health Statistics, Series 11, No. 124, Health Services and Mental Health Administration. Washington, D.C., U.S. Government Printing Office, 1973, pp. 282–288.)

TABLE A—12F-4. WEIGHT IN KILOGRAMS OF YOUTHS AGED 15 YEARS AT LAST BIRTHDAY BY SEX AND HEIGHT GROUP IN CENTIMETERS: SAMPLE SIZE, ESTIMATED POPULATION SIZE, MEAN, STANDARD DEVIATION, STANDARD ERROR OF THE MEAN, AND SELECTED PERCENTILES, UNITED STATES, 1966 TO 1970

SEX AND HEIGHT	n	N	$\bar{X}$	s	$s_{\bar{x}}$	PERCENTILE						
						5th	10th	25th	50th	75th	90th	95th
						in kilograms						
Male												
Under 130	—	—	—	—	—	—	—	—	—	—	—	—
130.0–134.9	—	—	—	—	—	—	—	—	—	—	—	—
135.0–139.9	—	—	—	—	—	—	—	—	—	—	—	—
140.0–144.9	—	—	—	—	—	—	—	—	—	—	—	—
145.0–149.9	1	2	*	*	*	*	*	*	*	*	*	*
150.0–154.9	10	30	45.72	8.582	3.550	35.7	39.2	42.6	44.7	46.0	48.7	76.1
155.0–159.9	34	99	52.81	10.552	1.695	40.3	43.1	46.7	49.2	56.7	69.6	76.3
160.0–164.9	71	206	53.01	8.417	0.986	42.7	44.1	46.9	51.5	56.3	65.3	68.8
165.0–169.9	132	404	57.72	8.503	0.819	48.0	48.8	53.1	56.4	61.3	67.1	73.3
170.0–174.9	176	574	62.88	8.464	0.633	51.6	53.4	56.7	61.9	67.2	72.9	78.1
175.0–179.9	118	374	65.80	9.457	1.045	53.1	55.6	59.7	64.3	69.5	80.2	89.2
180.0–184.9	51	144	72.00	11.928	1.724	54.6	60.3	64.4	70.2	78.4	84.4	96.6
185.0–189.9	14	48	74.21	15.035	5.200	58.3	58.5	62.9	70.7	84.6	92.4	110.8
190.0–194.9	6	15	83.39	16.431	10.332	66.4	66.7	69.6	73.8	103.0	105.7	106.2
195.0 and over	—	—	—	—	—	—	—	—	—	—	—	—

Female	n	N	X̄	s	s_x̄							
Under 130												
130.0–134.9	—	—	—	—	—	—	—	—	—	—	—	—
135.0–139.9	—	—	—	—	—	—	—	—	—	—	—	—
140.0–144.9	2	5	*	*	*	*	*	*	*	*	*	*
145.0–149.9	15	51	47.91	7.875	3.623	36.0	39.4	42.1	45.4	52.7	55.7	66.3
150.0–154.9	69	242	49.69	8.895	1.190	39.1	40.6	44.3	48.1	52.8	60.5	68.3
155.0–159.9	111	400	51.52	8.473	0.934	41.4	43.5	46.3	50.8	55.1	59.8	65.2
160.0–164.9	137	509	57.03	10.828	0.875	45.1	47.3	50.2	55.0	60.2	71.7	77.7
165.0–169.9	109	398	60.71	10.357	1.053	47.5	49.3	55.1	58.4	65.7	74.1	81.0
170.0–174.9	49	188	65.27	10.730	1.880	49.7	53.6	57.2	61.2	71.6	85.3	86.4
175.0–179.9	7	23	63.30	8.872	4.807	49.7	49.9	53.8	62.4	71.1	71.9	79.2
180.0–184.9	3	26	*	*	*	*	*	*	*	*	*	*
185.0–189.9	1	3	*	*	*	*	*	*	*	*	*	*
190.0–194.9	—	—	—	—	—	—	—	—	—	—	—	—
195.0 and over	—	—	—	—	—	—	—	—	—	—	—	—

n, Sample size; N, estimated number of youths in population in thousands; X̄, mean; s, standard deviation; s_x̄, standard error of the mean. (From National Center for Health Statistics: Height and weight of youths 12–17 years, United States. In Vital and Health Statistics, Series 11, No. 124, Health Services and Mental Health Administration. Washington, D.C., U.S. Government Printing Office, 1973, pp. 282–288.)

TABLE A—12F-5. WEIGHT IN KILOGRAMS OF YOUTHS AGED 16 YEARS AT LAST BIRTHDAY BY SEX AND HEIGHT GROUP IN CENTIMETERS: SAMPLE SIZE, ESTIMATED POPULATION SIZE, MEAN, STANDARD DEVIATION, STANDARD ERROR OF THE MEAN, AND SELECTED PERCENTILES, UNITED STATES, 1966 TO 1970

SEX AND HEIGHT	n	N	$\bar{X}$	s	$s_{\bar{x}}$	PERCENTILE						
						5th	10th	25th	50th	75th	90th	95th
						in kilograms						
Male												
Under 130	—	—	—	—	—	—	—	—	—	—	—	—
130.0–134.9	—	—	—	—	—	—	—	—	—	—	—	—
135.0–139.9	—	—	—	—	—	—	—	—	—	—	—	—
140.0–144.9	—	—	—	—	—	—	—	—	—	—	—	—
145.0–149.9	1	1	*	*	*	*	*	*	*	*	*	*
150.0–154.9	4	12	*	*	*	*	*	*	*	*	*	*
155.0–159.9	11	33	49.89	7.323	3.572	42.0	42.2	44.7	46.8	54.4	59.8	67.2
160.0–164.9	32	108	53.09	6.459	1.273	44.2	44.9	48.2	51.4	58.0	60.9	66.1
165.0–169.9	87	275	59.39	9.178	0.981	48.5	49.8	52.7	58.0	63.9	69.3	75.9
170.0–174.9	166	552	62.66	7.556	0.629	51.6	53.8	57.5	61.6	67.1	73.1	78.0
175.0–179.9	149	511	67.33	9.018	0.856	56.3	58.2	61.0	65.4	72.5	80.1	83.8
180.0–184.9	72	227	72.38	12.485	1.993	58.3	59.3	64.4	68.9	76.5	90.2	96.9
185.0–189.9	29	95	81.06	14.268	3.265	63.7	66.6	69.7	78.4	90.3	97.0	111.4
190.0–194.9	3	10	*	*	*	*	*	*	*	*	*	*
195.0 and over	2	7	*	*	*	*	*	*	*	*	*	*

Female

Under 130

Weight (lb)	n	N	$\bar{X}$	s	$s_{\bar{x}}$	5th	10th	25th	50th	75th	90th	95th
130.0–134.9	—	—	—	—	—	—	—	—	—	—	—	—
135.0–139.9	—	—	—	—	—	—	—	—	—	—	—	—
140.0–144.9	2	5	*	*	*	*	*	*	*	*	*	*
145.0–149.9	10	33	52.58	8.198	3.191	43.9	44.1	44.9	51.0	54.5	72.0	72.1
150.0–154.9	57	178	51.79	10.457	1.053	41.4	42.0	45.8	48.9	54.1	61.5	83.3
155.0–159.9	117	354	53.20	7.766	0.734	44.0	45.6	48.4	51.6	56.4	61.9	69.0
160.0–164.9	160	547	57.71	11.129	1.246	46.1	47.3	51.5	55.5	61.2	69.5	75.1
165.0–169.9	122	450	61.72	11.998	0.802	47.1	48.8	53.3	59.1	67.3	78.7	86.7
170.0–174.9	53	170	63.61	8.734	1.126	52.9	53.8	58.1	62.1	66.8	73.8	84.2
175.0–179.9	14	45	72.55	15.012	5.224	58.6	58.8	61.7	65.9	80.6	99.1	105.5
180.0–184.9	1	2	*	*	*	*	*	*	*	*	*	*
185.0–189.9	—	—	—	—	—	—	—	—	—	—	—	—
190.0–194.9	—	—	—	—	—	—	—	—	—	—	—	—
195.0 and over	—	—	—	—	—	—	—	—	—	—	—	—

n, Sample size; N, estimated number of youths in population in thousands; $\bar{X}$, mean; s, standard deviation; $s_{\bar{x}}$, standard error of the mean. (From National Center for Health Statistics: Height and weight of youths 12–17 years, United States. In Vital and Health Statistics, Series 11, No. 124, Health Services and Mental Health Administration. Washington, D.C., U.S. Government Printing Office, 1973, pp. 282–288.)

TABLE A—12F-6. WEIGHT IN KILOGRAMS OF YOUTHS AGED 17 YEARS AT LAST BIRTHDAY BY SEX AND HEIGHT GROUP IN CENTIMETERS: SAMPLE SIZE, ESTIMATED POPULATION SIZE, MEAN, STANDARD DEVIATION, STANDARD ERROR OF THE MEAN, AND SELECTED PERCENTILES, UNITED STATES, 1966 TO 1970

SEX AND HEIGHT	n	N	$\bar{X}$	s	$s_{\bar{x}}$	PERCENTILE						
						5th	10th	25th	50th	75th	90th	95th
						in kilograms						
Male												
Under 130	—	—	—	—	—	—	—	—	—	—	—	—
130.0–134.9	—	—	—	—	—	—	—	—	—	—	—	—
135.0–139.9	—	—	—	—	—	—	—	—	—	—	—	—
140.0–144.9	—	—	—	—	—	—	—	—	—	—	—	—
145.0–149.9	—	—	—	—	—	—	—	—	—	—	—	—
150.0–154.9	1	3	*	*	*	*	*	*	*	*	*	*
155.0–159.9	11	39	54.63	9.397	3.414	43.8	46.4	48.2	49.7	57.8	69.9	73.2
160.0–164.9	25	81	57.75	6.503	1.355	49.7	51.1	52.5	56.9	61.6	70.1	70.8
165.0–169.9	63	248	62.57	8.344	1.224	50.2	53.2	56.4	61.5	66.9	72.7	77.3
170.0–174.9	115	396	67.06	11.163	0.704	53.3	55.5	59.5	64.6	71.9	80.9	91.6
175.0–179.9	151	537	68.37	9.907	0.831	56.9	58.9	61.5	66.5	73.6	79.4	88.4
180.0–184.9	80	297	73.31	12.454	1.335	59.6	61.0	65.1	71.2	78.4	91.8	102.7
185.0–189.9	36	133	76.03	9.171	1.301	62.4	66.3	70.5	75.3	80.8	90.3	92.9
190.0–194.9	7	25	81.40	10.985	7.588	62.9	62.9	67.8	87.3	80.3	90.6	90.6
195.0 and over	—	—	—	—	—	—	—	—	—	—	—	—

Female

Height (cm)	n	N	$\bar{X}$	s	$s_{\bar{x}}$	5th	10th	25th	50th	75th	90th	95th
Under 130	—	—	—	—	—	—	—	—	—	—	—	—
130.0–134.9	—	—	—	—	—	—	—	—	—	—	—	—
135.0–139.9	—	—	—	—	—	—	—	—	—	—	—	—
140.0–144.9	2	5	*	*	*	*	*	*	*	*	*	*
145.0–149.9	8	26	43.49	3.939	1.604	38.6	38.8	40.1	45.1	45.7	51.1	51.2
150.0–154.9	43	151	49.96	6.508	0.827	41.6	42.3	44.6	48.9	53.5	59.2	64.1
155.0–159.9	103	385	54.71	9.903	0.775	44.4	45.5	48.7	53.2	57.7	61.6	76.2
160.0–164.9	133	506	57.79	10.620	1.028	46.8	48.0	50.2	55.4	61.5	72.3	82.3
165.0–169.9	116	433	60.63	10.117	1.182	47.9	50.3	55.1	59.3	65.1	69.4	71.6
170.0–174.9	51	186	62.18	9.132	1.407	50.6	52.9	55.5	60.2	65.7	76.1	82.7
175.0–179.9	12	47	65.76	8.405	2.229	54.9	56.7	60.1	61.7	75.2	75.9	83.0
180.0–184.9	1	2	*	*	*	*	*	*	*	*	*	*
185.0–189.9	—	—	—	—	—	—	—	—	—	—	—	—
190.0–194.9	—	—	—	—	—	—	—	—	—	—	—	—
195.0 and over	—	—	—	—	—	—	—	—	—	—	—	—

n, Sample size; N, estimated number of youths in population in thousands; $\bar{X}$, mean; s, standard deviation; $s_{\bar{x}}$, standard error of the mean. (From National Center for Health Statistics: Height and weight of youths 12–17 years, United States. *In* Vital and Health Statistics, Series 11, No. 124, Health Services and Mental Health Administration. Washington, D.C., U.S. Government Printing Office, 1973, pp. 282–288.)

TABLE A–13A. WEIGHT IN KILOGRAMS FOR WOMEN 18 TO 74 YEARS OF AGE: NUMBER EXAMINED, MEAN, STANDARD DEVIATION, AND SELECTED PERCENTILES BY RACE AND AGE, UNITED STATES, 1976 TO 1980*

RACE AND AGE (years)	NUMBER OF EXAMINED PERSONS	MEAN	STANDARD DEVIATION	PERCENTILE								
				5th	10th	15th	25th	50th	75th	85th	90th	95th
All races†												
18–74	6,588	65.4	14.6	47.7	50.3	52.2	55.4	62.4	72.1	79.2	84.4	93.1
18–24	1,066	60.6	11.9	46.6	49.1	50.6	53.2	58.0	65.0	70.4	75.3	82.9
25–34	1,170	64.2	15.0	47.4	49.6	51.4	54.3	60.9	69.6	78.4	84.1	93.5
35–44	844	67.1	15.2	49.2	52.0	53.3	56.9	63.4	73.9	81.7	87.5	98.9
45–54	763	68.0	15.3	48.5	51.3	53.3	57.3	65.5	75.7	82.1	87.6	96.0
55–64	1,329	67.9	14.7	48.6	51.3	54.1	57.3	65.2	75.3	82.3	87.5	95.1
65–74	1,416	66.6	13.8	47.1	50.8	53.2	57.4	64.8	73.8	79.8	84.4	91.3
White												
18–74	5,686	64.8	14.1	47.7	50.3	52.2	55.2	62.1	71.1	77.9	83.3	91.5
18–24	892	60.4	11.6	47.3	49.5	50.8	53.3	57.9	64.8	69.7	74.3	82.4
25–34	1,000	63.6	14.5	47.3	49.5	51.3	54.0	60.6	68.9	76.3	81.5	89.7
35–44	726	66.1	14.5	49.3	51.8	52.9	56.3	62.4	71.9	79.7	85.8	94.9
45–54	647	67.3	14.4	48.6	51.3	53.4	57.0	65.0	74.8	81.1	85.6	94.5
55–64	1,176	67.2	14.4	48.5	50.7	53.7	57.1	64.7	74.5	81.8	86.2	92.8
65–74	1,245	66.2	13.7	47.2	50.7	52.9	57.2	64.3	72.9	79.2	84.3	91.2
Black												
18–74	782	71.2	17.3	48.8	51.6	55.1	59.1	67.8	80.6	87.4	94.9	105.1
18–24	147	63.1	13.9	46.2	49.0	50.6	53.8	60.4	70.0	75.8	79.1	89.3
25–34	145	69.3	16.7	48.3	50.8	53.1	57.8	65.3	80.2	87.1	91.5	102.7
35–44	103	75.3	18.4	50.7	55.2	57.2	63.0	70.2	85.2	95.3	103.5	113.1
45–54	100	77.7	18.8	55.1	60.3	60.8	64.5	74.3	83.6	94.5	98.2	117.5
55–64	135	75.8	16.4	54.2	55.2	57.6	65.4	74.6	83.4	91.9	95.5	108.5
65–74	152	72.4	13.6	52.9	56.4	60.3	64.0	70.0	82.2	84.4	86.5	98.1

*Includes clothing weight, estimated as ranging from 0.09 to 0.28 kilogram.
†Includes all other races not shown as separate categories.
(From National Center for Health Statistics: Anthropometric Reference Data and Prevalence of Overweight, United States 1976–1980. DHHS Publication No. 87–1688. Hyattsville, MD, U.S. Department of Health and Human Services, Public Health Service, 1987.)

TABLE A–13B. WEIGHT IN KILOGRAMS FOR MEN 18 TO 74 YEARS OF AGE: NUMBER EXAMINED, MEAN, STANDARD DEVIATION, AND SELECTED PERCENTILES BY RACE AND AGE, UNITED STATES, 1976 TO 1980*

RACE AND AGE (years)	NUMBER OF EXAMINED PERSONS	MEAN	STANDARD DEVIATION	PERCENTILE								
				5th	10th	15th	25th	50th	75th	85th	90th	95th
All races[†]												
18–74	5,916	78.1	13.5	58.6	62.3	64.9	68.7	76.9	85.6	91.3	95.7	102.7
18–24	988	73.8	12.7	56.8	60.4	61.9	64.8	72.0	80.3	85.1	90.4	99.5
25–34	1,067	78.7	13.7	59.5	62.9	65.4	69.3	77.5	85.6	91.1	95.1	102.7
35–44	745	80.9	13.4	59.7	65.1	67.7	72.1	79.9	88.1	94.8	98.8	104.3
45–54	690	80.9	13.6	60.8	65.2	67.2	71.7	79.0	89.4	94.5	99.5	105.3
55–64	1,227	78.8	12.8	59.9	63.8	66.4	70.2	77.7	85.6	90.5	94.7	102.3
65–74	1,199	74.8	12.8	54.4	58.5	61.2	66.1	74.2	82.7	87.9	91.2	96.6
White												
18–74	5,148	78.5	13.1	59.3	62.8	65.5	69.4	77.3	85.6	91.4	95.5	102.3
18–24	846	74.2	12.8	56.8	60.5	62.0	65.0	72.4	80.6	85.5	91.0	100.0
25–34	901	79.0	13.1	59.9	63.7	65.9	69.8	78.0	85.6	91.3	95.3	102.7
35–44	653	81.4	12.8	62.3	66.6	68.8	72.9	80.1	88.2	94.6	98.7	104.1
45–54	617	81.0	13.4	62.0	66.1	67.3	71.9	79.0	89.4	94.2	99.0	104.5
55–64	1,086	78.9	12.4	60.5	64.5	66.6	70.6	78.2	85.6	90.4	94.5	101.7
65–74	1,045	75.4	12.4	55.5	59.5	62.5	67.0	74.7	83.0	87.9	91.2	96.0
Black												
18–74	649	77.9	15.2	58.0	61.1	63.6	67.2	75.3	85.4	92.9	98.3	105.4
18–24	121	72.2	12.0	58.3	60.9	62.3	64.9	70.8	77.1	81.8	83.7	93.6
25–34	139	78.2	16.3	58.7	63.4	64.9	68.4	75.3	84.4	90.6	92.2	106.3
35–44	70	82.5	15.4	*	61.7	65.2	69.7	83.1	94.8	100.4	104.2	*
45–54	62	82.4	14.5	*	64.7	67.0	73.2	81.8	93.0	100.0	102.5	*
55–64	129	78.6	14.7	56.8	61.4	64.3	68.0	77.0	86.5	93.8	98.6	104.7
65–74	128	73.3	15.3	52.5	56.7	58.0	61.0	71.2	81.1	90.8	97.3	105.1

*Includes clothing weight, estimated as ranging from 0.09 to 0.28 kilogram.
[†]Includes all other races not shown as separate categories.
(From National Center for Health Statistics: Anthropometric Reference Data and Prevalence of Overweight, United States 1976–1980. DHHS Publication No. 87–1688. Hyattsville, MD, U.S. Department of Health and Human Services, Public Health Service, 1987.)

TABLE A–13C. HEIGHT IN CENTIMETERS FOR WOMEN 18 TO 74 YEARS OF AGE: NUMBER EXAMINED, MEAN, STANDARD DEVIATION, AND SELECTED PERCENTILES BY RACE AND AGE, UNITED STATES, 1976 TO 1980*

RACE AND AGE (years)	NUMBER OF EXAMINED PERSONS	MEAN	STANDARD DEVIATION	PERCENTILE								
				5th	10th	15th	25th	50th	75th	85th	90th	95th
All races†												
18–74	6,588	161.8	6.6	150.9	153.6	155.2	157.4	161.7	166.3	168.6	170.3	172.6
18–24	1,066	163.4	6.6	152.9	155.2	156.7	159.0	163.7	167.6	170.0	171.6	174.0
25–34	1,170	163.1	6.3	153.2	155.2	156.6	158.7	163.1	167.6	169.9	171.3	173.7
35–44	844	162.8	6.3	152.6	155.5	156.7	158.5	162.5	167.0	169.3	171.0	173.5
45–54	763	161.3	6.4	150.5	152.9	154.5	156.6	161.3	165.6	167.7	169.4	171.8
55–64	1,329	160.1	6.4	149.2	151.8	153.7	155.9	160.3	164.5	166.7	168.0	170.3
65–74	1,416	158.1	6.2	147.9	150.0	151.7	154.1	158.4	162.2	164.5	166.0	167.7
White												
18–74	5,686	161.9	6.5	151.3	153.8	155.4	157.6	161.9	165.4	168.7	170.3	172.7
18–24	892	163.7	6.4	153.1	155.7	157.1	159.4	163.9	167.7	170.1	171.8	174.0
25–34	1,000	163.3	6.2	153.5	155.4	156.6	158.9	163.3	167.8	170.1	171.5	173.7
35–44	726	162.9	6.3	152.6	155.6	156.7	158.4	162.6	167.0	169.4	171.2	173.5
45–54	647	161.5	6.2	151.5	153.6	155.2	157.2	161.3	165.7	167.6	169.4	171.7
55–64	1,176	160.1	6.3	149.6	151.9	153.9	156.1	160.3	164.4	166.5	167.7	170.1
65–74	1,245	158.1	6.2	147.8	150.1	151.7	154.1	158.5	162.2	164.5	166.0	167.7
Black												
18–74	782	162.1	6.7	150.6	154.2	155.2	157.6	162.2	166.6	168.9	170.4	173.0
18–24	147	163.2	6.9	152.8	155.1	156.4	158.6	163.0	168.1	170.2	171.1	174.8
25–34	145	162.2	6.3	151.3	154.8	156.3	158.1	162.5	166.2	168.6	170.4	174.1
35–44	103	163.3	5.5	155.2	156.9	157.3	159.7	162.5	167.0	168.7	170.1	171.7
45–54	100	161.7	6.9	150.4	152.6	154.4	155.5	162.1	167.5	169.3	170.5	171.9
55–64	135	161.0	7.4	148.7	149.2	153.4	155.8	161.8	166.5	169.1	171.0	174.5
65–74	152	158.8	6.2	148.2	150.4	152.6	155.6	159.1	163.0	164.7	166.4	169.4

*Height without shoes.
†Includes all other races not shown as separate categories.

(From National Center for Health Statistics: Anthropometric Reference Data and Prevalence of Overweight, United States 1976–1980. DHHS Publication No. 87–1688. Hyattsville, MD, U.S. Department of Health and Human Services, Public Health Service, 1987.)

TABLE A–13D. HEIGHT IN CENTIMETERS FOR MEN 18 TO 74 YEARS OF AGE: NUMBER EXAMINED, MEAN, STANDARD DEVIATION, AND SELECTED PERCENTILES BY RACE AND AGE, UNITED STATES, 1976 TO 1980*

RACE AND AGE (years)	NUMBER OF EXAMINED PERSONS	MEAN	STANDARD DEVIATION	PERCENTILE								
				5th	10th	15th	25th	50th	75th	85th	90th	95th
All races†												
18–74	5,916	175.5	7.2	163.9	166.4	168.2	171.1	175.7	180.4	182.9	184.5	187.0
18–24	988	177.0	7.1	165.8	168.3	169.8	172.2	177.0	181.6	183.9	186.0	189.6
25–34	1,067	176.7	6.7	165.5	167.9	170.0	172.2	176.8	181.2	183.6	185.3	187.4
35–44	745	176.3	7.3	164.1	166.4	168.8	172.2	176.5	181.2	183.6	185.2	188.0
45–54	690	175.2	6.6	164.5	167.2	168.3	170.7	175.1	179.8	182.5	184.3	185.7
55–64	1,227	173.7	6.9	162.1	165.4	166.8	169.2	173.7	178.5	180.6	182.2	184.6
65–74	1,199	171.3	7.1	159.3	162.3	164.1	166.3	171.5	176.1	178.6	180.4	183.1
White												
18–74	5,148	175.7	7.1	164.2	166.7	168.6	171.2	175.9	180.5	183.0	184.6	187.2
18–24	846	177.2	7.0	166.3	168.6	170.1	172.4	177.1	181.9	184.1	186.4	189.7
25–34	901	177.0	6.6	165.8	168.2	170.6	172.5	177.0	181.4	183.8	185.4	187.7
35–44	653	176.7	7.3	164.5	166.7	169.6	172.6	176.8	181.7	183.7	185.8	188.0
45–54	617	175.4	6.8	164.6	167.3	168.9	171.2	175.3	179.8	182.5	184.3	185.7
55–64	1,086	173.8	6.8	163.1	165.6	167.2	169.5	173.6	178.5	180.7	182.2	184.5
65–74	1,045	171.6	6.9	159.6	162.9	164.6	166.9	171.6	176.4	178.7	180.5	183.3
Black												
18–74	649	175.5	7.0	164.3	166.5	168.1	171.1	175.7	180.3	183.0	184.5	186.5
18–24	121	176.7	7.0	165.1	167.6	169.9	172.5	177.9	181.0	183.8	185.0	186.4
25–34	139	176.7	6.9	165.5	168.5	169.6	172.4	177.1	181.8	183.2	184.7	187.1
35–44	70	176.5	6.4	*	167.6	170.7	172.8	175.2	179.9	181.9	185.1	*
45–54	62	174.2	6.7	*	167.6	167.7	169.1	172.8	178.4	183.2	184.5	*
55–64	129	174.2	6.9	162.7	165.3	166.8	168.6	174.6	178.8	180.7	182.8	186.8
65–74	128	171.2	6.5	161.2	162.6	163.8	165.9	171.6	175.3	177.7	180.8	182.2

*Height without shoes.
†Includes all other races not shown as separate categories.
(From National Center for Health Statistics: Anthropometric Reference Data and Prevalence of Overweight, United States 1976–1980. DHHS Publication No. 87–1688. Hyattsville, MD, U.S. Department of Health and Human Services, Public Health Service, 1987.)

TABLE A—13E. PROVISIONAL AGE- AND SEX-SPECIFIC REFERENCE VALUES FOR WEIGHT IN KILOGRAMS (POUNDS) IN ELDERLY SUBJECTS*,†

AGE GROUP (YEARS)	5%	50%	95%
Men			
65	62.6 (138.0)	79.5 (175.0)	102.0 (224.9)
70	59.7 (131.6)	76.5 (168.7)	99.1 (218.5)
75	56.8 (125.2)	73.6 (162.3)	96.3 (212.3)
80	53.9 (118.8)	70.7 (155.9)	93.4 (205.9)
85	51.0 (112.4)	67.8 (149.5)	90.5 (199.5)
90	48.1 (106.0)	64.9 (143.1)	87.6 (193.1)
Women			
65	51.2 (112.9)	66.8 (147.3)	87.1 (192.0)
70	49.0 (108.0)	64.6 (142.4)	84.9 (187.2)
75	46.8 (103.2)	62.4 (137.6)	82.8 (182.5)
80	44.7 (98.5)	60.2 (132.7)	80.6 (177.7)
85	42.5 (93.7)	58.0 (127.9)	78.4 (172.8)
90	40.3 (88.8)	55.9 (123.2)	76.2 (168.0)

*Data from 119 men and 150 women. The subjects were all ambulatory.
†See Tables A—14b-1 through A—14b-6 for data compiled by Frisancho (Am. J. Clin. Nutr., 40:808—819, 1984) from NHANES I and II.
(From Chumlea, W.C., Roche, A.F., Mukherjee, D.: Nutritional Assessment of the Elderly through Anthropometry. Ohio, Wright State University School of Medicine, 1984.)

TABLE A–14A-1. TRICEPS SKINFOLD THICKNESS: GIRLS, 1 TO 17 YEARS, UNITED STATES, 1971 TO 1974

RACE AND AGE IN YEARS	NUMBER IN SAMPLE	ESTIMATED POPULATION IN THOUSANDS	MEAN†	STANDARD DEVIATION	PERCENTILE								
					5th	10th	15th	25th	50th	75th	85th	90th	95th
					Triceps Skinfold in Millimeters								
All Races*													
1	267	1,620	10.1	2.8	6.0	6.5	7.0	8.0	10.0	12.0	13.0	14.0	15.0
2	272	1,708	10.5	2.5	7.0	7.5	8.0	9.0	10.0	12.0	13.5	14.0	15.0
3	292	1,701	10.9	2.7	6.0	7.0	8.0	9.0	11.0	12.5	13.5	14.0	15.0
4	281	1,599	10.5	2.7	7.0	7.5	8.0	8.0	10.0	12.0	13.0	14.0	15.0
5	314	1,695	10.5	3.8	6.0	7.0	7.0	8.0	10.0	12.0	13.0	15.0	17.5
6	176	1,787	10.3	3.3	6.0	6.5	7.0	8.0	10.0	12.0	13.0	13.5	15.0
7	169	1,754	10.8	4.2	4.0	6.0	7.0	8.0	10.5	12.0	15.0	16.0	18.0
8	152	1,800	12.3	4.8	6.5	8.0	8.0	9.0	11.0	15.0	17.0	18.0	22.5
9	171	2,017	13.2	4.8	7.0	7.5	8.0	10.0	12.5	16.0	18.0	20.0	22.0
10	197	2,173	13.1	5.0	7.0	8.0	8.0	9.5	12.0	15.5	19.0	20.0	23.0
11	166	1,911	14.5	6.2	7.0	8.0	8.5	10.0	13.0	18.0	20.5	23.5	28.5
12	177	1,812	15.0	5.9	7.5	8.0	9.0	10.5	14.0	18.5	20.0	23.0	27.0
13	198	2,175	16.2	6.8	7.0	8.0	10.0	11.5	15.0	20.0	24.0	25.0	30.0
14	184	2,036	17.5	7.3	8.5	9.5	10.0	13.0	16.0	21.0	24.0	27.0	33.0
15	171	2,163	17.0	7.0	8.0	10.0	11.0	12.0	16.0	20.5	23.0	25.0	28.5
16	175	2,145	18.2	6.7	10.0	10.5	12.0	13.5	17.0	21.0	24.0	26.0	32.5
17	157	1,804	19.6	8.1	10.0	11.5	12.0	13.0	19.0	24.0	26.5	29.5	35.0
White													
1	189	1,328	10.2	2.8	6.0	7.0	7.0	8.0	10.0	12.0	13.0	13.5	15.5
2	203	1,434	10.6	2.6	7.0	7.5	8.0	9.0	10.0	12.0	13.5	14.0	15.0
3	211	1,438	11.1	2.6	7.0	8.0	8.5	9.0	11.0	13.0	13.5	14.0	15.0
4	204	1,339	10.8	2.6	7.5	8.0	8.0	9.0	10.5	12.0	13.0	14.5	16.0
5	224	1,416	10.7	3.7	6.0	7.0	8.0	8.5	10.0	12.0	13.0	15.0	17.5
6	125	1,445	10.6	3.3	6.5	7.0	7.5	8.0	10.5	12.0	13.0	14.0	16.0
7	122	1,507	10.9	4.2	4.0	6.0	7.0	8.0	11.0	12.0	15.0	15.5	17.5
8	117	1,507	12.4	4.7	7.0	8.0	8.0	9.0	11.5	15.0	16.5	18.0	22.0
9	129	1,751	13.6	4.6	7.5	8.0	9.0	10.0	13.0	16.0	18.0	20.0	22.0
10	148	1,855	13.4	4.8	7.5	8.0	8.5	10.0	12.5	15.5	19.0	20.0	23.0

(Continued)

TABLE A–14A-1. (CONTINUED)

RACE AND AGE IN YEARS	NUMBER IN SAMPLE	ESTIMATED POPULATION IN THOUSANDS	MEAN†	STANDARD DEVIATION	PERCENTILE								
					5th	10th	15th	25th	50th	75th	85th	90th	95th
11	122	1,569	14.9	6.1	8.0	8.5	9.0	10.0	13.0	17.5	20.5	24.5	28.5
12	128	1,506	15.2	5.6	8.0	9.0	10.0	11.0	14.0	18.5	20.0	23.0	26.0
13	153	1,886	16.2	6.8	7.0	8.0	10.0	11.5	15.0	20.0	24.0	25.0	28.5
14	132	1,731	17.8	7.3	9.0	9.5	10.5	13.0	16.7	21.0	24.0	28.5	33.0
15	125	1,752	17.7	6.7	9.0	10.5	11.0	13.0	17.0	21.0	24.0	25.0	28.5
16	141	1,933	18.2	6.6	10.0	10.5	12.5	14.0	17.0	21.0	24.0	26.0	32.1
17	117	1,549	19.8	8.0	10.0	12.0	12.5	13.5	19.0	24.0	26.5	29.5	35.0
Black													
1	73	257	10.0	3.0	5.5	5.5	7.0	8.0	10.0	12.0	13.0	14.0	15.0
2	66	261	10.0	2.3	7.0	8.0	8.0	8.0	10.0	11.0	12.0	14.0	15.5
3	78	245	9.7	2.9	6.0	7.0	7.0	8.0	10.0	11.0	12.0	13.0	14.0
4	73	246	8.8	2.7	5.0	6.0	6.5	7.0	8.0	10.5	12.0	13.0	14.0
5	88	265	9.4	3.9	5.0	5.0	6.0	7.0	8.0	10.0	12.0	13.5	17.0
6	50	336	9.0	3.1	5.5	6.0	6.0	8.0	8.0	10.0	11.5	12.0	13.0
7	46	241	10.1	4.0	5.0	6.0	7.0	7.5	9.0	11.0	17.5	18.0	18.0
8	35	293	11.5	5.1	5.0	6.5	7.0	8.0	10.0	13.5	18.0	18.0	23.0
9	41	247	10.2	5.1	5.5	6.0	6.0	6.5	8.0	12.0	18.0	18.0	20.0
10	48	303	11.7	5.6	6.5	6.5	7.0	7.5	10.0	16.0	18.0	19.0	24.0
11	42	315	12.7	6.4	4.0	5.0	6.5	7.5	10.0	18.0	22.0	23.0	23.0
12	47	284	13.6	7.6	5.5	6.0	6.0	7.5	12.0	17.0	22.0	25.0	30.0
13	44	287	16.1	7.0	7.0	8.5	10.0	11.0	14.0	18.0	24.0	24.0	33.5
14	50	265	15.9	6.7	8.0	8.0	9.0	10.5	14.0	20.5	24.0	24.5	24.5
15	46	411	14.0	7.6	6.5	6.5	8.0	10.0	12.5	16.0	16.5	20.0	32.8
16	33	203	18.9	8.0	8.0	8.0	10.0	12.0	19.0	24.0	24.5	33.0	33.1
17	39	239	16.9	6.6	7.5	9.0	11.0	12.0	14.5	20.0	24.0	28.0	31.0

*Includes data for races that are not shown separately.
†Measurements made in the right arm.
(From the National Center for Health Statistics, Department of Health and Human Services. See also Bishop, C.W., Bowen, P.E., Ritchey, S.J.: Am. J. Clin. Nutr., *34*:2530–2539, 1981.)

TABLE A–14A-2. SUBSCAPULAR SKINFOLD THICKNESS: GIRLS, 1 TO 17 YEARS, UNITED STATES, 1971 TO 1974

RACE AND AGE IN YEARS	NUMBER IN SAMPLE	ESTIMATED POPULATION IN THOUSANDS	MEAN†	STANDARD DEVIATION	PERCENTILE								
					5th	10th	15th	25th	50th	75th	85th	90th	95th
					Subscapular Skinfold in Millimeters								
All Races*													
1	267	1,620	6.2	1.9	4.0	4.0	4.0	5.0	6.0	8.0	8.0	9.0	9.0
2	272	1,708	6.2	2.4	4.0	4.0	4.0	5.0	6.0	7.0	8.0	9.0	10.0
3	292	1,701	5.8	2.0	4.0	4.0	4.0	4.5	5.5	6.5	7.0	8.0	9.0
4	281	1,599	5.6	1.9	3.5	4.0	4.0	4.5	5.0	6.0	7.0	8.0	9.0
5	314	1,695	6.2	3.3	3.5	4.0	4.0	4.0	5.0	6.5	8.0	9.0	15.0
6	176	1,787	6.0	2.8	3.0	4.0	4.0	4.5	5.0	6.5	7.0	8.0	10.0
7	169	1,754	6.2	3.3	3.0	4.0	4.0	4.5	5.0	7.0	9.0	10.5	11.5
8	152	1,800	7.7	5.5	3.5	4.0	4.0	4.5	5.5	8.0	12.5	14.5	19.5
9	171	2,017	8.5	5.0	4.0	4.0	4.5	5.0	7.0	10.0	13.0	17.0	19.0
10	197	2,173	8.6	5.1	4.0	4.5	5.0	5.5	6.5	10.0	13.0	18.0	20.0
11	166	1,911	10.1	6.4	4.0	5.0	5.0	6.0	8.0	13.0	16.0	19.0	25.5
12	177	1,812	11.1	6.8	5.0	5.0	5.5	6.0	9.5	13.0	16.0	20.0	25.0
13	198	2,175	11.9	7.1	5.0	6.0	6.0	7.0	9.5	15.0	19.0	23.4	26.0
14	184	2,036	13.0	8.0	5.0	6.0	6.5	8.0	10.0	16.0	19.0	24.0	28.0
15	171	2,163	12.2	7.2	6.0	6.5	7.0	7.5	10.0	14.0	18.0	20.0	27.0
16	175	2,145	13.4	7.8	6.0	7.0	7.5	8.0	10.5	15.0	21.0	25.5	29.0
17	157	1,804	15.6	9.4	6.5	7.0	7.5	9.0	12.5	20.0	25.5	27.0	34.1
White													
1	189	1,328	6.3	1.9	3.5	4.0	4.0	5.0	6.0	8.0	8.0	9.0	9.5
2	203	1,434	6.0	2.1	4.0	4.0	4.0	5.0	6.0	7.0	8.0	8.5	10.0
3	211	1,438	5.8	1.9	4.0	4.0	4.0	5.0	5.5	6.5	7.0	8.0	9.0
4	204	1,339	5.7	1.9	3.5	4.0	4.0	4.5	5.0	6.0	7.0	8.0	9.0
5	224	1,416	6.2	3.2	3.5	4.0	4.0	4.5	5.5	6.5	8.0	10.0	15.0
6	125	1,445	6.0	2.7	3.0	3.5	4.0	4.5	6.0	6.5	7.0	8.0	10.0
7	122	1,507	6.2	3.4	3.0	3.5	4.0	4.5	5.0	7.0	8.5	10.0	12.5
8	117	1,507	7.6	5.6	3.5	4.0	4.0	4.5	6.0	8.0	10.0	13.0	21.0
9	129	1,751	8.5	4.7	4.0	4.5	5.0	5.0	7.0	10.0	13.0	16.0	18.0
10	148	1,855	8.8	5.1	4.0	4.5	5.0	5.5	7.0	10.0	13.0	18.0	20.0

(Continued)

TABLE A-14A-2. (CONTINUED)

RACE AND AGE IN YEARS	NUMBER IN SAMPLE	ESTIMATED POPULATION IN THOUSANDS	MEAN[†]	STANDARD DEVIATION	PERCENTILE								
					5th	10th	15th	25th	50th	75th	85th	90th	95th
11	122	1,569	10.3	6.7	4.0	5.0	5.0	6.0	8.0	13.0	16.5	20.5	25.5
12	128	1,506	11.1	6.4	5.0	5.0	6.0	6.5	9.5	13.5	17.0	20.0	22.0
13	153	1,886	11.6	6.9	5.0	5.5	6.0	7.0	9.0	15.0	19.0	21.0	25.0
14	132	1,731	13.2	8.2	5.0	6.0	6.5	8.0	10.5	16.0	20.0	24.0	30.0
15	125	1,752	12.4	6.9	6.0	7.0	7.0	8.0	10.0	14.5	18.0	20.0	27.0
16	141	1,933	12.9	7.3	6.0	7.0	7.5	8.0	10.0	15.0	20.5	25.0	28.5
17	117	1,549	15.2	9.3	6.0	7.0	7.5	8.0	12.5	18.0	25.0	26.5	34.0
Black													
1	73	257	6.1	2.0	4.0	4.0	4.0	5.0	5.5	8.0	8.5	9.0	9.0
2	66	261	6.8	3.3	4.0	4.0	4.5	5.0	6.0	7.5	9.5	12.0	15.5
3	78	245	5.5	2.0	4.0	4.0	4.0	4.5	5.0	6.0	7.0	7.0	8.0
4	73	246	5.2	1.7	3.0	3.5	4.0	4.0	5.0	6.0	6.0	8.0	8.5
5	88	265	5.8	3.5	4.0	4.0	4.0	4.0	5.0	6.0	6.5	7.0	13.0
6	50	336	6.0	3.3	3.0	4.0	4.0	4.5	5.0	7.0	7.5	7.5	10.0
7	46	241	6.4	2.6	3.0	4.0	4.0	5.0	5.5	8.0	11.0	11.0	11.0
8	35	293	8.2	5.2	4.0	4.0	4.0	4.5	5.0	14.0	15.0	16.0	17.5
9	41	247	8.3	6.4	4.0	4.0	4.0	4.5	5.5	7.5	14.5	24.0	24.0
10	48	303	8.1	5.5	4.0	4.0	4.5	5.0	6.0	8.0	12.5	14.3	22.0
11	42	315	9.2	4.5	4.0	5.0	5.0	5.5	8.0	11.0	14.5	14.5	15.5
12	47	284	10.7	8.6	4.5	5.0	5.0	5.5	7.0	11.5	16.0	28.0	31.0
13	44	287	13.9	8.1	6.0	6.0	6.5	8.0	12.0	15.0	26.0	26.0	28.4
14	50	265	12.5	7.3	6.0	6.0	6.5	7.0	10.0	16.5	23.0	23.0	25.0
15	46	411	11.2	8.4	5.5	5.5	6.0	6.5	7.5	10.5	19.0	20.0	33.4
16	33	203	17.8	10.7	6.0	7.0	8.0	10.5	15.0	24.5	31.0	38.0	38.0
17	39	239	16.4	8.4	7.0	7.5	8.0	9.0	12.5	23.5	27.0	28.0	30.0

*Includes data for races that are not shown separately.

[†]Measurements made in the right arm.

(From the National Center for Health Statistics, Department of Health and Human Services. See also Bishop, C.W., Bowen, P.E., Ritchey, S.J.: Am. J. Clin. Nutr., 34:2530-2539, 1981.)

RACE AND AGE IN YEARS	NUMBER IN SAMPLE	ESTIMATED POPULATION IN THOUSANDS	MEAN†	STANDARD DEVIATION	PERCENTILE								
					5th	10th	15th	25th	50th	75th	85th	90th	95th
					Triceps Skinfold in Millimeters								
All Races*													
1	286	1,693	10.4	3.1	6.0	7.0	7.5	8.0	10.0	12.0	14.0	15.0	16.0
2	298	1,747	10.0	2.7	6.0	6.5	7.0	8.0	10.0	12.0	12.5	13.5	15.0
3	308	1,807	9.9	2.7	6.5	7.0	7.0	8.0	10.0	11.0	12.5	13.1	14.5
4	304	1,815	9.4	2.5	5.0	6.5	7.0	8.0	9.0	11.0	12.5	12.5	14.0
5	273	1,563	9.5	3.3	5.0	6.0	7.0	7.0	9.0	11.0	12.5	13.5	15.0
6	179	1,673	8.6	3.0	5.0	5.5	6.0	6.5	8.0	10.0	12.0	12.0	14.0
7	164	1,979	8.9	3.5	4.0	5.0	6.0	6.5	8.0	10.0	12.0	13.0	15.5
8	152	1,861	9.0	3.3	5.0	5.5	6.0	6.5	8.0	10.0	12.0	13.0	16.0
9	169	2,019	10.6	4.8	5.0	6.0	6.5	7.0	9.0	14.0	17.0	17.0	19.0
10	184	2,205	10.9	4.4	5.5	6.0	6.0	8.0	10.0	13.5	17.0	17.0	19.5
11	178	2,177	11.9	6.4	5.0	6.0	6.0	7.5	10.0	14.5	18.0	20.0	24.0
12	200	2,304	11.9	6.3	4.5	6.0	6.5	8.0	10.5	13.5	16.5	20.0	27.0
13	174	1,978	11.2	6.6	5.0	5.0	5.5	7.0	10.0	13.0	19.0	22.0	25.0
14	174	2,030	10.3	6.2	4.0	5.0	5.5	6.5	8.0	12.0	16.5	19.0	22.5
15	171	2,093	10.0	6.1	4.0	5.0	5.0	6.0	8.0	11.5	15.0	19.0	23.5
16	169	2,019	9.7	5.2	4.0	5.0	5.0	6.0	8.0	12.0	14.0	17.0	22.0
17	176	2,095	9.2	5.4	4.0	5.0	5.0	6.0	7.5	11.0	12.5	15.0	19.0
White													
1	211	1,402	10.7	3.0	7.0	7.0	7.5	8.0	10.0	12.0	14.0	15.0	16.5
2	217	1,461	9.9	2.6	6.0	6.5	7.0	8.0	10.0	12.0	12.5	13.0	14.7
3	226	1,536	9.9	2.6	6.5	7.0	7.0	8.0	10.0	11.0	12.5	13.5	14.5
4	229	1,547	9.6	2.4	6.0	7.0	7.0	8.0	10.0	11.0	12.0	12.5	14.0
5	207	1,319	9.8	3.2	6.0	6.5	7.0	7.5	9.0	11.0	12.5	13.5	15.0
6	126	1,343	8.9	3.1	5.5	5.5	6.0	7.0	9.0	10.0	12.0	12.5	14.0
7	125	1,718	9.1	3.5	5.0	6.0	6.0	7.0	8.0	10.5	12.0	13.5	17.0
8	116	1,644	9.1	3.3	5.0	6.0	6.0	7.0	8.0	10.5	12.0	13.0	16.0
9	117	1,636	11.1	4.8	5.5	6.5	6.5	7.5	8.5	14.0	17.0	17.0	19.0
10	148	1,909	11.1	4.2	5.5	6.0	7.0	8.0	10.0	14.0	15.5	17.0	19.5

(Continued)

TABLE A-14A-3. (CONTINUED)

RACE AND AGE IN YEARS	NUMBER IN SAMPLE	ESTIMATED POPULATION IN THOUSANDS	MEAN†	STANDARD DEVIATION	PERCENTILE								
					5th	10th	15th	25th	50th	75th	85th	90th	95th
11	132	1,823	12.5	6.5	6.0	6.0	7.0	8.0	10.0	15.0	19.0	20.5	24.5
12	152	1,970	12.4	6.1	6.0	6.0	7.0	8.5	11.0	14.0	18.0	21.0	27.0
13	129	1,697	11.7	6.7	5.0	5.0	6.0	7.0	10.0	14.0	19.0	22.0	25.5
14	134	1,730	10.9	6.4	4.0	5.0	6.0	7.0	9.0	13.0	18.0	20.0	24.0
15	124	1,728	10.2	6.1	4.0	5.0	6.0	6.0	8.0	12.0	15.0	19.0	24.0
16	128	1,752	10.1	5.2	4.0	5.0	5.0	6.5	9.0	12.5	15.0	17.0	22.0
17	139	1,831	9.3	5.4	4.5	5.0	5.5	6.0	7.5	11.0	13.0	15.0	19.0
Black													
1	72	280	9.4	3.4	4.5	6.0	7.0	8.0	8.0	11.0	12.0	13.0	15.0
2	77	267	10.1	3.2	4.5	6.0	6.5	8.0	10.0	12.0	14.0	15.0	15.0
3	72	212	9.1	2.6	6.0	6.5	6.5	7.0	9.0	10.5	12.0	12.0	13.0
4	74	260	8.0	2.6	5.0	5.0	5.0	6.5	7.0	9.0	10.0	10.5	15.0
5	64	226	7.7	3.4	4.5	5.0	5.0	5.0	7.0	9.0	10.0	12.0	15.5
6	52	321	7.1	1.8	4.0	4.0	5.0	6.0	7.0	8.0	9.0	9.0	9.0
7	38	253	7.5	3.2	4.0	4.0	4.0	5.0	6.5	9.0	11.5	13.0	15.0
8	33	203	7.8	3.4	4.0	5.0	5.0	6.0	6.5	10.0	11.0	11.0	12.5
9	52	383	8.2	3.9	3.5	4.0	4.5	6.0	7.0	8.0	12.0	13.0	18.0
10	33	251	9.1	5.3	5.0	5.0	6.0	6.0	7.5	10.0	13.0	15.0	20.0
11	43	313	8.0	5.0	4.0	4.0	5.0	5.0	6.0	8.5	11.0	12.0	15.0
12	47	316	9.4	7.0	4.0	4.0	4.5	6.0	7.5	10.7	11.0	15.0	24.0
13	45	281	8.2	4.4	4.0	5.0	5.0	6.0	7.0	8.5	11.0	19.0	19.0
14	39	282	6.6	2.6	3.5	3.5	3.5	5.0	6.5	7.0	8.0	9.0	12.0
15	43	310	8.9	6.1	4.0	4.5	5.0	5.0	6.5	9.0	10.0	21.0	21.0
16	41	267	7.2	4.8	4.0	4.0	4.0	5.0	6.0	7.5	8.0	11.0	15.0
17	35	235	8.7	5.8	3.5	3.5	5.0	5.0	7.0	10.5	12.0	12.0	23.2

*Includes data for races that are not shown separately.

†Measurements made in the right arm.

(From the National Center for Health Statistics, Department of Health and Human Services. See also Bishop, C.W., Bowen, P.E., Ritchey, S.J.: Am. J. Clin. Nutr., 34:2530–2539, 1981.)

TABLE A–14A–4. SUBSCAPULAR SKINFOLD THICKNESS: BOYS, 1 TO 17 YEARS, UNITED STATES, 1971 TO 1974

RACE AND AGE IN YEARS	NUMBER IN SAMPLE	ESTIMATED POPULATION IN THOUSANDS	MEAN†	STANDARD DEVIATION	PERCENTILE								
					5th	10th	15th	25th	50th	75th	85th	90th	95th
					Subscapular Skinfold in Millimeters								
All Races*													
1	286	1,693	6.2	1.9	4.0	4.0	4.0	5.0	6.0	7.0	8.0	8.5	10.0
2	298	1,747	5.7	2.0	3.0	4.0	4.0	4.5	5.0	6.5	7.0	8.0	10.0
3	308	1,807	5.4	2.0	3.5	4.0	4.0	4.0	5.0	6.0	6.8	7.0	9.5
4	304	1,815	5.1	1.7	3.0	3.5	4.0	4.0	5.0	6.0	6.0	7.0	7.0
5	273	1,563	5.3	2.7	3.0	3.5	4.0	4.0	5.0	6.0	7.0	7.0	8.0
6	179	1,673	5.1	2.4	3.0	3.0	3.5	4.0	4.5	6.0	6.0	7.0	9.0
7	164	1,979	5.5	3.0	3.0	3.0	3.5	4.0	4.5	6.0	7.0	9.0	11.0
8	152	1,861	5.1	2.3	3.0	3.5	3.5	4.0	4.5	6.0	6.0	7.5	9.0
9	169	2,019	7.1	5.1	3.5	3.5	4.0	4.0	5.0	8.0	11.0	14.0	14.0
10	184	2,205	6.8	4.5	3.5	4.0	4.0	4.0	5.5	7.0	10.0	12.0	18.0
11	178	2,177	8.0	6.2	4.0	4.0	4.0	4.5	6.0	8.5	13.0	15.0	19.0
12	200	2,304	8.0	6.0	3.5	4.5	4.5	5.0	6.0	9.0	11.0	14.0	20.5
13	174	1,978	8.8	6.9	3.5	4.0	4.5	5.0	6.5	9.0	13.5	17.0	26.0
14	174	2,030	8.5	6.1	4.0	4.5	5.0	5.0	6.5	9.0	13.0	16.0	20.0
15	171	2,093	9.1	6.5	4.0	5.0	5.0	5.5	7.0	10.0	13.0	15.5	23.0
16	169	2,019	9.8	6.2	5.0	5.5	6.0	6.5	8.0	10.5	13.5	16.5	23.5
17	176	2,095	9.7	5.9	5.0	5.5	6.0	7.0	8.0	10.0	13.0	16.0	23.0
White													
1	211	1,402	6.3	2.0	4.0	4.0	4.0	5.0	6.0	7.0	8.0	8.5	10.0
2	217	1,461	5.6	1.9	3.0	3.5	4.0	4.0	5.0	6.0	7.0	7.5	10.0
3	226	1,536	5.4	2.0	3.5	4.0	4.0	4.0	5.0	6.0	6.5	7.0	10.0
4	229	1,547	5.2	1.8	3.0	4.0	4.0	4.0	5.0	6.0	6.0	7.0	7.0
5	207	1,319	5.3	2.7	3.0	3.5	4.0	4.0	5.0	6.0	7.0	7.0	8.0
6	126	1,343	5.1	2.4	3.0	3.5	4.0	4.0	4.5	5.5	6.0	7.0	10.0
7	125	1,718	5.6	3.1	3.0	3.0	3.5	4.0	5.0	6.0	7.0	8.0	11.5
8	116	1,644	5.1	2.3	3.0	3.0	3.0	4.0	4.5	6.0	6.0	7.5	11.0
9	117	1,636	7.2	4.7	3.5	4.0	4.0	4.0	5.0	8.5	11.5	14.0	14.0
10	148	1,909	6.8	4.5	3.0	4.0	4.0	4.0	5.5	7.0	9.5	12.0	18.0

(Continued)

TABLE A-14A-4. (CONTINUED)

RACE AND AGE IN YEARS	NUMBER IN SAMPLE	ESTIMATED POPULATION IN THOUSANDS	MEAN†	STANDARD DEVIATION	PERCENTILE								
					5th	10th	15th	25th	50th	75th	85th	90th	95th
11	132	1,823	8.2	6.4	3.5	4.0	4.0	4.5	6.0	9.0	14.0	15.0	20.0
12	152	1,970	8.1	5.8	3.5	4.0	4.0	5.0	6.0	9.0	11.5	14.0	21.0
13	129	1,697	9.0	7.1	3.5	4.0	4.0	5.0	6.5	9.0	14.0	17.0	27.0
14	134	1,730	9.0	6.5	4.0	5.0	5.0	5.5	6.5	9.0	14.0	16.0	20.0
15	124	1,728	8.8	6.4	4.0	5.0	5.0	5.5	7.0	9.0	13.0	15.0	22.0
16	128	1,752	9.9	6.4	5.0	5.0	6.0	6.5	8.0	11.0	13.5	17.0	23.5
17	139	1,831	9.7	6.1	5.0	5.5	6.0	6.5	8.0	10.0	13.0	16.0	23.0
Black													
1	72	280	6.0	1.6	4.0	4.0	4.0	5.0	6.0	7.0	7.5	8.0	9.0
2	77	267	6.5	2.4	4.0	4.0	4.0	5.0	5.5	7.0	10.0	11.5	11.5
3	72	212	5.3	1.6	3.5	4.0	4.0	4.0	5.0	6.0	6.5	6.5	9.0
4	74	260	4.8	1.2	3.0	3.0	3.5	4.0	4.5	5.1	6.0	6.0	8.0
5	64	226	5.1	2.5	2.5	3.0	3.5	4.0	5.0	5.0	7.0	7.0	8.5
6	52	321	4.9	2.1	3.0	3.0	3.0	4.0	4.0	5.0	5.5	7.0	7.0
7	38	253	5.2	2.4	3.0	3.0	3.5	3.5	5.0	6.0	8.0	10.0	11.0
8	33	203	5.5	2.1	3.5	3.5	3.0	4.0	5.0	6.0	7.5	9.0	9.0
9	52	383	6.6	6.3	3.0	3.0	4.0	4.0	5.0	6.0	8.0	8.0	30.0
10	33	251	6.7	3.8	4.0	4.0	4.0	4.5	5.0	7.0	9.0	12.0	18.5
11	43	313	6.7	4.9	4.0	4.0	4.0	5.0	5.5	6.5	8.0	8.0	12.5
12	47	316	7.4	6.9	4.0	4.0	4.5	4.5	5.0	7.0	7.0	17.0	19.0
13	45	281	7.6	5.9	4.0	4.5	4.5	5.0	6.0	7.0	8.0	18.5	26.0
14	39	282	6.1	2.1	4.0	4.0	5.0	5.0	6.0	7.0	7.0	7.5	12.0
15	43	310	10.6	6.7	4.0	5.0	5.5	7.0	9.0	12.0	12.0	24.0	24.0
16	41	267	8.5	4.2	5.5	5.5	6.5	6.5	7.0	9.0	9.5	10.0	16.0
17	35	235	9.6	5.2	6.0	6.0	6.0	7.0	8.0	10.0	12.0	16.0	16.0

*Includes data for races that are not shown separately.

†Measurements made in the right arm.

(From the National Center for Health Statistics, Department of Health and Human Services. See also Bishop, C.W., Bowen, P.E., Ritchey, S.J.: Am. J. Clin. Nutr., 34:2530–2539, 1981.)

TABLE A–14B-1. SELECTED PERCENTILES OF WEIGHT, TRICEPS AND SUBSCAPULAR SKINFOLDS, AND BONE-FREE UPPER ARM MUSCLE AREA (AMA) FOR UNITED STATES MEN AND WOMEN WITH SMALL FRAMES (25 TO 54 YEARS OLD)

HT (in)	cm	n	WT (kg)							TRICEPS (mm)							SUBSCAPULAR (mm)							BONE-FREE AMA (cm²)						
			5	10	15	50	85	90	95	5	10	15	50	85	90	95	5	10	15	50	85	90	95	5	10	15	50	85	90	95
Men																														
62	157	23	46*	50*	52*	64	71*	74*	77*				11							16							52			
63	160	43	48*	51*	53	61	70	75*	79*			5	10	17					8	12	20					32	48	54		
64	163	73	49*	53	55	66	76	76	80*		5	6	10	16	18			7	7	15	25	29			37	38	49	58	63	
65	165	112	52	53	58	66	77	81	84	4	5	6	11	17	19	21	7	8	9	14	25	28	35	31	35	37	47	60	63	71
66	168	129	56	57	59	67	78	83	84	5	6	6	11	18	18	20	7	8	8	14	26	26	32	31	36	38	49	60	62	71
67	170	132	56	60	62	71	82	83	88	5	6	6	11	18	18	22	6	7	9	15	23	25	30	35	39	41	49	58	60	62
68	173	107	56	59	65	71	79	82	85	5	6	6	10	15	20	20	7	8	7	13	24	30	40	33	37	40	49	59	62	69
69	175	97	57*	62*	67	74	84	87	88*		6	6	11	17	16			7	7	13	24	26			36	40	58	61	62	
70	178	46	59*	62*	67	75	87	86*	90*		7	7	10	17	20			7	9	14	23					35	48	57	63	
71	180	49	60*	64*	70	76	79	88*	91*			7	10	16					8	13	22					39	47	52		
72	183	21	62*	65*	67*	74	87*	89*	93*				10							14							45			
73	185	9	63*	67*	69*	79*	89*	91*	94*																					
74	188	6	65*	68*	71*	80*	90*	92*	96*																					
Women																														
58	147	53	37*	43	43	52	58	62	66*		12	13	24	30	33	37		10	12	23	34	38			22	24	29	36	44	43
59	150	108	42	43	44	53	63	69	72	8	11	14	21	29	36	33	6	9	10	18	29	32	34		20	22	28	38	39	44
60	152	142	42	45	45	53	63	65	70	8	11	12	21	28	29	34	6	7	8	18	27	32	39	17	21	22	28	36	40	42
61	155	218	44	46	47	54	64	66	72	11	12	14	21	28	31	34	7	8	9	16	28	32	36	19	21	23	28	38	39	37
62	157	255	44	47	48	55	63	64	70	10	12	14	20	28	31	34	6	7	8	14	22	27	32	20	21	21	27	33	35	37
63	160	239	46	48	49	55	65	68	79	10	11	13	20	27	30	36	6	7	7	14	27	29	31	20	21	22	27	33	35	38
64	163	146	49	50	51	57	67	68	74	10	13	13	20	28	30	34	6	7	8	13	24	27	34	22	23	23	28	34	35	42
65	165	113	50	52	53	60	70	72	80	12	13	14	22	29	31	34	7	8	8	15	26	30	33	21	22	23	28	37	38	47
66	168	47	46*	49*	54	58	65	71*	74*			12	19	30					9	12	25					23	27	35	39	
67	170	18	47*	50*	52*	59	70*	72*	76*				18							13							26			
68	173	18	48*	51*	53*	62	71*	73*	77*				20							15							25			
69	175	5	49*	52*	54*	63*	72*	74*	78*																					
70	178	1	50*	53*	55*	64*	73*	75*	79*																					

*Value estimated through linear regression equation.

(From Frisancho, A. R.: Am. J. Clin. Nutr., 4D:808–819, 1984, with permission.)

TABLE A–14B-2. SELECTED PERCENTILES OF WEIGHT, TRICEPS AND SUBSCAPULAR SKINFOLDS, AND BONE-FREE UPPER ARM MUSCLE AREA (AMA) FOR UNITED STATES MEN AND WOMEN WITH MEDIUM FRAMES (25 TO 54 YEARS OLD)

HT			WT (kg)							TRICEPS (mm)							SUBSCAPULAR (mm)							BONE-FREE AMA (cm²)						
in	cm	n	5	10	15	50	85	90	95	5	10	15	50	85	90	95	5	10	15	50	85	90	95	5	10	15	50	85	90	95
Men																														
62	157	10	51*	55*	58*	68	81*	83*	87*				15							13							58			
63	160	30	52*	56*	59*	71	82*	85*	89*				11							18							55			
64	163	71	54*	60	61	71	83	84	90*				12							17							56			
65	165	154	59	62	65	74	87	90	94	6	7	8	12	18	20	25	8	9	10	16	26	29	32	40	43	47	56	67	71	70
66	168	212	58	61	65	75	85	87	93	5	6	7	11	18	19	22	7	9	9	16	25	27	33	38	43	45	56	67	69	78
67	170	409	62	66	68	77	89	93	100	6	7	7	13	21	23	28	8	9	10	16	26	30	33	39	42	44	55	69	72	73
68	173	478	60	64	66	78	89	92	97	5	6	7	11	18	20	24	8	8	9	16	25	27	31	38	42	44	53	66	69	76
69	175	464	63	66	68	78	90	93	97	5	6	7	12	18	20	24	7	8	9	16	24	27	31	39	41	44	55	67	71	73
70	178	419	64	66	70	81	90	93	97	5	5	7	12	18	20	23	7	8	9	15	24	27	30	37	44	44	54	66	68	72
71	180	282	62	68	70	81	92	96	100	4	5	7	12	19	21	25	7	8	9	14	24	27	32	40	42	43	55	65	68	73
72	183	231	68	71	74	84	97	100	104	5	6	8	12	20	22	26	7	9	9	15	26	30	32	39	42	44	56	67	69	74
73	185	106	70	72	75	85	100	101	104	4	5	7	12	20	24	24	8	7	9	15	25	29	32		43	43	55	65	69	73
74	188	50	68*	76	77	88	100	100	104*	6		9	13	21	23	27				14							55	62	63	73
Women																														
58	147	40	41*	46*	50	63	77	75*	79*				25							23							35			
59	150	104	47	50	52	66	76	79	85	14	19	21	30	37	40	41	8	12	13	29	38	39	41	23	24	26	33	43	45	49
60	152	208	47	50	52	60	77	79	85	11	15	17	26	35	37	42	8	10	11	22	35	37	42	22	25	25	32	42	45	49
61	155	465	47	49	51	61	73	78	86	12	14	15	25	34	36	40	7	9	10	19	32	36	40	21	24	25	31	42	45	51
62	157	644	49	50	52	61	73	77	83	11	13	16	25	34	36	38	7	9	10	19	33	37	40	21	23	25	31	40	43	48
63	160	685	49	51	53	62	77	80	88	12	15	15	24	33	36	40	7	8	10	18	31	34	38	22	23	25	32	41	43	50
64	163	722	50	52	54	62	76	82	87	11	14	15	23	33	34	38	7	8	8	16	31	35	40	21	23	24	31	40	43	48
65	165	628	52	54	55	63	75	80	89	12	14	15	22	31	33	37	7	8	8	15	29	35	38	22	24	24	31	40	43	49
66	168	428	52	54	55	63	75	78	83	11	13	14	22	29	30	35	7	8	9	14	28	30	35	22	23	25	30	39	41	44
67	170	257	54	56	57	65	79	82	88	12	13	15	21	30	32	36	7	8	8	15	28	32	37	22	24	25	30	40	43	44
68	173	119	58	59	60	67	77	85	87	10	12	12	22	29	31	36	8	8	8	15	25	33	35	23	24	25	30	37	38	39
69	175	59	49*	58	60	68	79	82	87*				19							12							30			
70	178	15	50*	54*	57*	70	80*	83*	87*											20							32			

*Value estimated through linear regression equation.
(From Frisancho, A. R.: Am. J. Clin. Nutr., 40:808–819, 1984, with permission.)

TABLE A–14B-3. SELECTED PERCENTILES OF WEIGHT, TRICEPS AND SUBSCAPULAR SKINFOLDS, AND BONE-FREE UPPER ARM MUSCLE AREA (AMA) FOR UNITED STATES MEN AND WOMEN WITH LARGE FRAMES (25 TO 54 YEARS OLD)

HT in	cm	n	WT(kg) 5	10	15	50	85	90	95	TRICEPS(mm) 5	10	15	50	85	90	95	SUBSCAPULAR(mm) 5	10	15	50	85	90	95	BONE-FREE AMA(cm²) 5	10	15	50	85	90	95
Men																														
62	157	1	57*	62*	66*	82*	99*	103*	108*																					
63	160	1	58*	63*	67*	83*	100*	104*	109*																					
64	163	5	59*	64*	68*	84*	101*	105*	110*																					
65	165	15	60*	65*	69*	79	102*	106*	111*																		62			
66	168	37	60*	65*	75	84	103	106*	112*			9	14	30					13	21	36				50	48	58	76		
67	170	54	62*	70	71	84	102	111	113*		7	7	11	23	27			8	11	22	36	40			51	52	61	73		
68	173	84	63*	74	76	86	101	104	114*		9	10	14	22	23			12	14	20	31	35	38		48	53	65	78	78	
69	175	126	68	71	74	89	103	105	114	6	7	8	15	25	29	31	9	10	11	20	31	32	38	46	47	49	61	73	86	83
70	178	150	68	72	74	87	106	112	114		7	7	14	23	25	30	7	10	11	18	31	35	46	43	48	50	61	75	78	83
71	180	123	73	78	82	91	113	116	123	6	8	7	15	25	27	31	9	11	11	17	35	40	46	45	48	50	62	75	77	86
72	183	114	73	76	78	91	109	112	121	5	6	10	15	22	22	25	8	11	9	20	30	28	36	47	49	51	61	77	81	83
73	185	109	72	77	79	93	106	107	116	5	6	7	12	19	22	31	7	10	9	18	27	28	30			53	61	79	80	86
74	188	37	69*	74*	82	92	105	115*	120*			8	13	19				9	9	18	32						66	78	83	86
Women																														
58	147	6	56*	63*	67*	86*	105*	110*	117*				36							35							45			
59	150	19	56*	62*	67*	78	105*	109*	116*				38	48	50	50				42	48	53	55				44	62	74	72
60	152	32	55*	62*	66*	87	104*	109*	116*			26	36	48	48	51			17	35	48	51	50			33	41	56	63	77
61	155	92	54*	64	66	81	105	117	115*	16	25	22	34	46	48	49	13	17	18	32	44	48	50	26	29	31	44	60	65	63
62	157	135	59	61	65	81	103	107	113	19	19	22	34	43	45	48	11	16	16	28	42	46	50	27	28	32	43	50	55	67
63	160	162	58	63	67	83	105	109	119	18	20	21	32	43	46	48	10	14	15	29	42	48	52	26	30	29	39	56	59	69
64	163	196	59	62	63	79	102	104	112	16	20	21	31	40	43	45	10	12	14	25	36	40	45	27	28	29	39	49	53	55
65	165	242	59	61	63	81	103	109	114	17	20	18	30	41	43	49	8	12	11	25	41	46	55	23	28	27	35	50	53	
66	168	166	55	58	62	75	95	100	107	13	17	17	29	37	40		7	9	11	20	45	48		25	24	30	37	51	54	
67	170	144	58	60	65	80	100	108	114	13	16	20	30	42				10	12	16					28	30	38			
68	173	81	51*	66	66	76	104	105	111*	16		21	20					10	11						28	27	35			
69	175	39	50*	57*	68	79	105	104*	111*																		37			
70	178	17	50*	56*	61*	76	99*	104*	110*																					

*Value estimated through linear regression equation.
(From Frisancho, A. R.: Am. J. Clin. Nutr., 40:808–819, 1984, with permission.)

TABLE A–14B-4. SELECTED PERCENTILES OF WEIGHT, TRICEPS AND SUBSCAPULAR SKINFOLDS, AND BONE-FREE UPPER ARM MUSCLE AREA (AMA) FOR UNITED STATES MEN AND WOMEN WITH SMALL FRAMES (55 TO 74 YEARS OLD)

HT in	HT cm	n	WT (kg) 5	10	15	50	85	90	95	TRICEPS (mm) 5	10	15	50	85	90	95	SUBSCAPULAR (mm) 5	10	15	50	85	90	95	BONE-FREE AMA (cm²) 5	10	15	50	85	90	95
Men																														
62	157	47	45*	49*	56	61	68	73*	77*			6	9	12					11	16	23					38	46	52		
63	160	78	47*	49	51	62	71	71	79*		5	5	10	16	17				6	12	21	22			34	35	43	54		
64	163	107	47	50	54	63	72	74	80		4	4		20		22	6	7		14	24			26	30	31	44	53	55	56
65	165	132	48	54	59	70	80	90	90		6	7	11	18	19	24	6	8	8	16	28	25	29	26	30	35	48	57	54	
66	168	112	51	55	59	68	77	80	84		6	7	11	16	20	20	7	7	9	15	25	26	30	25	31	37	45	54	60	62
67	170	128	55	60	61	69	79	81	88		6	7	10	15	17	25	7	8	13	13	22	25	31	30	36	35	45	58	60	64
68	173	95	54*	54	58	70	79	81	86*		5	6	10	15	17			7	7	13	21				35	37	43	53	55	59
69	175	47	56*	59*	63	75	81	84*	88*			5	10	15					7	16	27					35	47	62	60	
70	178	29	57*	61*	63*	76	83*	86*	89*	4		8	11						10	16						38	48			
71	180	14	59*	62*	65*	69	85*	87*	91*	5										13							43			
72	183	6	60*	64*	66*	76*	86*	89*	92*	5										10										
73	185	1	62*	65*	68*	78*	88*	90*	94*	5			9																	
74	188	1	63*	67*	69*	77*	89*	92*	95*																				
Women																														
58	147	85	39*	46	48	54	63	65	71*		14	16	21	31	34			8	9	18	32	33			22	23	29	40	42	
59	150	122	41	45	48	55	66	68	74		13	15	21	30	31	33		7	9	19	29	30	33	22	23	24	30	39	40	44
60	152	157	43	45	47	54	67	70	73	10	11	13	20	29	31	35	6	5	8	15	27	32	36	20	22	23	30	37	41	44
61	155	145	43	43	45	56	65	70	71	11	11	13	22	29	32	34	7	7	8	17	29	31	34	18	21	23	28	36	40	42
62	157	158	47	49	52	58	67	69	73	11	11	12	21	29	30	32		8	9	17	25	26	30	20	23	24	30	37	40	40
63	160	89	42*	45	49	58	67	68	74*		12	13	20	29	30			6	7	14	25	27			19	20	27	35	36	43
64	163	50	43*	47	49	60	68	70	75*		12	13	21	27	29			6	7	18	24	25			21	21	28	37	42	
65	165	26	43*	47*	49*	60	69*	72*	75*			13	18							13							28			
66	168	12	44*	48*	50*	68	70*	72*	76*				23							13							33			
67	170	1	45*	48*	51*	61*	71*	73*	77*																				
68	173	1	45*	49*	51*	61*	71*	74*	77*																				
69	175	0	46*	49*	52*	62*	72*	74*	78*																				
70	178	0	47*	50*	52*	63*	73*	75*	79*																				

*Value estimated through linear regression equation.

(From Frisancho, A. R.: Am. J. Clin. Nutr., 40:808–819, 1984, with permission.)

TABLE A–14B-5. SELECTED PERCENTILES OF WEIGHT, TRICEPS AND SUBSCAPULAR SKINFOLDS, AND BONE-FREE UPPER ARM MUSCLE AREA (AMA) FOR UNITED STATES MEN AND WOMEN WITH MEDIUM FRAMES (55 TO 74 YEARS OLD)

HT (in)	HT (cm)	n	WT (kg)							TRICEPS (mm)							SUBSCAPULAR (mm)							BONE-FREE AMA (cm²)						
			5	10	15	50	85	90	95	5	10	15	50	85	90	95	5	10	15	50	85	90	95	5	10	15	50	85	90	95
Men																														
62	157	49	50*	54*	59	68	77	81*	85*			5	12	25					11	19	27					39	48	61		
63	160	89	51*	57	60	70	80	82	87*		7	6	11	20	23			8	10	15	26	28		35	36	38	50	60	63	71
64	163	210	55	59	62	71	82	83	91	5	6	6	10	17	20	26	6	7	9	15	25	27	35	35	39	40	51	64	66	72
65	165	335	56	60	64	72	83	86	89	5	6	7	11	17	19	24	7	8	9	17	25	29	31	34	38	41	52	63	65	67
66	168	405	57	62	66	74	83	84	89	6	6	7	12	18	19	22		9	10	16	25	28	31	35	39	42	51	60	62	67
67	170	509	59	64	66	78	87	89	94	5	6	7	12	18	20	23	7	9	10	17	26	29	34	37	40	42	52	65	67	70
68	173	413	62	66	68	78	89	95	101	6	7	8	12	18	21	23	7	9	10	17	26	29	32	31	36	40	51	65	67	70
69	175	366	62	66	68	77	90	93	99	5	6	7	11	19	22	25		8	9	16	25	28	30	36	41	42	53	62	65	72
70	178	248	62	68	71	80	90	95	101	6	6	7	11	16	19	21	6	9	10	16	25	27	30	36	42	44	56	63	67	68
71	180	146	68	70	72	84	94	97	101	5	7	8	11	16	17	20	7	8	10	15	25	26	31		27	39	50	58	59	71
72	183	81	66*	65	69	81	96	97	101*		6	8	11	16	20			8	10	16	25	28				43	56	67		
73	185	35	68*	72*	79	88	93	99*	103*		6	8	13	16					10	15	28	30					56			
74	188	11	69*	73*	76*	95	98*	101*	104*				11							18	26									
Women																														
58	147	105	40	44	49	57	72	82	85	5	13	17	28	40	40	41	3	7	10	25	37	43	48	21	23	25	32	46	47	51
59	150	198	47	49	52	62	74	78	86	12	15	18	26	34	38	41	8	9	11	23	32	36	43	24	26	27	35	44	48	48
60	152	358	47	50	52	65	76	79	86	13	17	18	25	33	34	38	8	10	12	22	34	36	40	21	24	26	35	45	49	57
61	155	543	49	51	54	64	78	81	86	13	16	18	25	33	37	42	8	10	10	22	33	36	42	22	26	26	34	44	44	52
62	157	576	49	53	54	64	78	82	88	13	15	17	24	33	36	39	8	8	10	20	33	36	38	24	25	27	35	45	47	54
63	160	551	52	54	55	65	79	83	89	12	14	16	24	32	35	38	8	8	10	18	32	33	41	24	26	26	33	44	45	51
64	163	406	51	54	57	66	78	81	87	12	14	16	25	33	34	37	7	9	10	17	30	34	38	21	24	26	34	44	46	49
65	165	307	54	56	59	67	78	84	88	14	16	17	24	33	35	39	7	8	9	17	30	35	37	24	25	27	34	44	45	50
66	168	119	54	57	57	66	79	85	88	12	13	16	24	33	33	36	6	7	8	16	30	31	39	24	26	27	33	41	43	49
67	170	63	51*	59	61	72	82	85	89*	17	17	17	27	35	35			9	10	19	35	35	36		27	28	32	41	43	49
68	173	28	52*	56*	59*	70	83*	86*	90*				25							16							36			
69	175	5	53*	57*	60*	72*	84*	87*	91*																					
70	178	1	54*	58*	61*	73*	85*	88*	92*																					

*Value estimated through linear regression equation.

(From Frisancho, A. R.: Am. J. Clin. Nutr., 40:808–819, 1984, with permission.)

TABLE A-14B-6. SELECTED PERCENTILES OF WEIGHT, TRICEPS AND SUBSCAPULAR SKINFOLDS, AND BONE-FREE UPPER ARM MUSCLE AREA (AMA) FOR UNITED STATES MEN AND WOMEN WITH LARGE FRAMES (55 TO 74 YEARS OLD)

HT in	cm	n	WT (kg)							TRICEPS (mm)							SUBSCAPULAR (mm)							BONE-FREE AMA (cm²)						
			5	10	15	50	85	90	95	5	10	15	50	85	90	95	5	10	15	50	85	90	95	5	10	15	50	85	90	95
Men																														
62	157	7	54*	59*	63*	77*	91*	95*	100*				15							20							57			
63	160	12	55*	60*	64*	80	92*	96*	101*				21							31							44			
64	163	20	57*	62*	65*	77	94*	97*	102*			11	14	22		25			14	20	27					44	59	66		
65	165	36	58*	63*	73	79	89	98*	103*		8	9	13	21	25			9	11	20	31	35	38		43	47	56	67	72	79
66	168	58	59*	67	73	80	101	102	105*		8	8	16	18	20	23	8	11	12	20	35	35	32		43	44	59	71	73	74
67	170	114	65	71	73	85	103	108	112	7	8	8	13	21	25	27	8	10	11	18	27	30	33	41	43	46	56	69	70	79
68	173	128	67	71	73	83	95	98	111	8	8	8	13	20	21	23	7	11	11	19	27	30	37	41	45	45	57	70	72	74
69	175	131	65	70	74	84	96	98	105	7	7	6	12	18	20	23	9		13	20	30	33		40	48	50	58	70	71	79
70	178	144	68	73	77	87	102	104	117	7	7	6	14	22	25	31				15	28	30		43	46	47	59	70	75	87
71	180	95	65*	70	70	84	102	109	111*	6	6	8	13						9	20		31				48	54	54	73	
72	183	72	67*	76	81	90	108	112	112*	6	6	8	13	23	22	26				19							59	59		
73	185	23	68*	73*	76*	88	105*	108*	113*	5			11							15										
74	188	15	69*	74*	78*	89	106*	109*	114*				12														54			
Women																														
58	147	14	53*	59*	63*	92	95*	99*	104*	18	25	26	45	44	45	46	13	19	21	44	42	45	48				50			
59	150	26	54*	59*	63*	78	95*	99*	105*	19	22	24	36	40	43	50	13	16	19	31	40	43	53				49			
60	152	72	54*	65	69	78	87	88	105*	20	24	24	35	44	43	45	13	19	22	31	39	48	51	31	28	33	41	58	60	71
61	155	117	64	68	69	79	94	95	106	18	24	25	33	40	43	43	10	15	16	29	41	45	55		32	34	44	59	61	76
62	157	126	59	61	63	82	93	101	111	15	25	23	32	41	46	45	8	12	16	29	42	46	48		29	34	43	59	63	67
63	160	154	61	65	67	80	100	102	118	18	23	20	33	42	44	50		9	12	24	41	46			32	33	41	56	60	67
64	163	147	60	65	67	77	97	102	119		17	18	29	43	44	46			12	26	34				29	32	42	54	62	78
65	165	117	60	66	69	80	98	102	111		18	20	30	35	40					26	46				32	31	41	53	57	65
66	168	64	57*	60	63	82	98	105	109*				27						14	25	46			29		30	40	58		
67	170	40	58*	64*	68*	79	100*	104*	109*	15	22	22	32	44						21					31	31	40	57	58	
68	173	17	58*	64*	68*	79	100*	104*	110*				26														25			
69	175	7	59*	65*	69*	85*	101*	105*	110*																					
70	178	2	60*	65*	69*	85*	101*	105*	111*																		48			

*Value estimated through linear regression equation.

(From Frisancho, A. R.: Am. J. Clin. Nutr., 40:808–819, 1984, with permission.)

TABLE A–14C-1. MIDARM MUSCLE CIRCUMFERENCE IN ADULTS (18 TO 74 YEARS), UNITED STATES*†

AGE GROUP (years)	SAMPLE SIZE	ESTIMATED POPULATION (millions)	MEAN (cm)	PERCENTILE 5th	10th	25th	50th	75th	90th	95th
Men										
18–74	5,261	61.18	28.0	23.8	24.8	26.3	27.9	29.6	31.4	32.5
18–24	773	11.78	27.4	23.5	24.4	25.8	27.2	28.9	30.8	32.3
25–34	804	13.00	28.3	24.2	25.3	26.5	28.0	30.0	31.7	32.9
35–44	664	10.68	28.8	25.0	25.6	27.1	28.7	30.3	32.1	33.0
45–54	765	11.15	28.2	24.0	24.9	26.5	28.1	29.8	31.5	32.6
55–64	598	9.07	27.8	22.8	24.4	26.2	27.9	29.6	31.0	31.8
65–74	1,657	5.50	26.8	22.5	23.7	25.3	26.9	28.5	29.9	30.7
Women										
18–74	8,410	67.84	22.2	18.4	19.0	20.2	21.8	23.6	25.8	27.4
18–24	1,523	12.89	20.9	17.7	18.5	19.4	20.6	22.1	23.6	24.9
25–34	1,896	13.93	21.7	18.3	18.9	20.0	21.4	22.9	24.9	26.6
35–44	1,664	11.59	22.5	18.5	19.2	20.6	22.0	24.0	26.1	27.4
45–54	836	12.16	22.7	18.8	19.5	20.7	22.2	24.3	26.6	27.8
55–64	669	9.98	22.8	18.6	19.5	20.8	22.6	24.4	26.3	28.1
65–74	1,822	7.28	22.8	18.6	19.5	20.8	22.5	24.4	26.5	28.1

*Measurements made in the right arm.
†See Tables A–14b-1 through A–14b-6 for data compiled by Frisancho (Am. J. Clin. Nutri., 40:808–819, 1984) from NHANES I and II.
(From Bishop, C. W., Bowen, P.E., Ritchey, S.J.: Am. J. Clin. Nutr., 34:2530–2539, 1981 [NHANES 1].)

TABLE A–14C-2. MIDARM MUSCLE AREA IN ADULTS (18 TO 74 YEARS), UNITED STATES*†

AGE GROUP (years)	SAMPLE SIZE	ESTIMATED POPULATION (millions)	MEAN (cm)	PERCENTILE						
				5th	10th	25th	50th	75th	90th	95th
Men										
18–74	5,261	61.18	62.4	45.1	49.0	55.1	62.0	69.8	78.5	84.1
18–24	773	11.78	59.8	44.0	47.4	53.0	58.9	66.5	75.5	83.1
25–34	804	13.00	63.8	46.6	51.0	55.9	62.4	71.7	80.0	86.2
35–44	664	10.68	66.0	49.8	52.2	58.5	65.6	73.1	82.0	86.7
45–54	765	11.15	63.3	45.9	49.4	55.9	62.9	70.7	79.0	84.6
55–64	598	9.07	61.5	41.4	47.4	54.7	62.0	69.8	76.5	80.5
65–74	1,657	5.50	57.2	40.3	44.7	51.0	57.6	64.7	71.2	75.0
Women										
18–74	8,410	67.84	39.2	27.0	28.7	32.5	37.8	44.3	53.0	59.8
18–24	1,523	12.89	34.8	24.9	27.2	30.0	33.8	38.9	44.3	49.4
25–34	1,896	13.93	37.5	26.7	28.4	31.8	36.5	41.8	49.4	56.3
35–44	1,664	11.59	40.3	27.2	29.4	33.8	38.5	45.9	54.2	59.8
45–54	836	12.16	41.0	28.1	30.3	34.1	39.2	47.0	56.3	61.5
55–64	669	9.98	41.4	27.5	30.3	34.4	40.7	47.4	55.1	62.9
65–74	1,822	7.28	41.4	27.5	30.3	34.4	40.3	47.4	55.9	62.9

*Measurements made in the right arm.
†See Tables A–14b-1 through A–14b-6 for data compiled by Frisancho (Am. J. Clin. Nutri., *40*:808–819, 1984) from NHANES I and II.
(From Bishop, C. W., Bowen, P.E., Ritchey, S.J.: Am. J. Clin. Nutr., *34*:2530–2539, 1981 [NHANES 1].)

TABLE A—14C-3. AGE CORRECTION FOR ESTIMATES OF WEIGHT, TRICEPS AND SUBSCAPULAR SKINFOLD THICKNESSES, AND BONE-FREE UPPER ARM MUSCLE AREA (AMA)

AGE GROUP: FRAME SIZE	MEDIAN AGE	WEIGHT	TRICEPS SKINFOLD	SUBSCAPULAR SKINFOLD	ARM MUSCLE AREA
Men					
25—54					
Small	39	0.074	0.016	0.080	0.030
Medium	39	0.080	0.005	0.083	0.055
Large	40	0.000	−0.024	0.049	0.026
55—74					
Small	66	−0.329	−0.036	−0.115	−0.407
Medium	67	−0.435	−0.040	−0.125	−0.521
Large	67	−0.562	−0.054	−0.185	−0.644
Women					
25—54					
Small	37	0.165	0.166	0.142	0.087
Medium	37	0.234	0.189	0.214	0.191
Large	37	0.284	0.191	0.233	0.270
55—74					
Small	67	−0.027	−0.072	−0.013	0.036
Medium	66	−0.196	−0.210	−0.221	−0.033
Large	67	−0.466	−0.370	−0.515	−0.378

(From Frisancho, A.R.: Am. J. Clin. Nutr., *40*:808—819, 1984, with permission.)

TABLE A—14D-1. PROVISIONAL PERCENTILES FOR TRICEPS SKINFOLD THICKNESS IN THE ELDERLY[*][†]

AGE GROUP (Years)	PERCENTILE		
	5th	50th	95th
Men			
65	8.6	13.8	27.0
70	7.7	12.9	26.1
75	6.8	12.0	25.2
80	6.0	11.2	24.3
85	5.1	10.3	23.4
90	4.2	9.4	22.6
Women			
65	13.5	21.6	33.0
70	12.5	20.6	32.0
75	11.5	19.6	31.0
80	10.5	18.6	30.0
85	9.5	17.6	29.0
90	8.5	16.6	28.0

*Data are from 119 men and 150 women. All subjects were ambulatory, and measurements were made in the recumbent position on the left side.

†See Tables A—14b-1 and A—14b-2 for data compiled by Frisancho (Am. J. Clin. Nutr., *40*:808—819, 1984) from NHANES I and II.

(From Chumlea, W.C., Roche, A.F., Mukherjee, D.: Nutritional Assessment of the Elderly Through Anthropometry. Ohio, Wright State University School of Medicine, 1984.)

TABLE A—14D-2. PROVISIONAL PERCENTILES FOR MIDARM MUSCLE AREA (cm^2) IN THE ELDERLY*†

AGE GROUP (Years)	PERCENTILE		
	5th	50th	95th
Men			
65	43.2	59.4	77.1
70	41.4	57.7	75.3
75	39.6	55.9	73.5
80	37.8	54.1	71.7
85	36.0	52.3	69.9
90	34.3	50.5	68.2
Women			
65	33.5	44.5	66.4
70	33.0	44.1	65.9
75	32.6	43.6	65.5
80	32.2	43.2	65.1
85	31.8	42.8	64.7
90	31.3	42.4	64.2

*Data are from 119 men and 150 women. All subjects were ambulatory, and measurements were made in the recumbent position on the left side.

†See Tables A—14b-1 and A—14b-2 for data compiled by Frisancho (Am. J. Clin. Nutr., *40*:808—819, 1984) from NHANES I and II.

(From Chumlea, W.C., Roche, A.F., Mukherjee, D.: Nutritional Assessment of the Elderly Through Anthropometry. Ohio, Wright State University School of Medicine, 1984.)

TABLES A—15A TO C. BODY FAT ESTIMATIONS FROM SKINFOLD DATA

Various investigators have developed equations for predicting the proportions of body fat by anthropometric measures of specific regions. Durnin and Womersley used four different skinfolds (Table A—15-a). Pollock, Schmidt, and Jackson have prepared tables based on three sites, including thigh skinfolds (Tables A—15-b and A—15-c). Because some technicians have difficulty in obtaining consistent results with thigh skinfold measurements, data also are available based on other equations that do not use this skinfold. These data are included in the following sources:

Golding, L.A., Meyers, C.R., Sinning, W.E.: Y's Way to Physical Fitness: The Complete Guide to Fitness Testing and Instruction. 3rd Ed. Champaign, IL, Human Kinetics Publishers, 1989.

Pollock, M.L., Schmidt, D.H., Jackson, A.S.: Compr. Ther., *6*:12—27, 1980.

Jackson, A.S. and Pollock, M.L.: Phys. Sportsmed., *13*:76—90, 1985.

TABLE A–15A. EQUIVALENT FAT CONTENT, AS PERCENTAGE OF BODY WEIGHT, FOR A RANGE OF VALUES FOR THE SUM OF FOUR SKINFOLDS*

SKINFOLDS (mm)	MEN (AGE IN YEARS)				WOMEN (AGE IN YEARS)			
	17–29	30–39	40–49	50+	16–29	30–39	40–49	50+
15	4.8				10.5			
20	8.1	12.2	12.2	12.6	14.1	17.0	19.8	21.4
25	10.5	14.2	15.0	15.6	16.8	19.4	22.2	24.0
30	12.9	16.2	17.7	18.6	19.5	21.8	24.5	26.6
35	14.7	17.7	19.6	20.8	21.5	23.7	26.4	28.5
40	16.4	19.2	21.4	22.9	23.4	25.5	28.2	30.3
45	17.7	20.4	23.0	24.7	25.0	26.9	29.6	31.9
50	19.0	21.5	24.6	26.5	26.5	28.2	31.0	33.4
55	20.1	22.5	25.9	27.9	27.8	29.4	32.1	34.6
60	21.2	23.5	27.1	29.2	29.1	30.6	33.2	35.7
65	22.2	24.3	28.2	30.4	30.2	31.6	34.1	36.7
70	23.1	25.1	29.3	31.6	31.2	32.5	35.0	37.7
75	24.0	25.9	30.3	32.7	32.2	33.4	35.9	38.7
80	24.8	26.6	31.2	33.8	33.1	34.3	36.7	39.6
85	25.5	27.2	32.1	34.8	34.0	35.1	37.5	40.4
90	26.2	27.8	33.0	35.8	34.8	35.8	38.3	41.2
95	26.9	28.4	33.7	36.6	35.6	36.5	39.0	41.9
100	27.6	29.0	34.4	37.4	36.4	37.2	39.7	42.6
105	28.2	29.6	35.1	38.2	37.1	37.9	40.4	43.3
110	28.8	30.1	35.8	39.0	37.8	38.6	41.0	43.9
115	29.4	30.6	36.4	39.7	38.4	39.1	41.5	44.5

(Continued)

SKINFOLDS (mm)	MEN (AGE IN YEARS)				WOMEN (AGE IN YEARS)			
	17–29	30–39	40–49	50+	16–29	30–39	40–49	50+
120	30.0	31.1	37.0	40.4	39.0	39.6	42.0	45.1
125	31.0	31.5	37.6	41.1	39.6	40.1	42.5	45.7
130	31.5	31.9	38.2	41.8	40.2	40.6	43.0	46.2
135	32.0	32.3	38.7	42.4	40.8	41.1	43.5	46.7
140	32.5	32.7	39.2	43.0	41.3	41.6	44.0	47.2
145	32.9	33.1	39.7	43.6	41.8	42.1	44.5	47.7
150	33.3	33.5	40.2	44.1	42.3	42.6	45.0	48.2
155	33.7	33.9	40.7	44.6	42.8	43.1	45.4	48.7
160	34.1	34.3	41.2	45.1	43.3	43.6	45.8	49.2
165	34.5	34.6	41.6	45.6	43.7	44.0	46.2	49.6
170	34.9	34.8	42.0	46.1	44.1	44.4	46.6	50.0
175	35.3					44.8	47.0	50.4
180	35.6					45.2	47.4	50.8
185	35.9					45.6	47.8	51.2
190						45.9	48.2	51.6
195						46.2	48.5	52.0
200						46.5	48.8	52.4
205							49.1	52.7
210							49.4	53.0

*Biceps, triceps, subscapular, and suprailiac of men and women of different ages.
(From Durnin, J.V.G.A., Womersley, J.: Br. J. Nutr., 32:77–97, 1974, with permission.)

TABLE A–15B. PERCENTAGE OF BODY FAT ESTIMATION FOR WOMEN FROM AGE AND TRICEPS, SUPRAILIUM, AND THIGH SKINFOLDS*

SUM OF SKINFOLDS (mm)	AGE TO THE LAST YEAR								
	Under 22	23 to 27	28 to 32	33 to 37	38 to 42	43 to 47	48 to 52	53 to 57	Over 58
23–25	9.7	9.9	10.2	10.4	10.7	10.9	11.2	11.4	11.7
26–28	11.0	11.2	11.5	11.7	12.0	12.3	12.5	12.7	13.0
29–31	12.3	12.5	12.8	13.0	13.3	13.5	13.8	14.0	14.3
32–34	13.6	13.8	14.0	14.3	14.5	14.8	15.0	15.3	15.5
35–37	14.8	15.0	15.3	15.5	15.8	16.0	16.3	16.5	16.8
38–40	16.0	16.3	16.5	16.7	17.0	17.2	17.5	17.7	18.0
41–43	17.2	17.4	17.7	17.9	18.2	18.4	18.7	18.9	19.2
44–46	18.3	18.6	18.8	19.1	19.3	19.6	19.8	20.1	20.3
47–49	19.5	19.7	20.0	20.2	20.5	20.7	21.0	21.2	21.5
50–52	20.6	20.8	21.1	21.3	21.6	21.8	22.1	22.3	22.6
53–55	21.7	21.9	22.1	22.4	22.6	22.9	23.1	23.4	23.6
56–58	22.7	23.0	23.2	23.4	23.7	23.9	24.2	24.4	24.7
59–61	23.7	24.0	24.2	24.5	24.7	25.0	25.2	25.5	25.7
62–64	24.7	25.0	25.2	25.5	25.7	26.0	26.2	26.4	26.7
65–67	25.7	25.9	26.2	26.4	26.7	26.9	27.2	27.4	27.7
68–70	26.6	26.9	27.1	27.4	27.6	27.9	28.1	28.4	28.6
71–73	27.5	27.8	28.0	28.3	28.5	28.8	29.0	29.3	29.5
74–76	28.4	28.7	28.9	29.2	29.4	29.7	29.9	30.2	30.4
77–79	29.3	29.5	29.8	30.0	30.3	30.5	30.8	31.0	31.3
80–82	30.1	30.4	30.6	30.9	31.1	31.4	31.6	31.9	32.1

(Continued)

TABLE A−15B. (CONTINUED)

SUM OF SKINFOLDS (mm)	AGE TO THE LAST YEAR								
	Under 22	23 to 27	28 to 32	33 to 37	38 to 42	43 to 47	48 to 52	53 to 57	Over 58
83–85	30.9	31.2	31.4	31.7	31.9	32.2	32.4	32.7	32.9
86–88	31.7	32.0	32.2	32.5	32.7	32.9	33.2	33.4	33.7
89–91	32.5	32.7	33.0	33.2	33.5	33.7	33.9	34.2	34.4
92–94	33.2	33.4	33.7	33.9	34.2	34.4	34.7	34.9	35.2
95–97	33.9	34.1	34.4	34.6	34.9	35.1	35.4	35.6	35.9
98–100	34.6	34.8	35.1	35.3	35.5	35.8	36.0	36.3	36.5
101–103	35.3	35.4	35.7	35.9	36.2	36.4	36.7	36.9	37.2
104–106	35.8	36.1	36.3	36.6	36.8	37.1	37.3	37.5	37.8
107–109	36.4	36.7	36.9	37.1	37.4	37.6	37.9	38.1	38.4
110–112	37.0	37.2	37.5	37.7	38.0	38.2	38.5	38.7	38.9
113–115	37.5	37.8	38.0	38.2	38.5	38.7	39.0	39.2	39.5
116–118	38.0	38.3	38.5	38.8	39.0	39.3	39.5	39.7	40.0
119–121	38.5	38.7	39.0	39.2	39.5	39.7	40.0	40.2	40.5
122–124	39.0	39.2	39.4	39.7	39.9	40.2	40.4	40.7	40.9
125–127	39.4	39.6	39.9	40.1	40.4	40.6	40.9	41.1	41.4
128–130	39.8	40.0	40.3	40.5	40.8	41.0	41.3	41.5	41.8

*Percentage of fat calculated by the formula of Siri: percentage of fat = $(4.95/D_b - 4.5) \times 100$, where D_b = body density.
(Reprinted with permission from Pollock, M.L., Schmidt, D.H., and Jackson, A.S.: Measurement of cardiorespiratory fitness and body composition in the clinical setting. Compr. Ther., 6:12–27, 1980.)

TABLE A–15C. PERCENTAGE OF BODY FAT ESTIMATION FOR MEN FROM AGE AND THE SUM OF CHEST, ABDOMINAL, AND THIGH SKINFOLDS*

SUM OF SKINFOLDS (mm)	AGE TO THE LAST YEAR								
	Under 22	23 to 27	28 to 32	33 to 37	38 to 42	43 to 47	48 to 52	53 to 57	Over 58
23–25	9.7	9.9	10.2	10.4	10.7	10.9	11.2	11.4	11.7
26–28	11.0	11.2	11.5	11.7	12.0	12.3	12.5	12.7	13.0
29–31	12.3	12.5	12.8	13.0	13.3	13.5	13.8	14.0	14.3
32–34	13.6	13.8	14.0	14.3	14.5	14.8	15.0	15.3	15.5
35–37	14.8	15.0	15.3	15.5	15.8	16.0	16.3	16.5	16.8
38–40	16.0	16.3	16.5	16.7	17.0	17.2	17.5	17.7	18.0
41–43	17.2	17.4	17.7	17.9	18.2	18.4	18.7	18.9	19.2
44–46	18.3	18.6	18.8	19.1	19.3	19.6	19.8	20.1	20.3
47–49	19.5	19.7	20.0	20.2	20.5	20.7	21.0	21.2	21.5
50–52	20.6	20.8	21.1	21.3	21.6	21.8	22.1	22.3	22.6
53–55	21.7	21.9	22.1	22.4	22.6	22.9	23.1	23.4	23.6
56–58	22.7	23.0	23.2	23.4	23.7	23.9	24.2	24.4	24.7
59–61	23.7	24.0	24.2	24.5	24.7	25.0	25.2	25.5	25.7
62–64	24.7	25.0	25.2	25.5	25.7	26.0	26.2	26.4	26.7
65–67	25.7	25.9	26.2	26.4	26.7	26.9	27.2	27.4	27.7
68–70	26.6	26.9	27.1	27.4	27.6	27.9	28.1	28.4	28.6
71–73	27.5	27.8	28.0	28.3	28.5	28.8	29.0	29.3	29.5
74–76	28.4	28.7	28.9	29.2	29.4	29.7	29.9	30.2	30.4
77–79	29.3	29.5	29.8	30.0	30.3	30.5	30.8	31.0	31.3
80–82	30.1	30.4	30.6	30.9	31.1	31.4	31.6	31.9	32.1

(Continued)

TABLE A-15C. (CONTINUED)

SUM OF SKINFOLDS (mm)	AGE TO THE LAST YEAR									
	Under 22	23 to 27	28 to 32	33 to 37	38 to 42	43 to 47	48 to 52	53 to 57	Over 58
83–85	30.9	31.2	31.4	31.7	31.9	32.2	32.4	32.7	32.9
86–88	31.7	32.0	32.2	32.5	32.7	32.9	33.2	33.4	33.7
89–91	32.5	32.7	33.0	33.2	33.5	33.7	33.9	34.2	34.4
92–94	33.2	33.4	33.7	33.9	34.2	34.4	34.7	34.9	35.2
95–97	33.9	34.1	34.4	34.6	34.9	35.1	35.4	35.6	35.9
98–100	34.6	34.8	35.1	35.3	35.5	35.8	36.0	36.3	36.5
101–103	35.3	35.4	35.7	35.9	36.2	36.4	36.7	36.9	37.2
104–106	35.8	36.1	36.3	36.6	36.8	37.1	37.3	37.5	37.8
107–109	36.4	36.7	36.9	37.1	37.4	37.6	37.9	38.1	38.4
110–112	37.0	37.2	37.5	37.7	38.0	38.2	38.5	38.7	38.9
113–115	37.5	37.8	38.0	38.2	38.5	38.7	39.0	39.2	39.5
116–118	38.0	38.3	38.5	38.8	39.0	39.3	39.5	39.7	40.0
119–121	38.5	38.7	39.0	39.2	39.5	39.7	40.0	40.2	40.5
122–124	39.0	39.2	39.4	39.7	39.9	40.2	40.4	40.7	40.9
125–127	39.4	39.6	39.9	40.1	40.4	40.6	40.9	41.1	41.4
128–130	39.8	40.0	40.3	40.5	40.8	41.0	41.3	41.5	41.8

*Percentage of fat calculated by the formula of Siri: percentage of fat = $(4.95/D_b - 4.5) \times 100$, where D_b = body density.
(Reprinted with permission from Pollock, M.L., Schmidt, D.H., and Jackson, A.S.: Measurement of cardiorespiratory fitness and body composition in the clinical setting. Compr. Ther., 6:12–27, 1980.)

TABLE A–16A. DIETARY RECOMMENDATIONS IN INDUSTRIALIZED AND DEVELOPING COUNTRIES, 1977 TO 1989*

Country/region or Source of Recommendation	Target Group(s)	Maintain Appropriate Body Weight, Exercise	Limit or Reduce Total Fat (% Energy)	Reduce Saturated Fatty Acids (% Energy)
Australia 1983	GP	Yes	Yes	NC
1987, targets for 1995	GP	Reduce obesity prevalence to 30%	35%	NS
1987, targets for 2000	GP	To 25%	33%	NS
Canada 1982	GP	Yes	35%	Yes
Czechoslovakia 1988	GP	Yes, reduce by 10–15%	Yes, reduce by 15 g/day	Yes
France 1981	GP	Yes	30–35%	Yes
Germany, Federal Republic of, 1985	GP	Yes	Yes	NS
Hungary 1988	GP	Yes	Avoid too much	Use vegetable oil
India 1988	HR (affluent people)	Yes	15–20%	NC
Ireland 1984	GP	Yes	≤35%	Yes
Japan 1985	GP	Yes	20–25%	Yes
Latin America 1988	GP	Yes	20–25%	≤8
Netherlands 1983–1984	GP	Yes	30–35%	Yes
1986	GP	Yes	30–35%	Yes

(Continued)

TABLE A–16A. (CONTINUED)

Country/region or Source of Recommendation	Target Group(s)	Maintain Appropriate Body Weight, Exercise	Limit or Reduce Total Fat (% Energy)	Reduce Saturated Fatty Acids (% Energy)
New Zealand 1982	GP HR	Yes	Yes	Yes
Norway 1981–1982	GP	NC	<35%	Yes
Poland 1988	GP	Yes	≈30%	Yes
Sweden 1981	GP	Yes	25–35%	Yes
1985	GP	Yes	Reduce by 5% energy by 1990; to ≈30% by 2000	NS
United Kingdom 1983	GP	Yes	30%	10
United States of America 1977	GP	Yes	27–33%	Yes
1979	GP	Yes	Yes	Yes
1985	GP	Yes	Yes	Yes
1988	GP HR	Yes	Yes	Yes
1989	GP	Balance energy intake and expenditure	≤30%	<10% for individuals, 7–8% population mean
WHO 1988				
Intermediate goals	GP	BMI	35%	15%
Ultimate goals		20–25	20–30%	10–15%

*BMI = Body-mass index; GP = General population; HR = High-risk groups; NC = No comment; NS = Not specified; P/S = Ratio of polyunsaturated to saturated fatty acids; RDA = Recommended dietary allowance.

(From Diet, Nutrition and the Prevention of Chronic Diseases. Report of a WHO Study Group. Technical Report Series No. 797. Geneva, WHO, 1990, pp. 180–181.)

TABLE A–16A. CONTINUED.

Increase Polyunsaturated Fatty Acids (% Energy)	Limit Cholesterol (mg/day)	Limit Free Sugars (% Energy)	Increase Complex Carbohydrates (% Energy for Total Carbohydrates)
NC	NC	Yes	Yes
NS	NS	<14%	Indirectly
NS	NS	<12%	Indirectly
Yes	No	Yes	Yes
No	NS	Yes	Yes, more plant foods, vegetables, cereals, legumes 50–55%
NS	NS	Yes	Yes; fresh fruits and vegetables, whole-grain cereals
NS	NS	Avoid excess	
NS	NS	Yes	Yes, fresh vegetables, salads, whole-grains
Balance $(n\text{-}3)/(n\text{-}6)$ ratio	NC	Yes	Yes; avoid refined and polished grains
NC	NC	Moderation; ≤7 g/day for weight reduction	Yes
Use vegetables and fish oils	NC	NC	NC
$P/S \approx 1.0$	<100 mg/1000 kcal$_{th}$ in children, up to 300 mg/day	Yes	Yes
Maximum 10%	Yes	Yes	NS
$P/S = 1.0$	<30 mg/MJ	Mono- and disaccharides 15–25%	45–55%

(Continued)

TABLE A–16A. (CONTINUED)

Increase Polyunsaturated Fatty Acids (% Energy)	Limit Cholesterol (mg/day)	Limit Free Sugars (% Energy)	Increase Complex Carbohydrates (% Energy for Total Carbohydrates)
NS	NS	Yes	Yes
P/S = 0.5	NS	<10%	Yes; 50–60%
NS	Yes, <300 mg	≤10%	Yes
P/S = 0.5	Yes	<10%	Yes; 50–60%
P/S = >0.5	NS	Decrease by 3% energy by 1990	Yes; increase starch to 45–50% energy by 2000
NS	No	To 20 kg/year	Through whole grains, vegetables, cereals, fruits
Yes	250–350	Yes	Yes
NS	Yes	Yes	Yes
No	Yes	Yes	Adequate starch and fiber
No	Yes	Yes	Yes
Up to 10 for individuals and ≈7 population mean	<300	Yes	≥55%; ≥5 servings/day vegetables and fruits; ≥6 daily servings cereals, breads, and legumes
P/S ≥0.5	<100 mg/ 1000 kcal$_{th}$	10%	>40%
P/S = 1.0			45–55%

TABLE A–16A. CONTINUED.

Increase Dietary Fiber (g/day)	Restrict Sodium Chloride (g/day)	Moderate Alcohol Intake (% energy)	Other Recommendations
Yes	Yes	Yes	Promote breast-feeding; variety
25	130 mmol/day	<5%	Promote water fluoridation, increase prevalence of breast-feeding
30	100 mmol/day	<5%	Exercise
Yes	Yes	Yes	Increase vitamin C intake; more plant foods; nutrition education; variety
Yes	Yes	<10%	Water fluoridation
Yes	Yes	Yes	Variety; small, frequent meals, proper cooking; sufficient protein
Yes	Yes	Yes	Variety; focus on cooking methods; consume milk and cheese as skimmed-milk products; 4 or 5 even meals daily; food labelling
Include grains, leafy vegetables, and whole grains	Yes	NC	Breast-feeding; water fluoridation upper limit 1 mg/L; different recommendation for general, poorer population
To 20–35	<9	<5%	Reduce protein to 1 g/kg of body weight daily; more vegetable protein
NC	<10	NC	Varied diet (at least 30 different foods daily); home cooking; pleasant eating environment
>8 g/1000 kcal$_{th}$	≤5; in profuse sweating, up to 10	NC	Protein 10–12% energy; variety; dietary interactions; vitamin C with iron-containing foods; calcium intake
NC	NC	Yes	Variety
3 g/MJ	Yes	<9 g/day	Variety

(Continued)

TABLE A–16A. (CONTINUED)

Increase Dietary Fiber (g/day)	Restrict Sodium Chloride (g/day)	Moderate Alcohol Intake (% energy)	Other Recommendations
Yes	Yes	Yes	Variety; less animal protein; water fluoridation
Yes	NC	NC	Maintain adequate nutrient intake
Yes	?	?	?
>30	≈7–8	Yes	Varied diet, exercise, regular meals
Increase by 7–8 g/day by 1990 and to 30–35 g by 2000	Reduce by 1–2 g/day by 1990 to 7–8 g by 2000	Yes	Year 1990 and year 2000 goals
To 30	Decrease by 3 g/day	<4%	Long-term proposals: food labeling; nutrition education; greater proportion of vegetable protein
Yes	<8	Yes	Limit additives and processed foods
NS	Yes	Yes	More fish, poultry, legumes; less red meat
Yes	Yes	Yes	Variety in diet; consider high-risk groups
Yes	Yes	Yes	Fluoridation of water; adolescent girls and women increase intake of calcium-rich foods; children, adolescents, and women of child-bearing age increase intake of iron-rich foods
Indirectly through vegetables, fruits, and cereals	≤6 with a goal of 4.5	<30 g of ethanol or <2 drinks/day	Population and individual goals; avoid dietary supplements in excess of RDAs; drink fluoridated water; limit protein intake to less than twice the RDA; comments on future goals
>30	7–8	Yes	Increase nutrient density of food; water fluoridation; iodine prophylaxis
	5		

TABLE A–16B. DIETARY RECOMMENDATIONS TO REDUCE CORONARY HEART DISEASE RISK IN INDUSTRIALIZED COUNTRIES*

COUNTRY/REGION OR SOURCE OF RECOMMENDATION	TARGET GROUP(S)	BODY WEIGHT/EXERCISE	TOTAL FAT (% ENERGY)
Australia 1979	HR	Avoid obesity	Reduce to 30–35
Canada 1977	GP	Maintain appropriate body weight	Reduce to 35
1988	GP HR	Adjust energy intake and expenditure	<30
Europe 1987	GP HR	Control obesity; increase exercise	≤30
Finland 1987	GP HR	Avoid excess weight; exercise	<30
Finland, Norway, Sweden 1968	GP	Reduce energy intake to avoid obesity; exercise	Reduce to 25–35
Germany, Federal Republic of 1975	GP	NC	Reduce
Japan 1983	GP	NC	20–25
Netherlands 1973	GP	Maintain appropriate body weight	33

(Continued)

TABLE A-16B. (CONTINUED)

COUNTRY/REGION OR SOURCE OF RECOMMENDATION	TARGET GROUP(S)	BODY WEIGHT/EXERCISE	TOTAL FAT (% ENERGY)
New Zealand			
1976	GP HR	Maintain appropriate body weight	35
United Kingdom			
1982	GP	Avoid obesity; increase exercise	30
1984	GP	Avoid obesity; exercise	Reduce to 35
United States of America			
1984	GP	Control obesity	<30
1985	GP HR	Maintain appropriate body weight	<30
1988	GP	Maintain appropriate body weight	<30
WHO			
1982	GP	Avoid obesity	Reduce to 20–30
1988	HR	BMI 20–25, regular exercise	20–30

*BMI = Body-mass index; GP = General population; HR = High-risk groups; NC = No comment; NS = Not specified; P:S = Ratio of polyunsaturated to saturated fatty acids.

(From Diet, Nutrition and the Prevention of Chronic Diseases. Report of a WHO Study Group. Technical Report Series No. 797. Geneva, WHO, 1990, pp. 182–183. With permission.)

TABLE A–16B. CONTINUED.

SATURATED FAT (% ENERGY)	POLYUNSATURATED FAT (% ENERGY)	CHOLESTEROL (MG/DAY)	COMPLEX CARBOHYDRATES AND FIBER
P:S = 1.0	P:S = 1.0	Restrict	Eat enough
10	10	NC	Increase
<10	<10	Restrict through less meats and egg yolks; for HR <300	Increase
<10	Increase oleic and linoleic acids	<300	Increase, especially vegetables, fruits, cereals, legumes
<10	P:S >0.5	Reduce	NC
Reduce	Increase	NC	Increase vegetables, fruits, potatoes
Reduce	Increase	Reduce	NC
NC	Cook with vegetable oil	NC	Increase

(Continued)

TABLE A–16B. (CONTINUED)

SATURATED FAT (% ENERGY)	POLYUNSATURATED FAT (% ENERGY)	CHOLESTEROL (MG/DAY)	COMPLEX CARBOHYDRATES AND FIBER
Restrict	10–13	250–300	Increase to make up energy need
Reduce especially for HR	HR should substitute for saturated fatty acids	Reduce	NC
<10	NC	NC	Increase
Reduce to 15	P/S≈0.45	NS	Increase breads, cereals, vegetables, fruits
8	<10	<250	Increase to make up energy loss
10	Up to 10	250–300	Endorsed earlier recommendations
<10	Up to 10	<300	Increase, ≥50% energy from total carbohydrates
<10	Up to 10	<300	Increase
10	Up to 10 P/S >1.0	<100 mg/1000 $kcal_{th}$	45–55% energy >30 g fiber/day

TABLE A–16B. CONTINUED.

FREE SUGARS	SODIUM CHLORIDE (G/DAY)	ALCOHOL INTAKE	OTHER RECOMMENDATIONS
Use less	Restrict	Moderation	Focus on HR groups; food labelling; recommendations safe for GP
NC	Restrict	NC	Variety of foods
NC	Limit	Limit	Focus on HR groups; limit protein to 10–15 % energy
Reduce	Moderation	Moderation, <25–30 g/day	Nutrition education; collaboration among government and other groups; food labelling
NC	Reduce; for HR <5	Moderation	Avoid trace element deficiencies; food labelling; focus on HR groups
Decrease	NC	NC	10–12% of energy from protein; 30–50% of animal origin
NC	NC	NC	NC
Reduce	Limit to <10	Avoid too much	Variety; eat enough protein, half from vegetables and half from animal sources; eat enough potassium, especially from green vegetables; eat lean meat and fish and fewer sweets

(Continued)

FREE SUGARS	SODIUM CHLORIDE (G/DAY)	ALCOHOL INTAKE	OTHER RECOMMENDATIONS
Use little	NC	NC	NC
Restrict to reduce weight	NC	Restrict to reduce weight	NC
NC	NC	NC	Special attention to children
Do not increase	Decrease	Avoid excess; <90 ml/day men; <65 ml/day women	Special recommendations for governments, professionals, industry
NC	5	NC	NC
NS	NC	NC	Guidelines for health professionals, industry, and public
NC	<3 (as sodium)	30–50 g ethanol/day	Protein to make up remainder of energy; wide variety of foods
NC	<5	Drink less	Emphasis on plant foods, fish, poultry, lean meats, low-fat dairy products, and fewer whole eggs
10% energy	<5	Limit	Increase nutrient density; water fluoridation 0.7–1.2 mg/L; iodine prophylaxis; intermediate and ultimate goals

TABLE A—16C. DIETARY RECOMMENDATIONS TO REDUCE CANCER RISK IN INDUSTRIALIZED COUNTRIES*

COUNTRY/ REGION	MAINTAIN APPROPRIATE BODY WEIGHT, EXERCISE	LIMIT OR REDUCE TOTAL FAT (% ENERGY)	MODIFY RATIO OF DIETARY FATS	PROMOTE FRUIT AND VEGETABLE INTAKE	INCREASE COMPLEX CARBOHYDRATE/ FIBER INTAKE
Canada 1985	Yes	Reduce	Decrease saturated fatty acids and cholesterol	Yes	More fiber- containing foods
Europe 1986	Yes	To ≈30	NC	Yes	Yes
Japan 1983	NC	Avoid excess	NC	Especially green/ yellow vegetables, oranges, carotene, and fungi	Unrefined cereal, seafood, fiber-rich legumes

(Continued)

TABLE A–16C. (CONTINUED)

COUNTRY/ REGION	MAINTAIN APPROPRIATE BODY WEIGHT, EXERCISE	LIMIT OR REDUCE TOTAL FAT (% ENERGY)	MODIFY RATIO OF DIETARY FATS	PROMOTE FRUIT AND VEGETABLE INTAKE	INCREASE COMPLEX CARBOHYDRATE/ FIBER INTAKE
United States of America					
1982	NC	To ≈30	NC	Especially citrus fruits, green and yellow and cruciferous vegetables	Whole-grain products, vegetables, and fruits
1984	Yes	To ≈30	NC	Especially vitamin A- and C-rich foods and cruciferous vegetables	High-fiber foods, whole-grain cereals
1987	Yes	To ≈30	NC	Vitamin A-rich, green and yellow vegetables, citrus fruits	Whole-grain products, 20–30 g fiber/day

*NC = No comment; NS = Not specified.
(From Diet, Nutrition and the Prevention of Chronic Diseases. Report of a WHO Study Group. Technical Report Series No. 797. Geneva, World Health Organization, 1990, pp. 184–185.)

TABLE A–16C. CONTINUED

RESTRICT SODIUM CHLORIDE	FOOD PREPARATION METHODS	ALCOHOL INTAKE	OTHER RECOMMENDATIONS
NS	Minimize cured, pickled, and smoked foods	Two or fewer drinks per day, if any	NC
To <5 g/day	As above; avoid frying and high-temperature cooking	Drink less, if at all	Varied diet; no food supplements; recommendations to government, scientists, and industry
Yes	Avoid hot drinks and burned foods	Drink less, if at all	Varied diet; chew food well
Minimize cured and pickled foods	Minimize cured, pickled, and smoked foods	Drink less, if at all	Avoid food supplements; monitor and test mutagens and carcinogens; recommendations to government, scientists, and industry
NS	As above	As above	NC
NS	As above, avoid frying and high-temperature cooking	As above	Balanced diet; read labels

TABLE A–16D. NATIONAL NUTRITION OBJECTIVES FOR THE YEAR 2000

A. *Health Status Objectives*

1. Reduce deaths from coronary heart disease to no more than 100 per 100,000 persons (age-adjusted baseline: 135 per 100,000 in 1987).

2. Reverse the rise in deaths from cancer to achieve a rate of no more than 130 per 100,000 persons (age-adjusted baseline: 133 per 100,000 in 1987).

3. Reduce the overweight population to no more than 20% among adults aged 20 years and older and no more than 15% among adolescents aged 12 through 19 years (baseline: 26% for adults aged 20 through 74 years in 1976 to 1980, 24% for men and 27% for women; 15% for adolescents aged 12 through 19 years in 1976 to 1980).

4. Reduce growth retardation among low-income children aged 5 years and younger to less than 10% (baseline: up to 16% among low-income children in 1988, depending on age and race/ethnicity).

B. *Risk Reduction Objectives*

5. Reduce dietary fat intake to an average of 30% of calories or less and reduce average saturated fat intake to less than 10% of calories among persons aged 2 years and older (baseline: 36% of calories from total fat and 13% from saturated fat for persons aged 20 through 74 years in 1976 to 1980; 36% and 13% for women aged 19 through 50 years in 1985).

6. Increase complex carbohydrates and fiber-containing foods in the diets of adults to 5 or more daily servings for vegetables (including legumes) and fruits, and to 6 or more daily servings for grain products (baseline: 2.5 servings of vegetables and fruits and 3 servings of grain products for women aged 19 through 50 years in 1985).

7. Increase to at least 50% the proportion of overweight persons aged 12 years and older who have adopted sound dietary practices combined with regular physical activity to attain an appropriate body weight (baseline: 30% of overweight women and 25% of overweight men for people aged 18 years and older in 1985).

8. Increase calcium intake so that at least 50% of youth aged 12 through 24 years and at least 50% of pregnant and lactating women are consuming 3 or more servings daily of foods rich in calcium, and at least 50% of adults aged 25 years and older are consuming 2 or more servings daily (baseline: 7% of women and 14% of men aged 19 through 24 years and 24% of pregnant and lactating women consumed 3 or more servings daily, and 15% of women and 23% of men aged 25 through 50 years consumed 2 or more servings daily in 1985 to 1986).

9. Decrease salt and sodium intake so that at least 65% of those who prepare home-cooked meals do so without adding salt, at least 80% of persons avoid using salt at the table, and at least 40% of adults regularly purchase foods modified or lower in sodium (baseline: 54% of women aged 19 through 50 years who prepared most of the meals did not use salt in food preparation, and 68% of women aged 19 through 50 years did not use salt at the table in 1985; 20% of all persons aged 18 years and older regularly purchased foods with reduced salt and sodium content in 1988).

10. Reduce iron deficiency to less than 3% among children aged 1 through 4 years and among women of childbearing age (baseline: 9% for children aged 1 through 2 years, 4% for children aged 3 through 4 years, and 5% for women aged 20 through 44 years in 1976 to 1980).

11. Increase to at least 75% the proportion of mothers who breast-feed their babies in the early postpartum period and to at least 50% the proportion who continue to breast-feed until their babies are 5 to 6 months old (baseline: 54% at discharge from birth site and 21% at 5 to 6 months in 1988).

12. Increase to at least 75% the proportion of parents and caregivers who use feeding practices that prevent baby-bottle tooth decay.

13. Increase to at least 85% the proportion of persons aged 18 years and older who use food labels to make nutritious food selections (baseline: 74% used labels to make food selections in 1988).

C. Service and Protection Objectives

14. Achieve useful and informative nutrition labeling for virtually all processed foods and for at least 40% of fresh meats, poultry, fish, fruits, vegetables, baked foods, and ready-to-eat carry-out foods (baseline: 60% of processed foods regulated by the Food and Drug Administration had nutrition labeling in 1988; baseline data on fresh and carry-out foods are unavailable).

15. Increase the available processed food products that are reduced in fat and saturated fat to at least 5000 brand items (baseline: 2500 brand items reduced in fat in 1986).

16. Increase to at least 90% the proportion of restaurants and institutional service operations than offer identifiable low-fat, low-calorie food choices, consistent with the nutrition principles in the Dietary Guidelines for Americans.

17. Increase to at least 90% the proportion of school lunch and breakfast services and child-care food services that offer menus consistent with the nutrition principles in the Dietary Guidelines for Americans.

18. Increase to at least 80% the receipt of home food services by people aged 65 years and older who cannot prepare their own meals or are otherwise in need of home-delivered meals.

19. Increase to at least 75% the proportion of schools in the United States that provide nutrition education from preschool through 12th grade, preferably as part of quality school health education.

20. Increase to at least 50% the proportion of worksites with 50 or more employees that offer nutrition education and/or weight management programs for employees (baseline: 17% offered nutrition education activities and 15% offered weight-control activities in 1985).

21. Increase to at least 75% the proportion of primary care providers who provide nutrition assessment and counseling and/or referral to qualified nutritionists or dietitians (baseline: physicians provided diet counseling for an estimated 40 to 50% of patients in 1988).

(From Nutrition in Healthy People 2000. In National Health Promotion and Disease Prevention Objectives. Washington, D.C., U.S. Government Printing Office, 1991.)

TABLE A—16E. RECOMMENDED DIET MODIFICATIONS TO LOWER BLOOD CHOLESTEROL

For Table A—16e, National Cholesterol Education Program (NCEP) Recommendations and Diets in the United States, see Table A—28, Recommendations for Phased Dietary Modification in the Prevention and Therapy of Hyperlipidemia (NCEP Step-One and Step-Two Diets).

BEVERAGE	CALORIES	SODIUM (mg)	SODIUM (mEq)	POTASSIUM (mg)	POTASSIUM (mEq)	PHOSPHORUS (mg)
Cola (avg.)	48.1–55.0[†]	0.8–4.7 (mg)[†]		0–4.4 (mg)[†]		18.1–25[†]
Diet cola (avg.)	0.1–0.5[†]	0.8–13.0 (mg)[†]		0–33.2 (mg)[†]		8.5–17.6[†]
Patio grape/orange	52	11.2	0.5	4.1	0.1	—
Mountain Dew	49	8.7	0.4	2.7	0.1	—
Teem	41	8.6	0.4	—	—	—
Root beer	45	1	0.1	3.9	0.1	0
Club soda	0	21.9	1.0	—	—	—
Sprite	48	15.4	0.7	0.4	—	—
Fanta (avg.)	53	6.4	0.3	0.6	—	—
Fresca	1	12.1	0.5	—	—	—
Fanta ginger ale	42	9.4	0.4	—	—	—
Slice	45	3	0.1	27.6	0.7	—
Apricot nectar	56	3	0.1	114	2.9	9
Apple juice	47	3	0.1	119	3	7
Cranberry juice	58	4	0.2	24	0.6	1
Grape juice, canned	61	3	0.1	132	3.4	11
Grapefruit juice, unsweetened	38	trace	—	153	3.9	11
Orange juice, unsweetened or fresh	45	1	0.1	200	5.1	17
Pear nectar	60	4	0.2	13	0.3	3
Peach nectar	54	7	0.3	40	1	6

(Continued)

BEVERAGE	CALORIES	SODIUM (mg)	SODIUM (mEq)	POTASSIUM (mg)	POTASSIUM (mEq)	PHOSPHORUS (mg)
Pineapple juice, unsweetened	56	trace	—	134	3.4	8
Tomato juice	20	200.7	8.7	227	5.8	16.5
Fruit-flavored beverage	45	—	—	—	—	—
Beer, regular	41	5.3	0.2	25	0.6	12.4
Beer, light	28	2.8	0.1	18.1	0.5	12.1
Gin, rum, vodka, whiskey (86 proof)	250	trace	—	3.6	0.1	—
Table wine, 12.2% alcohol/vol.	86	3.5	0.1	93.1	2.4	10.3
Dessert wine, 18.5% alcohol/vol.	137	3.3	0.1	76.7	2	—

Alcoholic beverages are customarily served in special glassware, the size of which tends to standardize the alcoholic content:

1 cordial glass	= 20 ml	1 burgundy glass	= 120 ml
1 brandy glass	= 30 ml	1 champagne glass	= 150 ml
1 jigger	= 45 ml	1 tumbler	= 240–360 ml
1 sherry glass	= 60 ml	1 mixing glass	= 360 ml
1 cocktail glass	= 90 ml		

*Brand name data supplied by the commercial producer of the product. Other data obtained from Composition of Foods, Fruits, and Fruit Juices: Raw, Processed, Prepared. Agriculture Handbook No. 8–9. Consumer Nutrition Center, Washington, U.S. Department of Agriculture, 1982.
†Range.

TABLE A—18A. DIETARY FIBER CONTENT OF SELECTED FOODS*,† (g/100 g EDIBLE PORTION)

FOOD ITEM	MOISTURE	TOTAL DIETARY FIBER (AOAC)‡
Breads, Crackers, and Cakes		
Bagels, plain	31.6	2.1
Biscuits, made from refrigerated		
dough, baked	28.7	1.5
Bread		
Bran	37.7	8.5
Cornbread mix, baked	34.4	2.4
Cracked-wheat	35.9	5.3
French	33.9	2.7
Hollywood-type, light	37.8	4.8
Italian	34.1	3.1
Mixed-grain	38.2	7.1
Oatmeal	36.7	3.9
Pita		
White	32.1	1.6
Whole-wheat	30.6	7.5
Pumpernickel	38.3	5.9
Reduced-calorie, high-fiber		
Wheat	43.7	11.3
White	41.8	9.3
Rye	37.0	6.2
Wheat	37.0	4.3
White	37.1	2.3
Whole-wheat	38.3	6.9
Bread crumbs, plain or		
seasoned	5.7	4.2
Bread stuffing, flavored, from		
dry mix	65.1	2.9
Cake mix		
Chocolate, prepared	33.3	2.2
Yellow, prepared	40.0	0.8
Cakes		
Boston cream pie	47.6	1.3
Coffeecake		
Crumb topping	22.3	3.3
Fruit	31.7	2.5
Fruitcake, commercial	22.0	3.5
Gingerbread, from dry mix	38.5	3.2
Cheesecake		
Commercial	44.6	2.1
From no-bake mix	44.4	1.9
Cookies		
Brownies	12.6	2.4
Brownies with nuts	12.6	2.6
Butter	4.7	2.4
Chocolate chip	4.0	2.7
Chocolate sandwich	2.2	3.0

(Continued)

FOOD ITEM	MOISTURE	TOTAL DIETARY FIBER (AOAC)‡
Fig bar	16.7	4.6
Fortune	8.0	1.6
Oatmeal	5.7	3.1
Oatmeal, soft-type	—	2.7
Peanut butter	6.7	1.8
Shortbread with pecans	3.3	1.8
Vanilla sandwich	2.1	1.5
Crackers		
Cheese, sandwich with peanut butter filling	4.0	1.1
Crisp bread, rye	6.1	16.2
Graham		
Regular	4.1	2.7
Honey	4.1	2.7
Matzoh		
Plain	6.1	3.0
Egg/onion	8.0	5.0
Whole-wheat	3.0	11.6
Melba toast		
Plain	5.6	6.5
Rye	6.7	8.0
Wheat	6.1	7.4
Rye	7.2	15.8
Saltines	—	2.7
Snack-type	4.2	2.0
Wheat	3.2	5.5
Whole-wheat	2.7	10.4
Croutons, plain or seasoned	5.6	5.0
Doughnuts		
Cake	19.7	1.7
Yeast-leavened, glazed	26.7	2.1
English muffin, whole-wheat	45.7	6.3
French toast, commercial, ready-to-eat	48.1	2.8
Ice cream cones		
Sugar, rolled-type	3.0	4.6
Wafer-type	5.3	4.1
Muffins, commercial		
Blueberry	37.3	3.6
Oat bran	35.0	7.5
Pancake, waffle mix, prepared	50.4	1.3
Pastry, Danish		
Fruit	27.6	1.9
Plain	19.3	1.2
Pies, commercial		
Apple	51.7	1.7
Cherry	46.2	0.8
Chocolate, cream	43.5	2.0
Egg custard	46.5	1.2
Fruit and coconut	—	0.9

FOOD ITEM	MOISTURE	TOTAL DIETARY FIBER (AOAC)‡
Lemon meringue	41.7	1.2
Pecan	19.8	3.5
Pumpkin	58.1	2.7
Rolls, dinner, egg	30.4	3.8
Taco shells	6.0	8.1
Toaster pastries	8.9	1.0
Tortillas		
Corn	43.6	5.2
Flour, wheat	26.2	3.1
Waffles, commercial, frozen,		
ready-to-eat	45.0	2.4
Breakfast Cereals, Ready-to-Eat		
Bran		
High-fiber	2.9	35.3
Extra fiber	—	45.9
Bran flakes	2.9	18.8
Bran flakes with raisins	8.3	13.4
Corn flakes		
Frosted or sugar-sparkled	1.9	2.2
Plain	2.8	2.0
Fiber cereal with fruit	—	14.8
Granola	3.3	10.5
Oat cereal	5.0	10.6
Oat flakes, fortified	3.1	3.0
Puffed wheat, sugar-coated	1.5	1.5
Rice, crispy	2.4	1.2
Wheat and malted barley		
Flakes	3.4	6.8
Nuggets	3.2	6.5
with raisins	—	6.0
Wheat flakes	4.3	9.0
Cereal Grains		
Barley	9.4	17.3
Bulgur, dry	8.0	18.3
Corn flour, whole-grain	10.9	13.4
Cornmeal		
Degermed	11.6	5.2
Whole-grain	10.3	11.0
Cornstarch	8.3	0.9
Farina, regular or instant,		
cooked	85.8	1.4
Hominy, canned	79.8	2.5
Millet, hulled, raw	—	8.5
Oat bran, raw	6.6	15.9
Oat flour	7.8	9.6
Oats, rolled or oatmeal, dry	8.8	10.3
Rice, brown, long-grain, cooked	73.1	1.7

(Continued)

FOOD ITEM	MOISTURE	TOTAL DIETARY FIBER (AOAC)‡
Rice, white		
glutinous, raw	10.0	2.8
Long-grain		
Parboiled, cooked	—	0.5
Precooked or instant,		
cooked	76.4	0.8
Rye flour, medium or light	9.4	14.6
Semolina	12.7	3.9
Tapioca, pearl, dry	12.0	1.1
Wheat bran, crude	9.9	42.4
Wheat flour		
White, all-purpose	11.8	2.7
Whole-grain	10.9	12.6
Wheat germ, toasted	2.9	12.9
Wild rice, raw	7.8	5.2
Fruits and Fruit Products		
Apples, raw:		
With skin	83.9	2.2
Without skin	84.5	1.9
Apple juice, unsweetened	87.9	0.1
Applesauce, unsweetened	88.4	1.5
Apricots, dried	31.1	7.8
Apricot nectar	84.9	0.6
Bananas, raw	74.3	1.6
Blueberries, raw	84.6	2.3
Cantaloupe, raw	89.8	0.8
Figs, dried	28.4	9.3
Fruit cocktail, canned in heavy		
syrup, drained	—	1.5
Grapefruit, raw	90.9	0.6
Grapes, Thompson, seedless,		
raw	81.3	0.7
Kiwifruit, raw	83.0	3.4
Nectarines, raw	86.3	1.6
Olives		
Green	—	2.6
ripe	—	3.0
Orange, raw	86.8	2.4
Orange juice, frozen		
concentrate, prepared	88.1	0.2
Peach		
Canned in juice, drained	—	1.0
Dried	31.8	8.2
Raw	87.7	1.6
Pears, raw	83.8	2.6
Pineapple		
Canned in heavy syrup,		
chunks, drained	79.0	1.1
Raw	86.5	1.2

FOOD ITEM	MOISTURE	TOTAL DIETARY FIBER (AOAC)‡
Prune		
Dried	32.4	7.2
Stewed	—	6.6
Prune juice	81.2	1.0
Raisins	15.4	5.3
Strawberries	91.6	2.6
Watermelon	91.5	0.4
Legumes, Nuts, and Seeds		
Almonds, oil-roasted	3.3	11.2
Baked beans, canned		
Barbecue-style	—	5.8
Sweet or tomato sauce, plain	72.6	7.7
Beans, Great Northern,		
canned, drained	69.9	5.4
Cashews, oil-roasted	5.4	6.0
Chickpeas, canned, drained	68.2	5.8
Coconut, raw	47.0	9.0
Cowpeas (black-eyed peas),		
cooked, drained	70.0	9.6
Hazelnuts, oil-roasted	1.2	6.4
Lima beans, cooked, drained	69.8	7.2
Miso	47.4	5.4
Mixed nuts, oil-roasted, with		
peanuts	—	9.0
Peanut		
Dry-roasted	1.6	8.0
Oil-roasted	2.0	8.8
Peanut butter		
Chunky	1.1	6.6
Smooth	1.4	6.0
Pecans, dried	4.8	6.5
Pistachio nuts	3.9	10.8
Sunflower seeds, oil-roasted	2.6	6.8
Tahini	3.0	9.3
Tofu	84.6	1.2
Walnuts, dried		
Black	4.4	5.0
English	3.6	4.8
Pasta		
Noodles, Chinese, chow mein	0.7	3.9
Noodles, egg, regular, cooked	68.7	2.2
Noodles, Japanese, dry		
Somen	9.2	4.3
Udon	8.7	5.4
Spaghetti and macaroni, cooked	64.7	1.6
Spaghetti, dry		
Spinach	8.7	10.6
Whole-wheat	7.1	11.8

(Continued)

FOOD ITEM	MOISTURE	TOTAL DIETARY FIBER (AOAC)‡
Snacks		
Banana chips	4.3	7.7
Corn cakes	4.6	1.9
Corn-based, extruded		
Chips		
Barbecue-flavor	1.2	5.2
Plain	1.0	4.4
Puffs or twists, cheese-flavor	1.5	1.0
CORNNUTS		
Barbecue-flavor	1.6	8.4
Nacho-flavor	2.1	8.0
Plain	1.3	6.9
Crisped rice bar		
Almond	6.7	3.6
Chocolate chip	7.0	2.2
Granola bars		
Hard		
Chocolate chip	2.4	4.4
Plain	3.9	5.3
Soft		
Milk-chocolate—coated, chocolate chip	3.6	3.4
Uncoated		
Chocolate chip	5.4	4.8
Chocolate chip, graham, and marshmallow	6.0	4.0
Nut and raisin	6.1	5.6
Peanut butter	7.3	4.3
Peanut butter and chocolate chip	5.9	4.2
Plain	6.4	4.6
Raisin	6.4	4.3
Popcorn		
Air-popped	4.1	15.1
Caramel-coated		
With peanuts	3.3	3.8
Without peanuts	2.8	5.2
Cheese-flavor	2.5	9.9
Oil-popped	2.8	10.0
Potato chips		
Barbecue-flavor	1.9	4.4
Plain	1.9	4.8
Sour-cream-and-onion—flavor	1.8	5.2
Potato chips, made from dried potatoes, plain	1.4	3.6
Potato sticks	2.2	3.4
Pretzels, hard, plain	3.3	2.8

TABLE A–18A. (CONTINUED)

FOOD ITEM	MOISTURE	TOTAL DIETARY FIBER (AOAC)‡
Rice cakes, brown rice		
Buckwheat	5.9	3.8
Corn	5.9	2.9
Multigrain	6.3	3.0
Plain	5.8	4.2
Rye	6.8	4.0
Tortilla chips		
Nacho-flavor	1.7	5.3
Plain	1.8	6.5
Sweets		
Baking chocolate, unsweetened, squares	1.3	15.4
Candies		
ALPINE WHITE Bar With Almonds	1.1	5.4
BABY RUTH Bar	5.0	2.9
BUTTERFINGER Bar	5.6	2.7
Caramels	8.5	1.2
CHUNKY Bar	2.9	4.8
Milk chocolate	1.3	2.8
Milk chocolate, with almonds	1.5	6.2
M&M's Plain Chocolate Candies	1.4	3.1
NESTLE CRUNCH Milk Chocolate With Crisp Rice	1.7	2.6
O'HENRY	5.9	3.5
Cocoa, dry powder, unsweetened	3.0	29.8
Jams and preserves	34.5	1.2
Jellies	28.4	0.6
Pie fillings, canned		
Apple	73.4	1.0
Cherry	69.7	0.6
Vegetables and Vegetable Products		
Artichokes, raw	84.4	5.2
Beans, snap		
Canned, drained, solids	93.3	1.3
Raw	90.3	1.8
Beets, canned, drained, solids	91.0	1.7
Broccoli		
Cooked	90.2	2.6
Raw	90.7	2.8
Brussel sprouts, boiled	87.3	4.3
Cabbage, Chinese		
Cooked	95.4	1.6
Raw	94.9	1.0
Cabbage, red		
Cooked	93.6	2.0
Raw	91.6	2.0

(Continued)

FOOD ITEM	MOISTURE	TOTAL DIETARY FIBER (AOAC)‡
Cabbage, white, raw	91.5	2.4
Carrots		
Canned, drained, solids	93.0	1.5
Raw	87.8	3.2
Cauliflower		
Cooked	92.5	2.2
Raw	92.3	2.4
Celery, raw	94.7	1.6
Chives	92.0	3.2
Corn, sweet		
Canned		
Brine pack, drained, solids	76.9	1.4
Cream-style	78.7	1.2
Cooked	69.6	3.7
Cucumbers		
Raw	96.0	1.0
Pared	—	0.5
Lettuce		
Butterhead or iceberg	95.7	1.0
Romaine	94.9	1.7
Mushrooms		
Boiled	91.1	2.2
Raw	91.8	1.3
Onions, raw	90.1	1.6
Parsley, raw	88.3	4.4
Peas, edible, podded		
Cooked	88.9	2.8
Raw	88.9	2.6
Peas, sweet, canned, drained, solids	81.7	3.4
Peppers, sweet, raw	92.8	1.6
Pickles		
Dill	93.8	1.2
Sweet	68.9	1.1
Potatoes		
Baked		
Flesh	75.4	1.5
Skin	47.3	4.0
Boiled	77.0	1.5
French-fried, home-prepared from frozen	52.9	4.2
Hashed brown	56.1	2.0
Spinach		
Boiled	91.2	2.2
Raw	91.6	2.6
Squash		
Summer, cooked	93.7	1.4
Winter, cooked	89.0	2.8

FOOD ITEM	MOISTURE	TOTAL DIETARY FIBER (AOAC)‡
Sweet potatoes		
Canned, drained, solids	72.5	1.8
Cooked	72.8	3.0
Tomato, raw	94.0	1.3
Tomato products		
Catsup	—	1.6
Paste	74.1	4.3
Puree	87.3	2.3
Sauce	89.1	1.5
Turnip greens		
Boiled	93.2	3.1
Raw	91.1	2.4
Turnips, boiled	93.6	2.0
Vegetables, mixed, frozen,		
cooked	83.2	3.8
Water chestnuts, canned,		
drained, solids	87.9	2.2
Watercress	95.1	2.3

*Modified from the Provisional Table on the Dietary Fiber Content of Selected Foods, HNIS/PT-106, 1988 and from updated Appendix Tables 8—19, Aug. 1991, and 8—20, Oct. 1989.

†Appreciation is expressed to the U.S. Department of Agriculture, Human Nutrition Information Service, Nutrition Monitoring Division for assistance in obtaining these data.

‡The total dietary fiber in foods is measured by the enzymatic-gravimetric method (the Association of Official Analytical Chemists (AOAC) official method of analysis). Duplicate samples of dried foods, with fat extracted if containing >10% fat, are gelatinized with Termamyl (heat-stable α-amylase) and then enzymatically digested with protease and amyloglucosidase to remove protein and starch. (When analyzing mixed diets, fat is always extracted prior to determining total dietary fiber.) Four volumes of ethyl alcohol (EtOH) are added to precipitated soluble dietary fiber. Total residue is filtered and then washed with 78% EtOH, 95% EtOH, and acetone. After drying, residue is weighed. One duplicate is analyzed for protein; the other is incinerated at 525° and ash is determined.

Total dietary fiber = weight residue − weight (protein + ash)

TABLE A—18B. NONSTARCH POLYSACCHARIDE CONTENT
OF SELECTED FOODS*

FOOD ITEM	TOTAL g/100g FRESH WEIGHT
Vegetables and Legumes	
Beans, baked, canned	3.5
Beans, French, cooked	3.1
Beans, red kidney, cooked	6.7
Cabbage, red, cooked	3.3
Carrots, raw	2.4
Lentils, red, cooked	1.9
Onion, cooked	1.8
Peas, garden, canned	4.0
Potato, boiled, fresh	1.1
Potato Crisps	4.9
Sprouts, Brussel, boiled	4.8
Fruits and Nuts	
Apple, Golden Delicious with skin	1.7
Apricots, fresh	2.3
Avocado, fresh	4.4
Canteloupe	0.6
Coconut, fresh	7.3
Figs, dried	7.5
Kiwi fruit, no skin	1.7
Peanuts, roasted	6.2
Raisins, dried	2.1
Cereal Products	
Bran flakes	11.3
Corn flakes	0.9
Oatmeal, coarse	7.0
Popcorn	9.8
Pumpernickel bread	7.5
Shredded wheat	9.8
Spaghetti, white, cooked	1.7
Spaghetti, whole-wheat, cooked	3.5
White bread	1.6
Wholemeal bread (average)	5.0

*Schwartz, SE, Levine RA, Singh A et al.: Gastroenterology 83:812-817, 1982 and Edwards CA: Physiological effects of fiber. In Dietary Fiber: Chemistry, Physiology and Health Effects. Edited by D. Kritchevsky, C. Bonfield and JW Anderson, New York, Plenum Press, 1990.
    Courtesy of Dr. Barbara Schneeman.

	FAT (g)	SFA (g)	MFA (g)	PFA (g)	M18:1 (g)	P18:2 (g)	P18:3 (g)	P:S	CHOL (mg)	S14:0 (g)	S16:0 (g)	S18:0 (g)	P20:5 (g)	P22:5 (g)	P22:6 (g)
Meats															
Liver, calf	6.90	2.56	1.49	1.09	1.28	0.61	0.08	0.43	561.00	0.00	1.40	1.16	0.00	0.00	0.00
Liver, pork	4.40	1.41	0.63	1.05	0.56	0.42	0.04	0.74	355.00	0.02	0.53	0.84	0.00	0.04	0.03
Kidney, beef	3.44	1.09	0.74	0.74	0.61	0.40	0.01	0.68	387.00	0.06	0.47	0.51	0.00	0.00	0.00
Kidney, pork	4.70	1.51	1.55	0.38	1.40	0.25	0.01	0.25	480.00	0.05	0.85	0.60	0.00	0.00	0.00
Brains, beef	12.53	2.92	2.50	1.44	2.00	0.03	0.00	0.49	2054.00	0.06	1.51	1.27	0.00	0.30	0.67
Brains, pork	9.51	2.15	1.72	1.47	1.10	0.09	0.12	0.68	2552.00	0.04	1.06	1.03	0.00	0.22	0.46
Beef, 5% fat, cooked	4.90	1.68	1.90	0.22	1.75	0.17	0.02	0.13	84.00	0.11	1.02	0.54	0.00	0.00	0.00
Beef, 26% fat, cooked	25.98	10.52	11.16	0.90	10.04	0.61	0.27	0.09	84.00	0.85	6.45	3.07	0.00	0.00	0.00
Lamb, 9% fat, cooked	9.17	3.28	4.02	0.60	3.72	0.49	0.05	0.18	92.00	0.29	1.76	1.13	0.00	0.00	0.00
Lamb, 36% fat, cooked	36.00	16.80	14.68	2.10	13.80	1.36	0.68	0.13	98.00	1.45	8.28	6.18	0.00	0.00	0.00
Veal, 6% fat, cooked	5.81	2.31	2.16	0.43	1.87	0.32	0.04	0.19	109.00	0.21	1.23	0.77	0.00	0.00	0.00
Veal, 25% fat, cooked	21.20	9.21	9.24	1.30	7.82	0.87	0.33	0.14	101.00	0.94	4.84	3.19	0.00	0.00	0.00
Chicken, light meat, unknown part, skin removed before cooking	3.87	1.15	1.05	0.92	0.88	0.66	0.02	0.80	77.00	0.03	0.67	0.32	0.00	0.03	0.03
Duck, domestic, skin removed before cooking	11.94	4.37	4.02	1.49	3.56	1.34	0.15	0.34	92.50	0.05	2.53	1.34	0.00	0.00	0.00
Ground beef, unknown % fat	22.56	8.86	9.88	0.84	8.63	0.62	0.09	0.09	89.00	0.64	5.10	2.66	0.00	0.00	0.00
Bologna, beef, regular	28.49	12.07	13.80	1.09	12.16	0.85	0.24	0.09	58.00	0.87	6.64	4.05	0.00	0.00	0.00
Pork, fresh, 25% fat, cooked	25.13	9.08	11.52	2.84	10.59	2.29	0.45	0.31	82.00	0.32	5.60	2.94	0.00	0.00	0.00
Frankfurter, all beef (Kosher), regular	28.54	12.05	13.62	1.38	11.99	1.11	0.27	0.11	61.00	0.94	6.52	3.96	0.00	0.00	0.00
Frankfurter, chicken	17.70	5.89	5.58	5.00	5.30	4.64	0.36	0.85	107.00	0.30	3.62	1.83	0.00	0.00	0.00
Frankfurter, regular, beef and pork	29.15	10.76	13.67	2.73	12.36	2.34	0.39	0.25	50.00	0.53	6.45	3.65	0.00	0.00	0.00
Pork, cured, 23% fat, cooked	23.48	8.38	11.03	2.51	10.15	2.15	0.36	0.30	67.00	0.25	5.12	2.93	0.00	0.00	0.00
Salami, pork	33.72	11.89	16.00	3.74	14.67	3.27	0.28	0.31	79.00	0.52	7.64	3.56	0.00	0.00	0.00
Bacon, regular cut	49.24	17.42	23.69	5.81	21.96	4.89	0.79	0.33	85.00	0.62	10.98	5.67	0.00	0.00	0.00
Fish															
Mussel, cooked from fresh or frozen	1.95	0.19	0.17	0.55	0.07	0.03	0.01	2.89	67.00	0.03	0.12	0.04	0.14	0.10	0.15
Fish, 0 to 2.9% fat	1.53	0.36	0.31	0.63	0.15	0.01	0.02	1.75	68.00	0.06	0.23	0.05	0.24	0.05	0.26
Fish, 3.0 to 6.9% fat	4.31	0.83	1.33	1.54	0.79	0.32	0.15	1.86	73.00	0.09	0.49	0.17	0.18	0.13	0.55
Fish, 7.0 to 10.9% fat	7.54	1.39	2.61	2.20	1.52	0.32	0.24	1.58	49.00	0.35	0.79	0.24	0.41	0.27	0.62
Fish, 11.0 to 14.9% fat	12.14	4.50	3.31	1.46	0.75	0.05	0.00	0.32	64.00	0.21	0.95	0.35	0.13	0.11	0.03
Herring, smoked/ kippered, canned and drained	12.37	2.79	5.11	2.92	2.07	0.18	0.14	1.05	82.00	0.76	1.85	0.15	0.97	0.07	1.18

(Continued)

	FAT (g)	SFA (g)	MFA (g)	PFA (g)	M18:1 (g)	P18:2 (g)	P18:3 (g)	P:S	CHOL (mg)	S14:0 (g)	S16:0 (g)	S18:0 (g)	P20:5 (g)	P22:5 (g)	P22:6 (g)
Salmon, canned, drained, with salt	6.05	1.53	1.81	2.05	1.07	0.06	0.06	1.34	55.00	0.05	1.35	0.13	0.84	0.05	0.81
Sardines, canned in oil, drained	11.45	1.53	3.87	5.15	2.14	3.54	0.50	3.37	142.00	0.19	0.99	0.34	0.47	0.00	0.51
Tuna, canned, oil pack, regular, drained	8.21	1.53	2.95	2.88	2.84	2.68	0.07	1.88	18.00	0.03	1.41	0.09	0.03	0.00	0.10
Tuna, canned, water pack, regular, drained, not rinsed	0.50	0.16	0.14	0.13	0.07	0.00	0.00	0.81	18.00	0.03	0.11	0.02	0.04	0.01	0.07
Clams, cooked from fresh or frozen	1.95	0.19	0.17	0.55	0.07	0.03	0.01	2.89	67.00	0.03	0.12	0.04	0.14	0.10	0.15
Crab, hardshell, Alaskan King	1.77	0.23	0.28	0.68	0.15	0.03	0.02	2.96	100.00	0.02	0.14	0.06	0.24	0.05	0.23
Lobster, cooked from fresh or frozen	0.59	0.11	0.16	0.09	0.09	0.00	0.00	0.82	72.00	0.01	0.08	0.02	0.05	0.00	0.03
Oyster, cooked from fresh or frozen, Pacific	4.95	1.26	0.50	1.48	0.19	0.10	0.07	1.17	109.00	0.22	0.87	0.12	0.42	0.10	0.46
Scallops	1.40	0.15	0.07	0.48	0.03	0.01	0.00	3.20	31.81	0.02	0.10	0.02	0.17	0.03	0.20
Shrimp, cooked from fresh or frozen	1.08	0.29	0.20	0.44	0.11	0.02	0.01	1.52	195.00	0.02	0.14	0.10	0.17	0.02	0.14
Caviar	17.90	4.21	5.86	5.66	2.94	0.99	0.55	1.34	588.00	0.90	1.87	0.72	1.03	0.81	1.35
Eggs Dairy															
Eggs, whole, cooked	10.02	3.10	3.81	1.36	3.47	1.15	0.03	0.44	425.00	0.03	2.23	0.78	0.00	0.00	0.04
Eggs, yolk only, cooked	30.87	9.55	11.74	4.20	10.70	3.54	0.10	0.44	1281.00	0.10	6.86	2.42	0.01	0.00	0.11
Eggs, white only, cooked	0.00	0.00	0.00	0.00	0.00	0.00	0.00	0.00	0.00	0.00	0.00	0.00	0.00	0.00	0.00
Cream, coffee creamer, liquid/frozen	9.97	9.30	0.11	0.00	0.11	0.00	0.00	0.00	0.00	1.00	0.43	0.60	0.00	0.00	0.00
Cream, coffee creamer, powder, regular	35.48	32.52	0.97	0.01	0.97	0.00	0.01	0.00	0.00	5.99	3.75	6.34	0.00	0.00	0.00
Cream, coffee creamer, liquid/frozen	11.28	1.68	4.85	4.25	4.79	3.94	0.29	2.53	0.00	0.01	1.10	0.56	0.00	0.00	0.00
Cream, half and half, 10 to 12% fat	11.50	7.16	3.32	0.43	2.89	0.26	0.17	0.06	36.90	1.16	3.02	1.39	0.00	0.00	0.00
Cream, light/coffee cream, 20% fat	19.31	12.02	5.58	0.72	4.86	0.44	0.28	0.06	66.10	1.94	5.08	2.34	0.00	0.00	0.00
Milk, buttermilk, 1% fat	0.88	0.55	0.25	0.03	0.22	0.02	0.01	0.05	3.50	0.09	0.23	0.11	0.01	0.00	0.00
Milk, skim	0.18	0.12	0.05	0.01	0.04	0.00	0.00	0.08	1.80	0.02	0.05	0.02	0.00	0.00	0.00
Milk, 1% fat	1.06	0.66	0.31	0.04	0.27	0.02	0.01	0.06	4.00	0.11	0.28	0.13	0.00	0.00	0.00
Milk, 2% fat	1.92	1.19	0.55	0.07	0.48	0.04	0.03	0.06	7.50	0.19	0.50	0.23	0.00	0.00	0.00
Milk, whole, 3.5 to 4% fat	3.34	2.08	0.96	0.12	0.84	0.07	0.05	0.06	13.60	0.34	0.88	0.40	0.00	0.00	0.00
Parmesan cheese, dry	30.02	19.07	8.73	0.66	7.74	0.32	0.34	0.03	78.70	3.38	8.10	2.67	0.00	0.00	0.00
American cheese, processed	31.25	19.69	8.95	0.99	7.51	0.61	0.38	0.05	94.40	3.21	9.10	3.80	0.00	0.00	0.00
Cottage cheese, lowfat, 2% fat	1.93	1.22	0.55	0.06	0.45	0.04	0.02	0.05	8.40	0.20	0.58	0.22	0.00	0.00	0.00
Cottage cheese, regular or creamed, 4% fat	4.51	2.85	1.28	0.14	1.06	0.10	0.04	0.05	14.90	0.47	1.36	0.51	0.00	0.00	0.00

Item															
Cream cheese, Neufchatel	23.43	14.80	6.77	0.65	5.66	0.45	0.20	0.04	76.10	2.35	6.88	2.98	0.00	0.00	0.00
Cheddar cheese, natural	33.14	21.09	9.39	0.94	7.90	0.58	0.36	0.04	104.90	3.33	9.80	4.01	0.00	0.00	0.00
Swiss cheese, natural	27.45	17.78	7.27	0.97	6.02	0.62	0.35	0.05	91.70	3.06	7.79	3.25	0.00	0.00	0.00
Monterey Jack cheese, natural	30.04	19.11	8.71	0.66	7.34	0.43	0.23	0.03	95.60	3.07	9.22	3.57	0.00	0.00	0.00
Mozzarella cheese, part skim milk	17.12	10.88	4.85	0.51	4.17	0.36	0.15	0.05	54.00	1.72	5.22	2.08	0.00	0.00	0.00
Brie cheese	24.26	15.26	7.02	0.72	5.75	0.45	0.27	0.05	72.00	2.69	7.23	2.52	0.00	0.00	0.00
Cheese, Kraft Light N' Lively Singles, American flavor	15.50	9.77	4.44	0.49	3.73	0.30	0.19	0.05	52.91	1.59	4.51	1.88	0.00	0.00	0.00
Cheese, Borden Lite-Line Singles, American flavor	8.20	4.99	2.34	0.26	1.94	0.19	0.07	0.05	45.00	0.82	2.47	0.88	0.00	0.00	0.00
Yogurt, frozen, fruit or vanilla, whole milk, 3 to 4% fat	3.24	2.10	0.90	0.09	0.75	0.06	0.03	0.04	9.74	0.33	0.87	0.30	0.00	0.00	0.00
Yogurt, frozen, fruit or vanilla, low fat, 1 to 2% fat	1.08	0.70	0.30	0.03	0.25	0.02	0.01	0.04	4.20	0.11	0.29	0.10	0.00	0.00	0.00
Yogurt, plain, lowfat, 1 to 2% fat	1.55	1.00	0.43	0.04	0.35	0.03	0.01	0.04	6.10	0.16	0.42	0.15	0.00	0.00	0.00
Yogurt, fruit, nonfat, <1% fat	0.20	0.12	0.05	0.01	0.00	0.00	0.00	0.08	2.00	0.00	0.00	0.00	0.00	0.00	0.00
Yogurt, fruit, whole milk, 3 to 4% fat	3.24	2.10	0.90	0.09	0.75	0.06	0.03	0.04	9.74	0.33	0.87	0.30	0.00	0.00	0.00
Ice cream and frozen desserts, regular, 10% fat, other flavors include chocolate chip	10.77	6.70	3.11	0.40	2.71	0.24	0.16	0.06	44.70	1.08	2.83	1.30	0.00	0.00	0.00
Sherbet, plain	1.98	1.23	0.57	0.07	0.50	0.04	0.03	0.06	7.30	0.20	0.52	0.24	0.00	0.00	0.00
Ice cream and frozen desserts, regular 5% fat, other flavors include chocolate chip	4.30	2.68	1.24	0.16	1.08	0.10	0.06	0.06	13.90	0.43	1.13	0.52	0.00	0.00	0.00
Fats/Oils															
Oils, canola	100.00	7.10	58.90	29.60	56.10	20.30	9.30	4.17	0.00	0.00	4.00	1.80	0.00	0.00	0.00
Oils, corn	100.00	12.70	24.20	58.70	24.20	58.00	0.00	4.62	0.00	0.00	10.90	1.80	0.00	0.00	0.00
Oils, sunflower	100.00	10.30	19.50	65.70	19.50	65.50	0.00	6.38	0.00	0.00	5.90	4.50	0.00	0.00	0.00
Oils, cottonseed	100.00	25.90	17.80	51.90	17.00	51.50	0.20	2.00	0.00	0.80	22.70	2.30	0.00	0.00	0.00
Oils, safflower	100.00	9.10	12.10	74.50	11.70	74.10	0.40	8.19	0.00	0.10	6.20	2.20	0.00	0.00	0.00
Oils, sesame	100.00	14.20	39.70	41.70	39.30	41.30	0.30	2.94	0.00	0.00	8.90	4.80	0.00	0.00	0.00
Oils, soybean (partially hydrogenated)	100.00	14.90	43.00	37.60	42.50	34.90	2.60	2.52	0.00	0.10	9.80	5.00	0.00	0.00	0.00
Oils, olive	100.00	13.50	73.70	8.40	72.50	7.90	0.60	0.62	0.00	0.10	11.00	2.20	0.00	0.00	0.00
Oils, peanut	100.00	16.90	46.20	32.00	44.80	32.00	0.00	1.89	0.00	0.10	9.50	2.20	0.00	0.00	0.00
Oils, coconut	100.00	86.50	5.80	1.80	5.80	1.80	0.00	0.02	0.00	16.80	8.20	2.80	0.00	0.00	0.00
Oils, palm	100.00	49.30	37.00	9.30	36.60	9.10	0.20	0.19	0.00	1.00	43.50	4.30	0.00	0.00	0.00

(Continued)

TABLE A–19A. (CONTINUED)

	FAT (g)	SFA (g)	MFA (g)	PFA (g)	M18:1 (g)	P18:2 (g)	P18:3 (g)	P:S	CHOL (mg)	S14:0 (g)	S16:0 (g)	S18:0 (g)	P20:5 (g)	P22:5 (g)	P22:6 (g)
Oils, palm kernel	100.00	81.40	11.40	1.60	11.40	1.60	0.00	0.02	0.00	16.40	8.10	2.80	0.00	0.00	0.00
Shortening, vegetable	100.00	25.00	44.50	26.10	44.50	24.50	1.60	1.04	0.00	0.40	14.10	10.60	0.00	0.00	0.00
Margarine, regular, stick, salted, corn oil	80.50	19.85	36.48	18.62	36.48	18.62	0.00	0.94	0.00	1.08	11.54	7.23	0.00	0.00	0.00
Lard	100.00	39.20	45.10	11.20	41.20	10.20	1.00	0.29	95.00	1.30	23.80	13.50	0.00	0.00	0.00
Butter, regular, salted	81.11	50.49	23.43	3.01	20.40	1.83	1.18	0.06	218.90	8.16	21.33	9.83	0.00	0.00	0.00
Oils, medium chain triglyceride	100.00	94.50	0.00	0.00	0.00	0.00	0.00	0.00	0.00	0.00	0.00	0.00	0.00	0.00	0.00
Mayonnaise/mayo-type dressing, real, regular, commercial	79.40	11.80	22.70	41.30	22.50	37.10	4.20	3.50	59.00	0.10	8.50	3.10	0.00	0.00	0.00
Oils, rapeseed	100.00	6.80	55.50	33.30	53.80	22.10	11.10	4.90	0.00	0.00	4.80	1.60	0.00	0.00	0.00
Miscellaneous															
Peanuts, peanut butter, with salt	49.98	9.59	23.58	14.36	22.96	14.10	0.08	1.50	0.00	0.05	5.50	2.14	0.00	0.00	0.00
Almonds, roasted, dry roasted, salted	56.53	5.27	36.71	11.86	36.03	11.36	0.40	2.25	0.00	0.32	3.74	1.11	0.00	0.00	0.00
Cashews, roasted, dry roasted, salted	48.21	9.70	28.41	8.15	27.89	7.97	0.17	0.84	0.00	0.36	4.53	3.09	0.00	0.00	0.00
Peanuts, roasted, dry roasted, salted	49.30	6.84	24.46	15.58	23.79	15.58	0.00	2.28	0.00	0.02	5.16	1.10	0.00	0.00	0.00
Walnuts	61.87	5.59	14.17	39.13	13.30	31.76	6.81	7.00	0.00	0.19	4.24	1.08	0.00	0.00	0.00
Olives, black	10.68	1.41	7.89	0.91	7.77	0.85	0.06	0.65	0.00	0.00	1.18	0.24	0.00	0.00	0.00
Candy, chocolate pieces, fudge, plain	10.78	4.93	4.53	0.93	4.48	0.86	0.06	0.19	3.92	0.10	2.29	2.35	0.00	0.00	0.00
Avocado, unknown type	15.32	2.44	9.61	1.95	8.96	1.84	0.11	0.80	0.00	0.00	2.40	0.03	0.00	0.00	0.00
Coconut, fresh	33.49	29.70	1.42	0.37	1.42	0.37	0.00	0.01	0.00	5.87	2.84	1.73	0.00	0.00	0.00
Soybeans, cooked from dried	8.97	1.30	1.98	5.06	1.96	4.46	0.60	3.89	0.00	0.02	0.95	0.32	0.00	0.00	0.00
Peas, black-eyed, cooked from dried	0.53	0.14	0.04	0.22	0.04	0.14	0.08	1.57	0.00	0.00	0.11	0.02	0.00	0.00	0.00
Split peas, yellow or green, cooked from dried	0.39	0.05	0.08	0.16	0.08	0.14	0.03	3.20	0.00	0.00	0.04	0.01	0.00	0.00	0.00

SFA = saturated fatty acid, MFA = monounsaturated fatty acid, PFA = polyunsaturated fatty acid, M18:1 = oleic acid, P18:2 = linoleic acid, P18:3 = linolenic acid, P:S = stearic acid, P20:5 = omega-3 (eicosapentaenoic acid), P22:5 = omega-3 (docosapentaenoic acid), P22:6 = omega-3 (docosahexaenoic acid). S14:0 = myristic acid, S16:0 = palmitic acid, S18:0 = stearic acid, CHOL = cholesterol. (With appreciation to the Nutrition Coding Center, University of Minnesota, Minneapolis, MN for the compilation and preparation of these tables. Data are based on Version 19 of the NCC Nutrient Data Base.)

TABLE A-19B. AVERAGE VALUES FOR TRIGLYCERIDES, FATTY ACIDS (FA), AND CHOLESTEROL OF MARINE FOODS AND OILS (INCLUDING OMEGA-3 FA)

FISH (100 g)	FAT (g)	CHOL (mg)	SFA (g)	MFA (g)	PFA (g)	M18:1 (g)	P18:2 (g)	P18:3 (g)	P20:5 (g)	P22:5 (g)	P22:6 (g)
Anchovy, European, raw	4.84	—	1.28	1.19	1.64	0.62	0.10	—	0.50	—	0.90
Bass, striped, raw	2.33	80.00	0.51	0.66	0.78	0.45	0.02	0.02	0.17	—	0.59
Bluefish, raw	4.24	58.82	0.92	1.79	1.06	0.68	0.06	trace	0.25	0.06	0.52
Burbot, raw	0.81	60.00	0.16	0.13	0.30	0.10	0.01	—	0.07	0.03	0.10
Carp, raw	5.60	65.88	1.08	2.33	1.44	1.15	0.52	0.27	0.24	0.08	0.11
Catfish, wild, raw	2.82	58.00	0.72	0.84	0.87	0.59	0.10	0.07	0.13	0.10	0.23
Catfish, farmed, raw	7.59	47.00	1.77	3.59	1.57	3.17	0.88	0.10	0.07	0.09	0.21
Cod, Atlantic, raw	0.67	43.53	0.13	0.09	0.23	0.06	0.01	trace	0.10	—	0.20
Eel, all varieties, raw	11.66	126.00	2.35	7.19	0.95	2.78	0.20	0.70	0.10	—	0.10
Flounder, unspecified, raw	1.00	46.00	0.20	0.30	0.30	—	—	trace	0.10	—	0.10
Haddock, raw	0.72	57.65	0.13	0.12	0.24	0.07	0.01	trace	0.10	—	0.10
Halibut, raw	2.29	31.77	0.33	0.65	0.84	0.36	0.03	0.07	0.07	0.09	0.29
Herring, Atlantic, raw	9.04	60.00	2.03	3.74	2.13	1.52	0.13	0.10	0.70	—	0.90
Mackerel, Atlantic, raw	13.87	70.07	3.26	4.06	4.76	2.28	0.22	0.16	0.90	0.21	1.40
Mussel, blue, raw	2.20	38.00	0.40	0.50	0.60	trace	—	—	0.20	1.03	0.37
Octopus, raw	1.01	—	0.30	0.10	0.30	—	—	—	0.10	—	0.10
Oyster, Eastern, wild, raw	2.46	53.00	0.77	0.31	0.97	0.12	0.06	0.05	0.27	0.06	0.29
Oyster, Eastern, farmed, raw	1.55	25.00	0.44	0.15	0.59	0.07	0.03	0.04	0.19	—	0.20
Perch, all varieties, raw	0.92	89.41	0.19	0.15	0.37	0.07	0.01	0.10	0.90	—	1.60
Pike, walleye, raw	1.21	85.88	0.25	0.29	0.45	0.20	0.03	0.01	0.09	0.04	0.23
Pollock, Atlantic, raw	0.98	71.06	0.14	0.11	0.48	0.07	0.01	—	0.07	0.02	0.35
Sablefish, raw	15.30	49.00	3.20	8.06	2.04	4.07	0.17	0.10	0.68	0.17	0.72
Salmon, Chinook, raw	10.45	65.88	2.51	4.48	2.08	2.80	0.11	0.09	0.79	0.23	0.57
Salmon, coho, wild, raw	5.93	45.00	1.26	2.13	1.99	1.20	0.21	0.16	0.43	0.23	0.66
Salmon, coho, farmed, raw	7.67	51.00	1.82	3.33	1.86	1.72	0.35	0.08	0.39	—	0.82

(Continued)

FISH (100 g)	FAT (g)	CHOL (mg)	SFA (g)	MFA (g)	PFA (g)	M18:1 (g)	P18:2 (g)	P18:3 (g)	P20:5 (g)	P22:5 (g)	P22:6 (g)
Sea bass, all, raw	2.00	41.18	0.51	0.42	0.74	0.29	0.02	trace	0.10	—	0.30
Smelt, rainbow, raw	2.58	75.00	0.48	0.68	0.94	0.43	0.05	0.10	0.30	—	0.40
Squid, short, finned, raw	1.50	0.40	0.42	0.09	0.52	—	—	trace	0.16	0.52	0.36
Red snapper, raw	1.34	37.06	0.29	0.25	0.46	0.17	0.02	trace	trace	—	0.20
Sole, European, raw	1.20	50.00	0.30	0.40	0.20	—	0.00	trace	trace	—	0.10
Sturgeon, all, raw	4.04	—	0.92	1.94	0.69	1.44	0.07	0.10	0.19	0.05	0.09
Swordfish, raw	4.01	38.82	1.10	1.54	0.92	1.09	0.03	—	0.10	0.00	0.10
Trout, rainbow, wild, raw	3.46	59.00	0.72	1.13	1.24	0.61	0.24	0.12	0.17	0.11	0.42
Trout, rainbow, farmed, raw	5.40	59.00	1.55	1.54	1.81	1.06	0.71	0.06	0.26	—	0.67
Tuna, bluefin, fresh, raw	4.91	37.65	1.26	1.37	1.67	0.92	0.05	—	0.40	—	1.20
Whitefish, all, raw	5.85	60.00	0.91	2.00	2.15	1.35	0.27	0.18	0.32	0.16	0.94
Cod liver oil	100.00	570.00	22.61	46.71	22.54	20.65	0.94	0.94	6.90	0.94	10.97
Herring oil	100.00	766.00	21.29	56.56	15.60	11.96	1.15	0.76	6.27	0.62	4.21
Menhaden oil	100.00	521.00	30.43	26.69	34.20	14.53	2.15	1.49	13.17	4.92	8.56
Max EPA conc fish body oil	100.00	600.00	25.40	28.30	41.10	—	—	0.00	17.80	—	11.60
Salmon oil	100.00	485.00	19.87	29.04	40.32	16.98	1.54	1.06	13.02	2.99	18.23

SFA = saturated fatty acid, MFA = monounsaturated fatty acid, PFA = polyunsaturated fatty acid, M18:1 = oleic acid, P18:2 = linoleic acid, P18:3 = linolenic acid, P20:5 = omega-3 (eicosapentaenoic acid), P22:5 = omega-3 (docosapentaenoic acid), P22:6 = omega-3 (docosahexaenoic acid).

(From Provisional Table on the Content of Omega-3 Fatty Acids and Other Fat Components in Selected Foods, U.S. Department of Agriculture, Human Nutrition Information Service, HNIS/PT-103, 1988. Other data obtained from Composition of Finfish and Shellfish Products, Agriculture Handbook No. 8-15, 1991 Supplement. Consumer Nutrition Center, Washington, U.S. Department of Agriculture, 1991.)

Trace is less than 0.05 g/100 g food.

— denotes Lack of reliable data for nutrient known to be present.

FOOD NAME	SERVING PORTION	Pro (g)	Na (mg)	K (mg)	Ca (mg)	PO$_4$ (mg)	Mg (mg)
Dairy Products							
Egg, whole, raw, large	1.0 Item	6.250	63.000	60.000	25.000	89.000	5.000
Cheese, cottage, uncreamed	1.0 Oz	4.888	3.715	9.189	8.994	29.523	1.173
Cream, coffee, table, light	1.0 Tbsp	0.405	5.937	18.250	14.437	12.000	1.312
Cream, sour, cultured	1.0 Tbsp	0.454	7.687	20.687	16.750	12.187	1.625
Milk, buttermilk, fluid	1.0 Cup	8.110	257.000	371.000	285.000	219.000	27.000
Milk, whole, 3.3% fat, fluid	1.0 Cup	8.030	120.000	370.000	291.000	228.000	33.000
Milk, nonfat/skim, fluid	1.0 Cup	8.350	126.000	406.000	302.000	247.000	28.000
Milk, whole, low sodium	1.0 Cup	7.560	6.000	617.000	246.000	209.000	12.000
Fats							
Butter, regular	1.0 Tbsp	0.119	116.000	3.640	3.360	3.220	0.280
Vegetable oil, corn	1.0 Tsp	0.000	0.000	0.000	0.000	0.000	0.000
Vegetable oil, olive	1.0 Tsp	0.000	0.002	0.000	0.008	0.055	0.000
Shortening, veg, soybn/cottnsd	1.0 Tsp	0.000	0.000	0.000	0.000	0.000	0.000
Margarine, reg, hard, unsalted	1.0 Tsp	0.000	0.100	1.160	0.820	0.630	0.070
Mayonnaise, soy, commercial	1.0 Tsp	0.067	26.133	1.667	0.667	1.333	0.047
Cereals							
Bran flakes, Kellogg's	0.5 Cup	2.455	152.000	124.000	9.550	96.000	35.500
Corn flakes, Kellogg's	0.5 Cup	0.920	116.000	10.450	0.341	7.150	1.360
Cream of rice, cooked	1.0 Cup	2.200	2.440	48.800	7.320	41.500	7.320
Cream of wheat, instant	1.0 Cup	4.400	6.000	48.000	59.000	43.000	14.000
Farina, cooked, enriched	1.0 Cup	3.260	0.000	30.300	4.660	28.000	4.660
Oatmeal, cooked	1.0 Cup	6.080	2.340	131.000	18.700	178.000	56.200
Wheat, puffed, plain	0.5 Cup	0.880	0.240	20.900	1.680	21.300	8.700
Wheat, shredded, biscuit	1.0 Item	2.600	0.472	77.000	9.680	86.000	40.100
Rice Krispies	0.5 Cup	0.965	170.000	14.750	1.990	17.200	5.100

(Continued)

TABLE A–20. (CONTINUED)

FOOD NAME	SERVING PORTION	Pro (g)	Na (mg)	K (mg)	Ca (mg)	PO₄ (mg)	Mg (mg)
Breads, Cookies, Crackers							
Bread, white, soft	1.0 Slice	2.070	129.000	28.000	31.500	27.000	5.250
Bread, whole-wheat, soft	1.0 Slice	2.690	178.000	49.300	20.200	72.800	26.000
Crackers, graham, plain	1.0 Item	0.500	33.000	27.500	3.000	10.500	3.570
Crackers, sodium free/whole wheat	1.0 Serving	1.000	1.000	35.000	—	—	—
Crackers, saltines	1.0 Item	0.250	36.800	3.250	0.500	2.500	0.770
Muffin, English, plain	0.5 Item	2.215	179.000	157.000	45.350	31.350	5.300
Bread, Italian, enriched	1.0 Slice	3.000	152.000	22.000	5.000	23.000	—
Roll, hard, enriched	0.5 Item	2.500	156.000	24.500	12.000	23.000	5.750
Roll, hamburger/hotdog	1.0 Item	3.430	241.000	36.800	53.600	32.800	7.600
Cookies, vanilla wafer	5.0 Items	1.000	50.000	14.500	8.000	12.500	3.400
Meat, Fish							
Pot roast, arm, beef, cooked	1.0 Oz	9.355	18.711	81.931	2.551	75.978	6.804
Hamburger patty, beef/lean	1.0 Oz	7.004	21.679	85.384	3.002	44.693	6.004
Steak, sirloin, lean, broiled	1.0 Oz	8.606	18.731	114.000	3.119	69.356	9.062
Chicken, leg, no skin, roasted	1.0 Oz	7.669	25.963	68.637	3.402	51.925	6.864
Chicken, breast, roasted	1.0 Oz	8.447	19.961	69.429	4.050	60.750	7.811
Lamb, all cuts, lean/fat, cooked	1.0 Oz	6.971	20.345	87.718	4.669	53.365	6.671
Turkey, dark meat, no skin	1.0 Oz	8.100	22.275	82.215	9.113	57.915	6.885
Turkey, light, no skin, roasted	1.0 Oz	8.485	18.023	86.265	5.468	62.168	7.898
Veal, all cuts, lean, cooked	1.0 Oz	9.039	25.348	96.056	6.671	71.042	8.005
Bluefish	1.0 Oz	5.689	17.010	105.000	1.890	64.449	9.450
Flatfish, raw	1.0 Oz	5.336	23.014	102.000	5.003	52.031	9.005
Cod, cooked, dry heat	1.0 Oz	6.473	22.050	69.143	3.969	39.060	11.970
Halibut, broiled, dry	1.0 Oz	7.571	19.578	163.000	17.010	80.714	30.351
Shrimp, raw, mixed species	1.0 Oz	5.751	42.525	52.650	15.188	58.725	10.125
Tuna, can/oil, drained	1.0 Oz	8.272	100.000	58.701	3.702	88.052	8.805
Tuna, diet, low sodium	1.0 Oz	7.656	11.380	73.670	1.418	62.390	9.074

	Serving						
Sweets							
Honey, strained/extracted	1.0 Tbsp	0.000	1.000	11.000	1.000	1.000	0.630
Ice milk, van, hard, 4.3% fat	0.5 Cup	2.580	52.500	133.000	88.000	64.500	9.500
Ice cream, van, hard, 10% fat	0.5 Cup	2.400	58.000	129.000	88.000	67.000	9.000
Ice cream, van, hard, 16% fat	0.5 Cup	2.065	54.000	111.000	75.500	57.500	8.000
Jams/preserves, regular	1.0 Tbsp	0.000	2.000	18.000	4.000	2.000	—
Sherbet, orange, 2% fat	0.5 Cup	1.080	44.000	99.000	51.500	37.000	7.500
Sugar, brown, pressed down	0.5 Cup	0.000	33.000	379.000	93.500	21.000	—
Sugar, white, granulated	1.0 Tbsp	0.000	0.120	0.000	0.000	0.000	—
Juices							
Apple juice, can and bottle	3.5 Fl ozs	0.066	3.062	129.000	7.612	7.875	3.500
Apricot nectar, can	3.5 Fl ozs	0.402	3.937	125.000	7.700	9.887	5.687
Cranberry juice, bottle	3.5 Fl ozs	0.000	4.375	19.906	3.321	2.214	2.214
Grape juice, can	3.5 Fl ozs	0.000	0.000	38.500	3.500	3.500	—
Grapefruit juice, can, unsweetened	3.5 Fl ozs	0.560	1.081	165.000	7.569	11.900	10.806
Lemon juice, can and bottle	3.5 Fl ozs	0.427	22.400	109.000	11.725	9.625	8.531
Orange juice, can	3.5 Fl ozs	0.643	2.179	191.000	8.706	15.268	11.987
Pear nectar, can	3.5 Fl ozs	0.120	4.375	14.219	5.469	3.281	3.281
Pineapple juice, can	3.5 Fl ozs	0.350	1.094	147.000	18.593	8.750	14.219
Prune juice, can and bottle	3.5 Fl ozs	0.682	4.462	309.000	13.431	28.000	15.662
Tomato juice, can	3.5 Fl ozs	0.809	385.000	235.000	9.625	20.300	11.725
Tomato juice, low sodium	3.5 Fl ozs	0.809	10.675	235.000	9.625	20.300	11.725
Vegetables							
Asparagus, can, spears	0.5 Cup	2.590	472.000	208.000	19.350	52.000	12.100
Asparagus, can, low sodium	0.5 Cup	2.195	425.000	187.000	17.100	46.350	11.000
Beans, snap, green, can, cuts	0.5 Cup	0.775	170.000	73.500	17.550	12.850	8.800
Beans, green, can, low sodium	0.5 Cup	0.780	1.360	74.000	16.000	13.000	9.000
Beans, snap, wax, raw, boiled	0.5 Cup	1.180	1.875	187.000	28.750	24.000	15.650
Beets, can, whole	0.5 Cup	1.025	324.000	175.000	17.200	19.700	19.700
Beets, can, diet, low sodium	0.5 Cup	1.025	324.000	175.000	17.200	19.700	19.700
Broccoli, raw, boiled, drained	0.5 Cup	2.310	20.150	227.000	35.650	45.750	18.600
Cabbage, common, boiled, drained	0.5 Cup	0.695	13.800	149.000	23.950	18.150	10.900

(Continued)

TABLE A-20. CONTINUED

FOOD NAME	SERVING PORTION	Pro (g)	Na (mg)	K (mg)	Ca (mg)	PO$_4$ (mg)	Mg (mg)
Carrots, can, sliced, drained	0.5 Cup	0.467	176.000	131.000	18.250	17.500	5.850
Carrots, can, low sodium	0.5 Cup	0.750	47.950	213.000	30.750	24.600	11.050
Carrot, raw, whole, scraped	1.0 Item	0.740	25.200	233.000	19.400	31.700	10.800
Cauliflower, raw, boiled, drained	0.5 Cup	1.160	4.000	200.000	17.000	22.000	7.000
Celery, Pascal, raw, stalk	1.0 Item	0.300	34.800	115.000	16.000	10.000	4.400
Corn, sweet, can, drained	0.5 Cup	2.160	267.000	161.000	4.125	53.500	16.500
Corn, sweet, can, low sodium	0.5 Cup	2.480	3.840	196.000	5.100	65.500	20.500
Cucumber, raw, sliced	0.5 Cup	0.281	1.040	77.500	7.300	8.850	5.700
Peas, green, can, drained	0.5 Cup	3.755	186.000	147.000	17.000	57.000	14.450
Peas, green, can, low sodium	0.5 Cup	3.755	1.700	147.000	17.000	57.000	14.450
Tomato, raw, red, ripe	1.0 Item	1.050	11.100	273.000	6.150	29.500	13.500
Tomato, red, can, stewed	0.5 Cup	1.185	324.000	305.000	42.100	25.500	15.300
Tomato, can, low sodium, diet	0.5 Cup	1.115	15.600	265.000	31.200	22.800	14.400
Potato, boiled, peeled before cooked	1.0 Item	2.310	6.750	443.000	10.800	54.000	27.000
Noodles, egg, enriched, cooked	0.5 Cup	3.500	1.500	35.000	8.000	47.000	21.600
Rice, white, parboiled, cooked	0.5 Cup	2.005	2.625	32.400	16.650	36.750	10.500

Fruits

	Pro	Na	K	Ca	PO₄	Mg
Apples, raw, unpeeled	1.0 Item	0.262	1.000	159.000	10.000	10.000	6.000
Apples, raw, peeled	1.0 Item	0.190	0.000	144.000	5.000	9.000	4.000
Applesauce, can, unsweetened	0.5 Cup	0.208	2.440	91.500	3.660	8.550	3.660
Apricots, can, light syrup	0.5 Cup	0.675	5.000	175.000	13.900	17.000	10.500
Bananas, raw, peeled	1.0 Item	1.170	1.140	451.000	6.840	22.000	33.000
Blueberries, raw	0.5 Cup	0.486	4.350	64.500	4.350	7.250	3.625
Cherries, sweet, can/juice	0.5 Cup	1.140	3.750	164.000	17.500	27.500	15.000
Grapefruit, red/pnk/wht, raw	0.5 Cup	0.725	0.500	161.000	13.500	10.000	9.500
Oranges, raw, all varieties	1.0 Item	1.230	0.000	237.000	52.400	18.300	13.100
Peaches, raw, whole	1.0 Item	0.609	0.000	171.000	4.350	10.400	6.090
Peaches, can, light syrup	0.5 Cup	0.565	6.500	122.000	4.500	13.500	6.000
Pears, raw, bartlett, unpeeled	1.0 Item	0.647	0.000	208.000	18.300	18.300	9.960
Pineapple, can/juice	0.5 Cup	0.525	2.000	153.000	17.500	7.500	17.500
Strawberries, raw, whole	0.5 Cup	0.455	0.745	124.000	10.450	14.150	7.450

Pro = protein, Na = sodium, K = potassium, Ca = calcium, PO₄ = phosphorus, Mg = magnesium.

(Created on Nutritionist III, Version 7, N-Squared Computing, 1991. Data compiled from U.S. Department of Agriculture Handbook 8- Series, manufacturers' data, published journals, and industry sources. Appreciation expressed to Ms. Lori Cohen, M.S., R.D., for her assistance in preparing this table.)

TABLE A–21A. VITAMIN A, VITAMIN E, α-TOCOPHEROL (TOC), VITAMIN C, THIAMIN, RIBOFLAVIN, NIACIN, VITAMIN B_6, VITAMIN B_{12}, AND FOLATE CONTENT OF SELECTED COMMON FOODS PER SERVING PORTION

FOOD NAME	SERVING PORTION	A* (RE)	E† (mg)	α-TOC (mg)	C (mg)	THIAMIN (mg)	RIBO (mg)	NIACIN (mg)	B_6 (mg)	B_{12} (µg)	FOLATE (µg)
Dairy Products											
Egg, whole, raw, large	1.0 Item	95.200	0.700	0.350	0.000	0.031	0.254	0.037	0.070	0.500	23.000
Cheese, cottage, uncreamed	1.0 Oz	2.581	—	0.181	0.000	0.007	0.040	0.044	0.023	0.235	4.106
Cream, coffee, table, light	1.0 Tbsp	32.437	0.094	—	0.114	0.005	0.022	0.009	0.005	0.033	0.375
Cream, sour, cultured	1.0 Tbsp	34.124	—	—	0.124	0.005	0.021	0.010	0.002	0.043	1.562
Milk, buttermilk, fluid	1.0 Cup	24.300	0.980	—	2.400	0.083	0.377	0.142	0.083	0.537	12.300
Milk, whole, 3.3% fat, fluid	1.0 Cup	92.200	0.220	0.146	2.290	0.093	0.395	0.205	0.102	0.871	12.000
Milk, nonfat/skim, fluid	1.0 Cup	150.000	0.221	0.147	2.400	0.088	0.343	0.216	0.098	0.926	13.000
Milk, whole, low sodium	1.0 Cup	95.200	0.220	0.146	2.290	0.049	0.256	0.105	0.083	0.876	12.200
Fats											
Butter, regular	1.0 Tbsp	105.000	0.221	0.221	0.000	0.001	0.005	0.006	0.000	0.018	0.420
Vegetable oil, corn	1.0 Tsp	0.000	3.771	0.650	0.000	0.000	0.000	0.000	0.000	0.000	0.000
Vegetable oil, olive	1.0 Tsp	0.000	0.569	0.535	0.000	0.000	0.000	0.000	0.000	0.000	0.000
Shortening, veg, soybn/cottnsd	1.0 Tsp	0.000	2.771	0.342	0.000	0.000	0.000	0.000	0.000	0.000	0.000
Margarine, reg, hard, unsalted	1.0 Tsp	47.000	2.710	0.423	0.004	0.000	0.001	0.000	0.000	0.003	0.030
Mayonnaise, soy, commercial	1.0 Tsp	3.900	2.667	0.967	0.000	0.000	0.000	0.000	0.027	0.012	0.360
Cereals											
Bran flakes, Kellogg's	0.5 Cup	258.000	0.412	0.082	0.000	0.254	0.293	3.430	0.351	1.050	69.000
Corn flakes, Kellogg's	0.5 Cup	150.000	—	0.012	6.000	0.148	0.171	2.000	0.205	0.000	40.050
Cream of rice, cooked	1.0 Cup	0.000	—	—	0.000	0.000	0.000	0.976	0.066	0.000	7.320

Food	Amount										
Cream of wheat, instant	1.0 Cup	0.000	—	—	0.000	0.200	0.100	1.800	0.029	0.000	11.000
Farina, cooked, enriched	1.0 Cup	—	2.190	—	0.000	0.186	0.117	1.280	0.023	0.000	4.660
Oatmeal, cooked	1.0 Cup	4.680	5.400	3.530	0.000	0.257	0.047	0.304	0.047	0.000	9.360
Wheat, puffed, plain	0.5 Cup	0.000	—	0.040	0.000	0.012	0.014	0.650	0.010	0.000	1.920
Wheat, shredded, biscuit	1.0 Item	0.000	0.508	0.085	0.000	0.070	0.060	1.080	0.060	0.000	12.000
Rice Krispies	0.5 Cup	188.000	0.040	0.006	7.550	0.185	0.213	2.500	0.256	0.000	50.000
Breads, Cookies, Crackers											
Bread, white, soft	1.0 Slice	0.000	0.298	0.030	0.000	0.118	0.078	0.938	0.009	0.000	8.750
Bread, whole-wheat, soft	1.0 Slice	0.000	0.252	0.028	0.000	0.098	0.059	1.070	0.052	0.000	15.400
Crackers, graham, plain	1.0 Item	0.000	0.128	0.026	0.000	0.010	0.040	0.250	0.006	0.000	0.910
Crackers, sodium free/whole-wheat	1.0 Serving	—	—	—	—	—	—	—	—	—	—
Crackers, saltines	1.0 Item	0.000	0.050	0.010	0.000	0.125	0.013	0.100	0.001	0.000	0.495
Muffin, English, plain	0.5 Item	0.000	—	—	0.000	0.129	0.090	1.050	0.011	0.000	8.950
Bread, Italian, enriched	1.0 Slice	0.000	0.357	0.036	0.000	0.120	0.070	1.000	0.016	0.000	10.500
Roll, hard, enriched	0.5 Item	0.000	0.133	0.010	0.000	0.100	0.060	0.850	0.009	0.000	14.750
Roll, hamburger/hotdog	1.0 Item	0.000	0.212	0.016	0.000	0.196	0.132	1.580	0.014	—	14.800
Cookies, vanilla wafer	5.0 Items	5.000	1.090	0.515	0.000	0.050	0.045	0.400	—	—	—
Meat, Fish											
Pot roast, arm, beef, cooked	1.0 Oz	0.000	—	0.040	0.000	0.023	0.082	1.055	0.094	0.964	3.118
Hamburger patty, beef, lean	1.0 Oz	3.005	0.172	0.101	0.000	0.014	0.060	1.464	0.073	0.667	2.668
Steak, sirloin, lean, broiled	1.0 Oz	1.519	0.156	0.037	0.000	0.036	0.084	1.215	0.128	0.810	2.835
Chicken, leg, no skin, roasted	1.0 Oz	5.372	0.156	0.099	0.000	0.021	0.066	1.791	0.104	0.093	2.387

(Continued)

TABLE A–21A. CONTINUED

FOOD NAME	SERVING PORTION	A* (RE)	E† (mg)	α-TOC (mg)	C (mg)	THIAMIN (mg)	RIBO (mg)	NIACIN (mg)	B_6 (mg)	B_{12} (µg)	FOLATE (µg)
Meat, Fish											
Chicken, breast, roasted	1.0 Oz	7.912	0.156	0.099	0.000	0.019	0.034	3.602	0.156	0.093	0.868
Lamb, all cuts, lean/ fat, cooked	1.0 Oz	—	—	—	—	0.027	0.073	1.888	0.037	0.724	5.003
Turkey, dark meat, no skin	1.0 Oz	0.000	0.181	0.000	0.000	0.018	0.070	1.035	0.101	0.105	2.552
Turkey, light, no skin, roasted	1.0 Oz	0.000	0.026	0.000	0.000	0.017	0.037	1.938	0.152	0.105	1.620
Veal, all cuts, lean, cooked	1.0 Oz	—	—	—	—	0.017	0.097	2.388	0.093	0.470	4.336
Bluefish	1.0 Oz	33.831	—	0.016	—	0.016	0.023	1.688	0.114	1.529	0.454
Flatfish, raw	1.0 Oz	2.668	—	—	—	0.025	0.022	0.820	0.059	0.430	—
Cod, cooked, dry heat	1.0 Oz	3.969	—	0.283	—	0.025	0.022	0.712	0.080	0.298	2.300
Halibut, broiled, dry	1.0 Oz	15.309	—	0.000	—	0.020	0.026	2.021	0.112	0.387	3.902
Shrimp, raw, mixed species	1.0 Oz	—	—	—	—	0.008	0.012	0.725	0.028	0.328	0.810
Tuna, can/oil, drained	1.0 Oz	6.537	—	0.474	0.000	0.011	0.034	3.502	0.031	0.624	1.504
Tuna, diet, low sodium	1.0 Oz	6.898	0.799	—	—	0.009	0.014	3.514	0.105	0.397	0.000
Sweets											
Honey, strained/ extracted	1.0 Tbsp	0.000	—	—	0.000	0.000	0.010	0.100	0.004	0.000	—
Ice milk, van, hard, 4.3% fat	0.5 Cup	26.000	0.230	0.040	0.380	0.038	0.174	0.059	0.043	0.438	1.500
Ice cream, van, hard, 10% fat	0.5 Cup	66.500	0.233	0.040	0.350	0.026	0.165	0.067	0.031	0.313	1.500
Ice cream, van, hard, 16% fat	0.5 Cup	104.000	0.259	0.045	0.305	0.022	0.142	0.058	0.027	0.269	1.000

Food	Measure										
Jams/preserves, regular	1.0 Tbsp	0.000	—	0.018	0.000	0.000	0.010	0.000	0.004	0.000	1.600
Sherbet, orange, 2% fat	0.5 Cup	19.500	—	—	1.930	0.016	0.045	0.066	0.013	0.079	7.000
Sugar, brown, pressed down	0.5 Cup	0.000	—	—	0.000	0.010	0.035	0.200	—	—	—
Sugar, white, granulated	1.0 Tbsp	0.000	—	—	0.000	0.000	0.000	0.000	—	—	—
Juices											
Apple juice, can and bottle	3.5 Fl ozs	0.087	—	0.011	1.006	0.023	0.018	0.108	0.032	0.000	0.108
Apricot nectar, can	3.5 Fl ozs	144.000	—	—	0.661	0.010	0.015	0.286	—	0.000	1.426
Cranberry juice, bottle	3.5 Fl ozs	0.000	—	—	39.199	0.010	0.010	0.039	0.021	0.000	0.221
Grape juice, can	3.5 Fl ozs	0.000	—	—	17.500	0.010	0.010	0.109	0.021	0.000	1.050
Grapefruit juice, can, unsweetened	3.5 Fl ozs	0.787	0.195	0.043	31.543	0.045	0.021	0.250	0.021	0.000	11.244
Lemon juice, can and bottle	3.5 Fl ozs	1.619	—	—	26.468	0.044	0.010	0.210	0.046	0.000	10.762
Orange juice, can	3.5 Fl ozs	19.118	0.218	0.044	37.493	0.065	0.031	0.342	0.096	0.000	19.731
Pear nectar, can	3.5 Fl ozs	0.044	—	—	1.203	0.002	0.014	0.140	0.015	0.000	1.312
Pineapple juice, can	3.5 Fl ozs	0.525	—	—	11.725	0.060	0.024	0.281	0.105	0.000	25.287
Prune juice, can and bottle	3.5 Fl ozs	0.394	—	—	4.594	0.018	0.078	0.879	0.244	0.000	0.446
Tomato juice, can	3.5 Fl ozs	59.936	0.757	0.234	19.556	0.050	0.033	0.717	0.119	0.000	21.262
Tomato juice, low sodium	3.5 Fl ozs	59.936	0.757	0.235	19.556	0.050	0.033	0.717	0.119	0.000	21.262
Vegetables											
Asparagus, can, spears	0.5 Cup	64.000	—	0.460	22.250	0.074	0.121	1.155	0.133	0.000	116.000
Asparagus, can, low sodium	0.5 Cup	57.500	—	0.464	20.000	0.066	0.109	1.040	0.120	0.000	104.000

(Continued)

TABLE A–21A. CONTINUED

FOOD NAME	SERVING PORTION	A* (RE)	E† (mg)	α-TOC (mg)	C (mg)	THIAMIN (mg)	RIBO (mg)	NIACIN (mg)	B6 (mg)	B12 (µg)	FOLATE (µg)
Vegetables											
Beans, snap, green, can, cuts	0.5 Cup	23.650	0.034	0.021	3.240	0.010	0.038	0.135	0.025	0.000	21.450
Beans, green, can, low sodium	0.5 Cup	—	0.034	0.021	3.200	0.010	0.038	0.137	—	0.000	21.600
Beans, snap, wax, raw, boiled	0.5 Cup	41.900	—	0.182	6.050	0.047	0.061	0.384	0.035	0.000	20.800
Beets, can, whole	0.5 Cup	1.238	—	0.037	4.795	0.013	0.047	0.186	0.068	0.000	35.650
Beets, can, diet, low sodium	0.5 Cup	1.238	—	0.037	4.795	0.013	0.047	0.186	0.068	0.000	35.650
Broccoli, raw, boiled, drained	0.5 Cup	108.000	0.496	0.357	58.000	0.043	0.088	0.445	0.111	0.000	38.750
Cabbage, common, boiled drained	0.5 Cup	6.550	1.210	1.210	17.600	0.042	0.040	0.165	0.047	0.000	14.700
Carrots, can, sliced, drained	0.5 Cup	1005.000	0.336	0.307	1.970	0.013	0.022	0.403	0.082	0.000	6.700
Carrots, can, low sodium	0.5 Cup	1620.000	0.565	0.515	3.445	0.024	0.033	0.520	0.138	0.000	9.950
Carrot, raw, whole, scraped	1.0 Item	2025.000	0.367	0.317	6.700	0.070	0.042	0.668	0.106	0.000	10.100
Cauliflower, raw, boiled, drained	0.5 Cup	0.900	0.057	0.019	34.300	0.039	0.032	0.342	0.125	0.000	31.700
Celery, Pascal, raw, stalk	1.0 Item	5.200	0.292	0.144	2.800	0.018	0.018	0.129	0.035	0.000	11.200
Corn, sweet, can, drained	0.5 Cup	13.200	0.510	0.033	7.000	0.027	0.065	0.990	0.039	0.000	40.100

Corn, sweet, can, low sodium	0.5 Cup	15.350	0.795	0.051	8.600	0.033	0.078	1.200	0.048	0.000	48.750
Cucumber, raw, sliced	0.5 Cup	2.600	0.161	0.078	2.445	0.016	0.010	0.156	0.027	0.000	7.250
Peas, green, can, drained	0.5 Cup	65.500	2.235	0.017	8.150	0.103	0.066	0.620	0.055	0.000	37.650
Peas, green, can, low sodium	0.5 Cup	65.500	2.235	0.017	8.150	0.103	0.066	0.620	0.055	0.000	37.650
Tomato, raw, red, ripe	1.0 Item	76.300	0.603	0.418	23.500	0.073	0.059	0.772	0.098	0.000	18.500
Tomato, red, can, stewed	0.5 Cup	70.000	0.905	0.281	16.950	0.059	0.045	0.910	0.022	0.000	6.900
Tomato, can, low sodium, diet	0.5 Cup	72.000	—	0.264	18.150	0.054	0.037	0.880	0.108	0.000	9.350
Potato, boiled, peeled before cooked	1.0 Item	0.000	0.081	0.041	9.990	0.132	0.026	1.770	0.363	0.000	12.000
Noodles, egg, enriched cooked	0.5 Cup	5.500	—	—	0.000	0.110	0.065	0.950	0.071	0.000	9.600
Rice, white, parboiled, cooked	0.5 Cup	0.000	0.342	0.097	0.000	0.219	0.016	1.225	0.016	0.000	3.000
Fruit											
Apple, raw, unpeeled	1.0 Item	7.400	0.911	0.814	7.800	0.023	0.019	0.106	0.066	0.000	3.900
Apple, raw, peeled	1.0 Item	5.600	0.845	0.346	5.120	0.022	0.013	0.116	0.059	0.000	0.500
Applesauce, can, unsweetened	0.5 Cup	3.500	—	0.110	1.465	0.016	0.031	0.230	0.032	0.000	0.730
Apricots, can, light syrup	0.5 Cup	167.000	—	1.125	3.415	0.020	0.026	0.385	0.069	0.000	2.150
Bananas, raw, peeled	1.0 Item	9.200	0.365	0.308	10.400	0.051	0.114	0.616	0.659	0.000	21.800
Blueberries, raw	0.5 Cup	7.250	—	—	9.450	0.035	0.037	0.261	0.026	0.000	4.640
Cherries, sweet, can/juice	0.5 Cup	15.650	—	—	3.125	0.023	0.030	0.510	0.038	0.000	5.250
Grapefruit, red/pnk/wht, raw	0.5 Cup	14.500	—	—	39.550	0.042	0.023	0.288	0.049	0.000	11.700

(Continued)

TABLE A-21A. CONTINUED

FOOD NAME	SERVING PORTION	A* (RE)	E† (mg)	α-TOC (mg)	C (mg)	THIAMIN (mg)	RIBO (mg)	NIACIN (mg)	B$_6$ (mg)	B$_{12}$ (µg)	FOLATE (µg)
Oranges, raw, all varieties	1.0 Item	26.900	0.314	0.314	69.700	0.114	0.052	0.369	0.079	0.000	39.700
Peaches, raw, whole	1.0 Item	46.500	—	0.087	5.740	0.015	0.036	0.861	0.016	0.000	2.960
Peaches, can, light syrup	0.5 Cup	44.500	—	—	2.950	0.012	0.032	0.745	0.024	0.000	4.100
Pears, raw, bartlet, unpeeled	1.0 Item	3.300	—	0.820	6.640	0.033	0.066	0.166	0.030	0.000	12.100
Pineapple, can/juice	0.5 Cup	4.750	0.125	0.125	11.900	0.119	0.024	0.355	0.093	0.000	6.000
Strawberries, raw, whole	0.5 Cup	2.050	0.194	0.090	42.250	0.015	0.049	0.172	0.044	0.000	13.200

*RE = µg retinol + µg β-carotene (0.167) + µg other carotenes (0.083)

    1 RE = 3.33 IU from vitamin A (retinol)

          10 IU from β-carotene

†mg of vitamin E represents mg of total tocopherol including α-tocopherol.

— denotes Lack of reliable data for nutrient to be present.

(Created on Nutritionist III, Version 7, N-Squared Computing, 1991. Data compiled from U.S. Department of Agriculture Handbook 8- Series, manufacturers' data, published journals, and industry sources. Appreciation expressed to Ms. Lori Cohen, M.S., R.D., for her assistance in preparing this table.)

TABLE A–21B. RETENTION OF NUTRIENTS IN COOKED VEGETABLES[1]

	ASCORBIC ACID (%)	THIAMIN (%)	RIBOFLAVIN (%)	NIACIN (%)	PANTOTHENIC ACID[6] (%)	VITAMIN B6 (%)	FOLACIN[7] (%)	VITAMIN A (%)
Potatoes								
Prepared from raw								
Baked in skin	80	85	95	95	90	95	90	—[8]
Boiled in skin	75	80	95	95	90	95	90	—
Boiled without skin	75	80	95	95	90	95	75	—
Fried	80	80	95	95	90	95	75	—
Hashed-brown[2]	25	40	85	80	—	—	65	—
Mashed	75	80	95	95	90	95	75	—
Scalloped and au gratin	80	80	95	95	90	95	75	—
Prepared from frozen								
French fried, heated	50	75	95	95	90	95	75	—
Baked, stuffed, heated	80	85	95	95	90	95	80	—
Hashed-brown	80	80	95	95	90	95	80	—
Sweet Potatoes								
Prepared from raw								
Baked in skin	80	85	95	95	90	95	90	90
Boiled in skin	75	80	95	95	90	95	90	85
Prepared from frozen								
Baked	80	80	95	95	90	95	80	90
Boiled	75	80	95	95	90	95	80	85
Tomatoes (prepared from raw, baked, boiled, or stewed)	95	95	95	95	95	95	70	95

(Continued)

TABLE A–21B. (CONTINUED)

	ASCORBIC ACID (%)	THIAMIN (%)	RIBOFLAVIN (%)	NIACIN (%)	PANTOTHENIC ACID[6] (%)	VITAMIN B6 (%)	FOLACIN[7] (%)	VITAMIN A (%)
Other Vegetables (cooked in small or moderate amount of water until tender)								
Prepared from raw, drained								
Greens, dark and leafy[3]	60	85	95	90	95	90	65	95
Roots, bulbs, other vegetables of high starch and/or sugar content[4]	70	85	95	95	90	95	70	90
Other[5]	80	85	95	90	90	90	70	90
Prepared from frozen, drained								
Greens, dark and leafy[3]	60	90	95	90	95	90	55	95
Roots, bulbs, other vegetables of high starch and/or sugar content[4]	70	90	95	95	90	95	70	90
Other[5]	80	90	95	90	90	90	70	90

[1]% True Retention = $\dfrac{\text{Nutrient content per g of cooked food} \times \text{g of food after cooking}}{\text{Nutrient content per g of raw food} \times \text{g of food before cooking}} \times 100$

[2]Potatoes were pared, boiled, and held overnight before hashed-browning.

[3]Vegetables such as beet greens, Chinese cabbage, collards, mustard greens, spinach, Swiss chard, turnip greens, and other wild greens.

[4]Vegetables such as beets, carrots, green peas, lima beans, onions, parsnips, rutabagas, salsify, turnips, summer and winter squash, and other immature seeds of the legume group.

[5]Vegetables such as asparagus, bean sprouts, broccoli, brussels sprouts, cabbage, cauliflower, eggplant, kohlrabi, okra, and sweet peppers.

[6]Because of limited data, values are based on nutrient retention data from other cooked plant products.

[7]Values are based on limited data.

[8]Dashes denote lack of reliable data.

(From Composition of Foods, Raw, Processed, Prepared. 1990 Supplement. Washington, D.C., U.S. Department of Agriculture, Human Nutrition Information Service, Agriculture Handbook No. 8.)

TABLE A–22. IRON, ZINC, COPPER, SELENIUM, AND MANGANESE CONTENT OF SELECTED FOODS, IN MG (100 g = 3½ oz)*

FOOD NAME	Fe	Zn	Cu	Se	Mn
Dairy Products					
Egg, whole, raw, large	1.440	1.100	0.014	0.044	0.024
Cheese, cottage, uncreamed	0.228	0.469	0.028	0.023	0.003
Cream, coffee, table, light	0.042	0.271	0.008	0.000	0.001
Cream, sour, cultured	0.061	0.270	0.019	—	0.003
Milk, buttermilk, fluid	0.049	0.420	0.011	0.001	0.002
Milk, whole, 3.3% fat, fluid	0.049	0.381	0.010	0.001	0.004
Milk, nonfat/skim, fluid	0.041	0.400	0.011	0.003	0.002
Milk, whole, low sodium	0.050	0.380	0.010	0.001	0.004
Fats					
Butter, regular, tablespoon	0.157	0.050	0.014	0.000	0.007
Vegetable oil, corn	0.000	0.000	0.000	—	0.000
Vegetable oil, olive	0.384	0.060	0.074	—	—
Shortening, veg, soybn/cottnsd	0.000	0.000	0.000	—	0.000
Margarine, reg, hard, unsalted	0.000	0.000	—	0.000	—
Mayonnaise, soy, commercial	0.714	0.143	0.243	—	—
Cereals					
Bran flakes, Kellogg's	63.590	13.205	0.741	0.010	4.333
Corn flakes, Kellogg's	6.300	0.282	0.066	0.004	0.084
Cream of rice, cooked	0.200	0.160	0.034	—	0.144
Cream of wheat, instant	4.979	0.170	0.038	—	—
Farina, cooked, enriched	0.502	0.070	0.011	—	—
Oatmeal, cooked	0.679	0.491	0.055	0.009	0.585
Wheat, puffed, plain	4.733	2.358	0.408	—	1.758
Wheat, shredded, biscuit	3.136	2.500	0.500	—	3.072
Rice Krispies	6.303	1.690	0.250	0.014	0.989

(Continued)

TABLE A–22. CONTINUED.

FOOD NAME	Fe	Zn	Cu	Se	Mn
Breads, Cookies, Crackers					
Bread, white, soft	2.840	0.620	0.140	0.028	0.280
Bread, whole-wheat, soft	3.373	1.655	0.338	0.046	—
Crackers, graham, plain	3.571	0.757	0.857	0.014	—
Crackers, sodium free/ whole-wheat	—	—	—	—	—
Crackers, saltines	4.545	0.618	0.182	0.145	—
Muffin, English, plain	2.821	0.720	0.311	0.027	—
Bread, Italian, enriched	2.333	—	—	0.027	—
Roll, hamburger/hotdog	2.975	0.620	0.165	0.030	—
Cookies, vanilla wafer	1.500	—	—	0.000	—
Meat, Fish					
Pot roast, arm, beef, cooked	3.790	8.660	0.164	0.006	0.019
Hamburger patty, beef/lean	2.106	5.365	0.066	0.024	0.014
Steak, sirloin, lean, broiled	3.357	6.518	0.146	0.034	0.018
Chicken, leg, no skin, roasted	1.305	2.853	0.080	0.014	0.021
Chicken, breast, roasted	1.061	1.020	0.050	0.027	0.018
Lamb, all cuts, lean/fat, cooked	1.871	4.459	0.119	—	0.022
Turkey, dark meat, no skin	2.336	4.464	0.160	0.025	0.023
Turkey, light, no skin, roasted	1.343	2.036	0.042	—	0.020
Veal, all cuts, lean, cooked	1.165	5.094	0.120	—	0.038
Bluefish	0.480	0.807	0.053	—	0.021
Flatfish, raw	0.353	0.459	0.032	—	0.016
Cod, cooked, dry heat	0.490	0.578	0.036	0.045	0.020
Halibut, broiled, dry	1.071	0.529	0.035	0.060	0.020
Shrimp, raw, mixed species	2.400	1.114	0.271	—	0.057
Tuna, can/oil, drained	1.388	0.900	0.071	0.072	0.015
Tuna, diet, low sodium	1.201	0.500	0.060	0.116	0.039

Food					
Sweets					
Honey, strained/extracted	0.476	0.095	0.038	0.005	0.029
Ice milk, van, hard, 4.3% fat	0.137	0.420	0.023	0.002	0.009
Ice cream, van, hard, 10% fat	0.090	1.060	0.019	0.002	0.006
Ice cream, van, hard, 16% fat	0.068	0.818	0.019	0.002	0.006
Jams/preserves, regular	1.000	—	0.310	0.000	—
Sherbet, orange, 2% fat	0.161	0.689	0.030	—	0.011
Sugar, brown, pressed down	3.409	—	0.350	0.001	—
Sugar, white, granulated	0.000	0.050	0.017	0.000	—
Juices					
Apple juice, can and bottle	0.371	0.028	0.022	0.001	0.113
Apricot nectar, can	0.382	0.092	0.073	—	0.032
Cranberry juice, bottle	0.150	0.070	0.018	0.000	0.193
Grape juice, can	0.096	—	—	—	—
Grapefruit juice, can, unsweetened	0.200	0.090	0.038	0.000	0.020
Lemon juice, can and bottle	0.130	0.060	0.037	0.000	0.020
Orange juice, can	0.442	0.070	0.057	0.000	0.014
Pear nectar, can	0.260	0.070	0.067	0.000	0.030
Pineapple juice, can	0.260	0.110	0.090	0.001	0.992
Prune juice, can and bottle	1.180	0.210	0.068	0.000	0.151
Tomato juice, can	0.582	0.140	0.101	0.000	0.077
Tomato juice, low sodium	0.582	0.140	0.101	0.000	0.077
Vegetables					
Asparagus, can, spears	1.831	0.400	0.096	0.004	0.170
Asparagus, can, low sodium	0.582	0.471	0.107	0.001	0.152
Beans, snap, green, can, cuts	0.904	0.290	0.038	0.001	0.200
Beans, green, can, low sodium	0.897	0.294	0.038	0.001	0.200
Beans, snap, wax, raw, boiled	1.280	0.360	0.103	0.001	0.294
Beets, can, whole	0.671	0.230	0.097	0.000	0.241
Beets, can, diet, low sodium	0.671	0.230	0.097	0.001	0.241
Broccoli, raw, boiled, drained	0.839	0.380	0.043	0.002	0.218

(Continued)

TABLE A-22. (CONTINUED)

FOOD NAME	Fe	Zn	Cu	Se	Mn
Cabbage, common, boiled, drained	0.390	0.160	0.028	0.002	0.129
Carrots, can, sliced, drained	0.640	0.260	0.104	0.001	0.450
Carrots, can, low sodium	0.610	0.290	0.103	0.001	0.451
Carrot, raw, whole, scraped	0.500	0.200	0.047	0.003	0.142
Cauliflower, raw, boiled, drained	0.419	0.242	0.090	0.001	0.177
Celery, pascal, raw, stalk	0.400	0.130	0.035	0.000	0.035
Corn, sweet, can, drained	0.861	0.390	0.058	0.001	0.173
Corn, sweet, can, low sodium	0.350	0.359	0.056	0.000	0.033
Cucumber, raw, sliced	0.280	0.230	0.040	0.001	0.061
Peas, green, can, drained	0.953	0.712	0.082	0.001	0.303
Peas, green, can, low sodium	0.953	0.712	0.082	0.001	0.303
Tomato, raw, red, ripe	0.450	0.089	0.074	0.001	0.105
Tomato, red, can, stewed	0.729	0.170	0.112	0.001	0.059
Tomato, can, low sodium, diet	0.608	0.160	0.110	0.001	—
Potato, boiled, peeled before cooked	0.310	0.270	0.167	0.001	0.140
Noodles, egg, enriched, cooked	0.875	—	0.169	0.059	—
Rice, white, parboiled, cooked	1.126	0.310	0.094	0.020	0.260

Fruits

Fruits	Fe	Zn	Cu	Se	Mn
Apples, raw, unpeeled	0.181	0.036	0.041	0.001	0.045
Apple, raw, peeled	0.070	0.039	0.031	0.001	0.023
Applesauce, can, unsweetened	0.119	0.030	0.026	0.000	0.075
Apricots, can, light syrup	0.391	0.107	0.079	0.000	0.052
Bananas, raw, peeled	0.307	0.160	0.104	0.001	0.152
Blueberries, raw	0.170	0.110	0.061	0.001	0.282
Cherries, sweet, can/juice	0.580	0.100	0.073	0.000	0.061
Grapefruit, red/pnk/wht, raw	0.087	0.070	0.047	—	0.012
Oranges, raw, all varieties	0.100	0.069	0.045	0.002	0.025
Peaches, raw, whole	0.110	0.140	0.068	0.001	0.047
Peaches, can, light syrup	0.359	0.088	0.052	—	0.046
Pears, raw, Bartlet, unpeeled	0.250	0.120	0.113	0.001	0.076
Pineapple, can/juice	0.280	0.100	0.086	0.001	1.120
Strawberries, raw, whole	0.380	0.130	0.049	0.001	0.290

*Values for five trace elements have been provided in this table. Other trace elements have been analyzed and can be found in the following article by Hunt and Mullen: Concentration of boron and other elements in human foods and personal-care products. J. Am. Diet Assoc., *91*:558–568, 1991. These authors report the analyzed concentrations of boron and molybdenum, as well as of calcium, copper, iron, magnesium, and manganese in selected foods and personal-care products (analgesics, antibiotics, decongestants, antihistamines, dental hygiene products, gastric antacids, and laxatives). For those interested in obtaining data on these nutrients, this article may serve as a helpful reference.

Fe = iron, Zn = zinc, Cu = copper, Se = selenium, Mn = manganese.

— denotes Lack of reliable data for nutrient known to be present.

(Created on Nutritionist III, Version 7, N-Squared Computing, 1991. Data compiled from U.S. Department of Agriculture Handbook 8- Series, manufacturers' data, published journals, and industry sources. Appreciation expressed to Ms. Lori Cohen, M.S., R.D., for her assistance in preparing this table.)

TABLE A-23A. STANDARD EXCHANGE LISTS*,†

The reason for dividing food into six different groups is that foods vary in their carbohydrate, protein, fat, and calorie content. Each exchange list contains foods that are alike; each choice contains about the same amount of carbohydrate, protein, fat, and calories.

The following chart shows the amount of these nutrients in one serving from each exchange list.

Exchange List	Carbohydrate (g)	Protein (g)	Fat (g)	Calories
Starch/bread	15	3	trace	80
Meat (lean)	—	7	3	55
(medium-fat)	—	7	5	75
(high-fat)	—	7	8	100
Vegetable	5	2	—	25
Fruit	15	—	—	60
Milk (skim)	12	8	trace	90
(low-fat)	12	8	5	120
(whole)	12	8	8	150
Fat	—	—	5	45

As you read the exchange lists, you will notice that one choice often is a larger amount of food than another choice from the same list. Because foods are so different, each food is measured or weighed so the amount of carbohydrate, protein, fat, and calories is the same in each choice.

*The exchange lists are based on material in the *Exchange Lists for Meal Planning* prepared by Committees of the American Diabetes Association, Inc., and the American Dietetic Association in cooperation with the National Institute of Arthritis, Metabolism, and Digestive Diseases and the National Heart and Lung Institutes of Health, Public Health Service, U.S. Department of Health and Human Services.
†From the American Diabetes Assoc., 1986, with permission.

TABLE A–23A. CONTINUED

STARCH/BREAD LIST

Each item in this list contains about 15 g of carbohydrate, 3 g of protein, a trace of fat, and 80 calories.

Whole-grain products average about 2 g of fiber per serving. Some foods are higher in fiber. Those foods that contain 3 or more g of fiber per serving are identified with the fiber symbol.†

You can choose your starch servings from any of the items on this list. If you want to eat a starch food that is not on this list, the general rule is that:

- ½ cup of cereal, grain, or pasta is one serving
- 1 ounce of a bread product is one serving

Cereals/Grains/Pasta

Bran cereals†, flaked	½ cup
Bran cereals†, concentrated (such as Bran Buds, All Bran	⅓ cup
Puffed cereal	1½ cup
Grapenuts	3 Tbsp
Shredded wheat	½ cup
Other ready-to-eat unsweetened cereals	¾ cup
Cooked cereals	½ cup
Bulgur (cooked)	½ cup
Grits (cooked)	½ cup
Pasta (cooked)	½ cup
Rice, white or brown (cooked)	⅓ cup
Cornmeal (dry)	2½ Tbsp
Wheat germ†	3 Tbsp

Dried Beans, Peas/Lentils

Beans† and peas† (cooked), e.g., kidney, white, split, blackeye	⅓ cup
Lentils† (cooked)	⅓ cup
Baked beans†	¼ cup

Crackers/Snacks

Animal crackers	8
Graham crackers, 2½" square	3
Matzoth	¾ oz
Melba toast	5 slices
Oyster crackers	24
Popcorn (popped, no fat added)	3 cups
Pretzels	¾ oz
Rye crisp, 2" × 3½"	4
Saltine-type crackers	6
Whole-wheat crackers, no fat added (crispbreads, such as Finn, Kavli, Wasa)	2–4 slices (¾ oz)

Starch Foods Prepared With Fat

(Count as 1 starch/bread serving plus 1 fat serving)

Biscuit, 2½" across	1
Chow mein noodles	½ cup
Cornbread, 2" cube	1 (2 oz)
Cracker, round butter type	6

(Continued)

TABLE A–23A. (CONTINUED)

STARCH/BREAD LIST

Starchy Vegetables			
Corn	½ cup	French fried potatoes, 2″ to 3½″ long	10 (1½ oz)
Corn on cob†, 6″ long	1	Muffin, plain, small	1
Lima beans†	½ cup	Pancake, 4″ across	2
Peas, green† (canned or frozen)	½ cup	Waffle, 4½″ square	1
Plantain†	½ cup	Stuffing, bread (prepared)	¼ cup
Potato, baked	1 small (3 oz)	Taco shell, 6″ across	2
Potato, mashed	½ cup	Whole-wheat crackers, fat added	4–6 (1 oz)
Squash, winter† (acorn, butternut)	¾ cup	(such as Triscuits)	
Yam, sweet potato, plain	⅓ cup		
Bread			
Whole wheat	1 slice (1 oz)		
Pita, 6″ across	½		
Raisin, unfrosted	1 slice (1 oz)		
Rye†, pumpernickel†	1 slice (1 oz)		
White (including French, Italian)	1 slice (1 oz)		
Bagel	½ (1 oz)		
Bread sticks, crisp, 4″ long × ½″	2 (⅔ oz)		
Croutons, low-fat	1 cup		
English muffin	½		
Plain roll, small	1 (1 oz)		
Frankfurter or hamburger bun	½ (1 oz)		
Tortilla, 6″ across	1		

†3 g or more of fiber per serving.

TABLE A–23A. CONTINUED

MEAT LIST

Each serving of meat and substitutes on this list contains varying amounts of fat and calories. The list is divided into three parts based on the amount of fat and calories: lean meat, medium-fat meat, and high-fat meat. One ounce (one meat exchange) of each of these includes:

	Carbohydrate (g)	Protein (g)	Fat (g)	Calories
Lean	0	7	3	55
Medium-fat	0	7	5	75
High-fat	0	7	8	100

You are encouraged to use more lean and medium-fat meat, poultry, and fish in your meal plan. This will help decrease your fat intake, which may help decrease your risk for heart disease. The items from the high-fat group are high in saturated fat, cholesterol, and calories. You should limit your choices from the high-fat group to three (3) times per week. Meat and substitutes do not contribute any fiber to your meal plan. Meat and meat substitutes that have 400 mg or more of sodium are identified with a § symbol.

Tips:

1. Bake, roast, broil, grill, or boil these foods rather than frying them with added fat.
2. Use a nonstick pan spray or a nonstick pan to brown or fry these foods.
3. Trim off visible fat before and after cooking.
4. Do not add flour, bread crumbs, coating mixes, or fat to these foods when preparing them.
5. Weigh meat after removing bones and fat, and after cooking. Three ounces of cooked meat is about equal to 4 ounces of raw meat. Some examples of meat portions are:

   2 oz meat (2 meat exchanges) = 1 small chicken leg or thigh
   ½ cup cottage cheese or tuna

   3 oz meat (3 meat exchanges) = 1 medium pork chop
   1 small hamburger
   ½ chicken breast (1 side)
   1 unbreaded fish fillet
   cooked meat, about the size of a deck of cards

6. Restaurants usually serve prime cuts of meat, which are high in fat and calories.

(Continued)

TABLE A–23A. CONTINUED

Lean Meat and Substitutes
(One exchange is equal to any one of the following items)

Beef:	USDA Good or Choice grades of lean beef, such as round, sirloin, and flank steak, tenderloin, and chipped beef§	1 oz
Pork:	Lean pork, such as fresh ham; canned, cured, or boiled ham; Canadian bacon§, tenderloin	1 oz
Veal:	All cuts are lean except for veal cutlets (ground or cubed).	1 oz
	Examples of lean veal are chops and roasts.	
Poultry:	Chicken, turkey, Cornish hen (without skin)	1 oz
Fish:	All fresh and frozen fish	1 oz
	Crab, lobster, scallops, shrimp, clams (fresh, or canned in water§)	2 oz
	Oysters	6 medium
	Tuna§ (canned in water)	¼ cup
	Herring (uncreamed or smoked)	1 oz
	Sardines (canned)	2 medium
Wild Game:	Venison, rabbit, squirrel	1 oz
	Pheasant, duck, goose (without skin)	1 oz
Cheese:	Any cottage cheese	¼ cup
	Grated Parmesan	2 Tbsp
	Diet cheese§ with less than 55 calories per oz	1 oz
Other:	95% fat-free luncheon meat§	1 oz
	Egg whites	3 whites
	Egg substitutes with less than 55 calories per ¼ cup	¼ cup

Medium-Fat Meat and Substitutes
(One exchange is equal to any one of the following items)

Beef:	Most beef products fall into this category. Examples are all ground beef, roast (rib, chuck, rump), steak (cubed, Porterhouse, T-bone), and meatloaf	1 oz
Pork:	Most pork products fall into this category. Examples are chops, loin roast. Boston butt, cutlets	1 oz

Lamb:	Most lamb products fall into this category. Examples are chops, leg, and roast	1 oz
Veal:	Cutlet (ground or cubed, unbreaded)	1 oz
Poultry:	Chicken (with skin), domestic duck or goose (well-drained of fat), ground turkey	1 oz
Fish:	Tuna§ (canned in oil and drained), salmon§ (canned)	¼ cup
Cheese:	Skim or part-skim milk cheeses, such as	
	Ricotta	¼ cup
	Mozzarella	1 oz
	Diet cheeses§ with 56–80 calories per oz	1 oz
Other:	86% fat-free luncheon meat§	1 oz
	Egg (high in cholesterol, limit to 3 per week)	1
	Egg substitutes with 56–80 calories per ¼ cup	¼ cup
	Tofu (2½" × 2¾" × 1")	4 oz
	Liver, heart, kidney, sweetbreads (high in cholesterol)	1 oz

High-Fat Meat and Substitutes

Remember, these items are high in saturated fat, cholesterol, and calories, and should be used only three (3) times per week.

(One exchange is equal to any one of the following items)

Beef:	Most USDA Prime cuts of beef, such as ribs, corned beef§	1 oz
Pork:	Spareribs, ground pork, pork sausage§ (patty or link)	1 oz
Lamb:	Patties (ground lamb)	1 oz
Fish:	Any fried fish product	1 oz
Cheese:	All regular cheese,§ such as American, Blue, Cheddar, Monterey, Swiss	1 oz
Other:	Luncheon meat,§ such as bologna, salami, pimento loaf	1 oz
	Sausage,§ such as Polish, Italian, knockwurst, smoked	1 oz
	Bratwurst§	1 oz
	Frankfurter§ (turkey or chicken)††	1 frank (10/lb)
	Peanut butter (contains unsaturated fat)	1 Tbsp

§400 mg or more of sodium per exchange.
††Frankfurter (beef, pork or combination). Count as one high-fat meat plus one fat exchange: 1 frank (10/lb).

TABLE A–23A. CONTINUED

VEGETABLE LIST

Each vegetable serving on this list contains about 5 g of carbohydrate, 2 g of protein, and 25 calories. Vegetables contain 2–3 g of dietary fiber. Vegetables that contain 400 mg or more of sodium per serving are identified with a § symbol.

Vegetables are a good source of vitamins and minerals. Fresh and frozen vegetables have more vitamins and less added salt. Rinsing canned vegetables will remove much of the salt.

Unless otherwise noted, the serving size for vegetables is:
- ½ cup of cooked vegetables or vegetable juice
- 1 cup of raw vegetables

Artichoke (½ medium)	Eggplant	Rutabaga
Asparagus	Greens (collard, mustard, turnip)	Sauerkraut§
Beans (green, wax, Italian)	Kohlrabi	Spinach, cooked
Bean sprouts	Leeks	Summer squash (crookneck)
Beets	Mushrooms, cooked	Tomato (1 large)
Broccoli	Okra	Tomato/vegetable juice§
Brussels sprouts	Onions	Turnips
Cabbage, cooked	Pea pods	Water chestnuts
Carrots	Peppers (green)	Zucchini, cooked
Cauliflower		

Starchy vegetables, such as corn, peas, and potatoes, are found on the Starch/Bread list.
For free vegetables, see Free Food list.

FRUIT LIST

Each item on this list contains about 15 g of carbohydrate and 60 calories. Fresh, frozen, and dry fruits have about 2 g of fiber per serving. Fruits that have 3 g or more of fiber per serving have a † symbol. Fruit juices contain very little dietary fiber.

The carbohydrate and calorie contents for a fruit serving are based on the usual serving of the most commonly eaten fruits. Use fresh fruits, or fruits frozen or canned without sugar added. Whole fruit is more filling than fruit juice, and may be a better choice for those who are trying to lose weight. Unless otherwise noted, the serving size for fruit is:
- ½ cup of fresh fruit or fruit juice
- ¼ cup of dried fruit

Fresh, frozen, and unsweetened canned fruit

Apple (raw, 2" across)	1 apple
Applesauce (unsweetened)	½ cup
Apricots (medium, raw)	4 apricots
Apricots (canned)	½ cup, or 4 halves
Banana (9" long)	½ banana
†Blackberries (raw)	¾ cup
†Blueberries (raw)	¾ cup
Cantaloupe (5" across)	⅓ melon
(cubes)	1 cup
Cherries (large, sweet, raw)	12 cherries
Cherries (canned)	½ cup
Figs (raw, 2" across)	2 figs
Fruit cocktail (canned)	½ cup
Grapefruit (medium)	½ grapefruit
Grapefruit (segments)	¾ cup
Grapes (small)	15 grapes
Honeydew melon (medium) (cubes)	⅛ melon
	1 cup
Kiwi (large)	1 kiwi
Mandarin oranges	¾ cup
Mango (small)	½ mango
†Nectarine (1½" across)	1 nectarine
Orange (2½" across)	1 orange
Papaya	1 cup
Peach (2¾" across)	1 peach, or ¾ cup
Peaches (canned)	½ cup, or 2 halves
Pear	½ large, 1 small
Pears (canned)	½ cup, or 2 halves
Persimmon (medium, native)	2 persimmons
Pineapple (raw)	¾ cup
Pineapple (canned)	⅓ cup
Plum (raw, 2" across)	2 plums
†Pomegranate	½ pomegranate
†Raspberries (raw)	1 cup
†Strawberries (raw, whole)	1¼ cup
†Tangerine (2½" across)	2 tangerines
Watermelon (cubes)	1¼ cup

Dried Fruit

†Apples	4 rings
†Apricots	7 halves
Dates	2½ medium
†Figs	1½
†Prunes	3 medium
Raisins	2 Tbsp

Fruit Juice

Apple juice/cider	½ cup
Cranberry juice cocktail	⅓ cup
Grapefruit juice	½ cup
Grape juice	⅓ cup
Orange juice	½ cup
Pineapple juice	½ cup
Prune juice	⅓ cup

$400 mg or more of sodium per serving.
†3 g or more of fiber per serving.

TABLE A–23A. CONTINUED

MILK LIST

Each serving of milk or milk products on this list contains about 12 g of carbohydrate and 8 g of protein. The amount of fat in milk is measured in percent (%) of butterfat. The calories vary, depending on what kind of milk you choose. The list is divided into three parts based on the amount of fat and calories: skim/very low-fat milk, low-fat milk, and whole milk. One serving (one milk exchange) of each of these includes:

	Carbohydrate (g)	Protein (g)	Fat (g)	Calories
Skim/Very low-fat	12	8	trace	90
Low-fat	12	8	5	120
Whole	12	8	8	150

Milk is the body's main source of calcium, the mineral needed for growth and repair of bones. Yogurt is also a good source of calcium. Yogurt and many dry or powdered milk products have different amounts of fat. If you have questions about a particular item, read the label to find out the fat and calorie content.

Milk is good to drink, but it can also be added to cereal and to other foods. Many tasty dishes, such as sugar-free pudding, are made with milk (see the Combination Foods list). Plain yogurt is delicious with one of your fruit servings mixed with it.

Skim and Very Low-Fat Milk

- 1 cup skim milk
- 1 cup ½% milk
- 1 cup 1% milk
- 1 cup low-fat buttermilk
- ½ cup evaporated skim milk
- ⅓ cup dry nonfat milk
- 8-oz carton plain nonfat yogurt

Low-Fat Milk

- 1 cup fluid 2% milk
- 8-oz carton plain low-fat yogurt (with added nonfat milk solids)

Whole Milk

The whole milk group has much more fat per serving than the skim and low-fat groups. Whole milk has more than 3¼% butterfat. Try to limit your choices from the whole milk group as much as possible.

- 1 cup whole milk
- ½ cup evaporated whole milk
- 8-oz carton whole milk plain yogurt

FAT LIST

Each serving on the fat list contains about 5 g of fat and 45 calories.

The foods on the fat list contain mostly fat, although some items may also contain a small amount of protein. All fats are high in calories and should be carefully measured. Everyone should modify their fat intake by eating unsaturated fats instead of saturated fats. The sodium content of these foods varies widely. Check the label for sodium information.

Unsaturated Fats

Avocado	⅛ medium
Margarine	1 tsp
Margarine, diet#	1 Tbsp
Mayonnaise	1 tsp
Mayonnaise, reduced-calorie#	1 Tbsp
Nuts and seeds:	
Almonds, dry roasted	6 whole
Cashews, dry roasted	1 Tbsp
Pecans	2 whole
Peanuts	20 small, 10 large
Walnuts	2 whole
Other nuts	1 Tbsp
Seeds, pine nuts, sunflower (without shells)	1 Tbsp
Pumpkin seeds	2 tsp
Oil (corn, cottonseed, safflower, soybean, sunflower, olive, peanut)	1 tsp
Olives#	10 small, 5 large
Salad dressing, mayonnaise-type	2 tsp
Salad dressing, mayonnaise-type, reduced-calorie	1 Tbsp
Salad dressing (all varieties)#	1 Tbsp
Salad dressing, reduced-calorie	2 Tbsp
(2 Tbsp of low-calorie is a free food)§	

Saturated Fats

Butter	1 tsp
Bacon	1 slice
Chitterlings	½ oz
Coconut, shredded	2 Tbsp
Coffee whitener, liquid	2 Tbsp
Coffee whitener, powder	4 tsp
Cream (light, coffee, table)	2 Tbsp
Cream, sour	2 Tbsp
Cream (heavy, whipping)	1 Tbsp
Cream cheese	1 Tbsp
Salt pork	¼ oz

#If more than one or two servings are eaten, foods have 400 mg or more of sodium.
§400 mg or more of sodium per serving.

FREE FOODS

A free food is any food or drink that contains 20 calories or less per serving. You can eat as much as you want of those items that have no serving size specified. You may eat 2 or 3 servings per day of those items that have a specific serving size. Be sure to spread them out through the day.

Drinks
Bouillon§ or broth without fat†
Bouillon, low-sodium
Carbonated drinks, sugar-free
Carbonated water
Club soda
Cocoa powder, unsweetened (1 Tbsp)
Coffee/Tea
Drink mixes, sugar-free
Mineral water
Tonic water, sugar-free

Nonstick pan spray
Fruit
Cranberries, unsweetened (½ cup)
Rhubarb, unsweetened (½ cup)

Seasonings can be very helpful in making food taste better. Be careful of how much sodium you use. Read the label and choose those seasonings that do not contain sodium or salt.

Basil (fresh)
Celery seeds
Cinnamon
Chili powder
Chives
Curry
Dill
Flavoring extracts (e.g., vanilla, lemon, almond, walnut, peppermint, butter)

Vegetables (raw, 1 cup)
Cabbage
Celery
Chinese cabbage†
Cucumber
Green onion
Hot peppers
Mushrooms
Radishes
Zucchinit
Salad greens
Endive
Escarole
Lettuce
Romaine
Spinach

Garlic
Garlic powder
Herbs
Hot pepper sauce
Lemon
lemon juice
Lemon pepper
Lime
Lime juice
Mint

Sweet Substitutes
Candy, hard, sugar-free
Gelatin, sugar-free
Gum, sugar-free
Jam/jelly, sugar-free (2 tsp)
Pancake syrup, sugar-free (¼ cup)
Sugar substitutes (saccharin, Equal)
Whipped topping, low calorie
Condiments
Catsup (1 Tbsp)
Horseradish
Mustard
Pickles§, dill, unsweetened
Salad dressing, low-calorie (2 Tbsp)
Taco sauce (1 Tbsp)
Vinegar

Onion powder
Oregano
Paprika
Pepper
Pimento
Spices
Soy sauce§
Soy sauce, low-sodium
Wine, used in cooking (¼ cup)
Worcestershire sauce

COMBINATION FOODS

Much of the food we eat is mixed together in various combinations. These combination foods do not fit into only one exchange list. It can be difficult to tell what is in a certain casserole dish or baked food item. This is a list of average values for some typical combination foods. This list will help you fit these foods into your meal plan. Ask your dietitian for information about any other foods you would like to eat. The *American Diabetes Association/American Dietetic Association Family Cookbooks* and the *American Diabetes Association Holiday Cookbook* have many recipes and further information about many foods, including combination foods. Check your library or local bookstore.

Food	Amount	Exchanges
Casseroles, homemade	1 cup (8 oz)	2 starch, 2 medium-fat meat, 1 fat
Cheese pizza§ thin crust	¼ of 15 oz or ¼ of 10″	2 starch, 1 medium-fat meat, 1 fat
Chili with beans†§ (commercial)	1 cup (8 oz)	2 starch, 2 medium-fat meat, 2 fat
Chow mein† (without noodles or rice)	2 cups (16 oz)	1 starch, 2 vegetable, 2 lean meat
Macaroni and cheese§	1 cup (8 oz)	2 starch, 1 medium-fat meat, 2 fat
Soup		
Bean†	1 cup (8 oz)	1 starch, 1 vegetable, 1 lean meat
Chunky, all varieties	10¾ oz can	1 starch, 1 vegetable, 1 medium-fat meat
Cream§ (made with water)	1 cup (8 oz)	1 starch, 1 fat
Vegetable§ or broth§	1 cup (8 oz)	1 starch
Spaghetti and meatballs§ (canned)	1 cup (8 oz)	2 starch, 1 medium-fat meat, 1 fat
Sugar-free pudding (made with skim milk)	½ cup	1 starch
If beans are used as a meat substitute:		
Dried beans,† peas,† lentils†	1 cup (cooked)	2 starch, 1 lean meat

†3 g or more of fiber per serving.
§400 mg or more of sodium per serving.

FOODS FOR OCCASIONAL USE

Moderate amounts of some foods can be used in your meal plan, in spite of their sugar or fat content, as long as you can maintain blood glucose control. The following list includes average exchange values for some of these foods. Because they are concentrated sources of carbohydrate, you will notice that the portion sizes are very small. Check with your dietitian for advice on how often and when you can eat them.

Food	Amount	Exchanges
Angel food cake	1/12 cake	2 starch
Cake, no icing	1/12 cake, or a 3" square	2 starch, 2 fat
Cookies	2 small (1¾" across)	1 starch, 1 fat
Frozen fruit yogurt	1/3 cup	1 starch
Gingersnaps	3	1 starch
Granola	1/4 cup	1 starch, 1 fat
Granola bars	1 small	1 starch, 1 fat
Ice cream, any flavor	1/2 cup	1 starch, 2 fat
Ice milk, any flavor	1/2 cup	1 starch, 1 fat
Sherbet, any flavor	1/4 cup	1 starch
Snack chips, § all varieties	1 oz	1 starch, 2 fat
Vanilla wafers	6 small	1 starch, 1 fat

MANAGEMENT TIPS

Some food you buy uncooked will weigh less after you cook it. This is true of most meats. Starches often swell in cooking, so a small amount of uncooked starch will become a much larger amount of cooked food. The following table shows some of the changes:

Food (Starch Group)	Uncooked	Cooked
Oatmeal	3 level Tbsp	½ cup
Cream of wheat	2 level Tbsp	½ cup
Grits	3 level Tbsp	½ cup
Rice	2 level Tbsp	⅓ cup
Spaghetti	¼ cup	½ cup
Noodles	⅓ cup	½ cup
Macaroni	¼ cup	½ cup
Dried beans	3 Tbsp	⅓ cup
Dried peas	3 Tbsp	⅓ cup
Lentils	2 Tbsp	⅓ cup
Food (Meat Group)		
Hamburger	4 oz	3 oz
Chicken	1 small drumstick	1 oz
	½ breast (1 side)	3 oz

- Read food labels. Remember—*dietetic* does not mean *diabetic!* When you see the word "dietetic" on a food label, it means that something has been changed or replaced. It may have less salt, less fat, or less sugar. It does not mean that the food is sugar-free or calorie-free. Some dietetic foods may be useful. Those that contain 20 calories or less per serving may be eaten as many as 3 times a day as free foods.
- Know your sweeteners. Two types of sweeteners are on the market: those with calories and those without calories. Sweeteners with calories, such as fructose, sorbitol, and mannitol, when used in large amounts, may cause cramping and diarrhea. Remember, these sweeteners do have calories that add up. Sweeteners without calories include saccharin and aspartame (Equal, Nutrasweet) and may be used in moderation.

§If more than one serving is eaten, these foods have 400 mg or more of sodium.

TABLE A-23B. DIABETIC EXCHANGES FOR AFRICAN-AMERICAN (SOUTHERN) COOKERY

FOOD EXCHANGE GROUP	FOOD	PORTION	SODIUM CONTENT
Starch/Bread			
(80 calories per exchange)	Biscuit, 2" diameter	1 (add 2 fat)	262 mg
	Cornbread, 2" × 2" × 1"	1 (add 1 fat)	220 mg
	Corn muffin, 2" diameter	1 (add 1 fat)	250 mg
	Crackling bread, 2" × 2" × 1"	1 (add 2 fat)	High
	CooCoo (cornmeal, okra, butter, salt, and water)	(equals 1 veg/1 fat)	High
	Cornmeal	2 Tbsp	Low
	Black-eyed peas	½ cup (add ½ lean meat)	6 mg
	Pinto beans	¼ cup (add ½ lean meat)	2 mg
	Baked beans (no pork)	¼ cup	239 mg
	Grits (instant/cooked)	½ cup	385 mg
	Hoe cake, 2" × 2" × 1"	1 (add 2 fat)	Medium
	Hominy (canned)	½ cup	720 mg
	Hoppin john (frozen)	½ cup (add 1 fat, ½ bread)	High
	Hush puppies	2 small pieces (add 2 fats)	High
	Spoon bread	½ cup (add 1 lean meat, 1 fat)	High
	Pound cake, 3½" × 3" × ½"	1 (add 2 fat)	Low
	Custard (baked)	½ cup (add 1 lean meat, ½ fat)	Medium
Meat			
Lean Meat	Chicken gizzard	1 oz	19 mg
(55 calories per ounce)	Pork		
	Hog maw, stomach	⅓ cup	30 mg
	Souse meat	3" × 2" × ¼"	High
	Pig ear	1 medium	Low

	Amount	
Medium-Fat Meat *(75 calories per ounce)*		
Fish		
Catfish, *4" × 2" × ¼"*	1	Low
Mullet, *4" × 2" × ¼"*	1	Low
Perch, *4" × 2" × ¼"*	1	Low
Snapper, *4" × 2" × ¼"*	1	Low
Sardines	3 drained	High
Pork		
Chipped ham	1 oz	High
Fresh butt	1 oz	High
Neck bones	½ cup	High
Pork cubes (lean)	1 oz	High
Tongue	1 oz	High
Organ meats		
Heart (beef)	1 oz	35 mg
Kidney	1 oz	71 mg
Liver (pork)	1 oz	14 mg
Sweetbreads	1 oz	32 mg
High-Fat Meat *(100 calories per ounce)*		
Fish		
Eel, American (fresh)	1 oz	25 mg
Mackerel (fresh)	1 oz	17 mg
Barbecued ribs	1 oz	High
Country ham	1 oz	High
Devild ham (canned)	1 oz	High
Pork belly (fresh)	1 oz	
Hock (smoked)	1 oz	
Pig's feet	1 (equals 2 exchanges)	
Pork shank	1 oz	
Pork tail	1 oz	
Sausage (bulk, patties, link)	1 oz	High
Pig snout	1 (equals 2 exchanges)	

(Continued)

TABLE A-23B. CONTINUED

FOOD EXCHANGE GROUP	FOOD	PORTION	SODIUM CONTENT
Luncheon Meats (100 calories per ounce)	Bologna	1 oz	High
	Frankfurter (hot dogs)	1 oz	High
	Sausage link (canned or frozen)	1 oz (add 1 fat)	215 mg
	Sausage links (brown and serve)	1 oz (add 1 fat)	High
	Small Vienna sausage	3 (add 1 fat)	High
	Spam	1 oz	High
	Treat	1 oz	High
	Scrapple	1 oz	High
Organ Meats	Brains	¼ cup	70 mg
Combination Meats	Chicken and dumplings	3 oz (equals 2 lean meat, 1 veg, 1 bread, 1 fat)	High
	Chili, 1 cup	(equals 2 medium-fat meat, 2 bread, 2 fat)	
	Smothered chicken (no skin)	¼ broiler (equals 4 lean meat, ½ bread)	High
	Steamed fish with butter	3 oz (equals 4 lean meat, ½ fat)	Low

Vegetable
(25 calories per exchange)

Food	Serving	
Collard (cooked without fat)	½ cup	25 mg
Kale (cooked without fat)	½ cup	29 mg
Mustard (cooked without fat)	½ cup	18 mg
Turnip (cooked withou fat)	cup	8.5 mg
Poke salad (cooked without fat)	1 cup	High
Rape	½ cup (add 2 fat)	High
Greens (cooked with fat)	½ cup	High
Okra	8-9 pods	High
Chickory (raw)	1 cup	6 mg
Cressie greens (raw)	1 cup	5 mg per 10 sprigs

Fruit
(60 calories per exchange)

No additions

Milk
(90 calories per exchange)

Food	Serving	
Buttermilk (skim milk)	1 cup	257 mg
Buttermilk (whole milk)	1 cup (omit 2 fat)	250 mg

Fats
(Saturated)
(45 calories per teaspoon)

Food	Serving	
Bacon (thick sliced, crisp)	1 strip	High
Bacon (thin/medium sliced, crisp)	1 strip	High
Bacon grease	1 tsp	High
Chitterlings, fried	2 Tbsp	High
Crackling, pork	1½ tsp	High
Fat back	¾" cube	High
Salt pork	¾" cube	High
Slab of bacon, 1" × 1" × ¼"	1 slice	High
Streak o'lean, 1" × 1" × ¼"	1 slice	High

(Adapted with permission from The American Diabetes Association, Washington, D.C. Area Affiliate, Inc.: Exchange Lists for Meal Planning: Black American Cookery. 1987.)

TABLE A-23C. SUPPLEMENTARY EXCHANGE LISTS FOR CHINESE-AMERICAN FOODS

FOOD EXCHANGE GROUP	FOOD	PORTION
Starch/Bread	Cellophane or mung bean noodles (cooked)	¾ cup
	Ginkgo seeds	½ cup
	Lotus root, ¼"-thick slice, 2½" diameter	10 slices
	Mung beans or green gram beans (cooked)	⅓ cup
	Red beans (cooked)	⅓ cup
	Rice congee or soup	¾ cup
	Rice vermicelli or noodles (cooked)	½ cup
	Taro (cooked)	⅓ cup
Meat and Meat Substitutes		
Lean Meat	Beef jerky, 3½" × 1"*	½ oz
	Dried scallop	1 large
	Dried shrimp	1 Tbsp or 10 medium shrimp
	Soybeans (cooked)	3 Tbsp
	Squid	2 oz
	Tripe (beef)	2 oz
	Beef tongue	1 oz
Medium-fat Meat and Substitutes	Tofu or soybean curd, 2½" × 2¾" × 1"†	4 oz or ½ cup
High-fat Meat	Salted duck egg‡§	1
	Thousand-year-old or preserved limed duck egg‡§	1
High-fat Meat + 1 Fat	Chinese sausage (pork and spices and/or liver)*§	1 (2 oz)
Vegetables (½ cup cooked or 1 cup raw unless indicated otherwise)	Amaranth or Chinese spinach (cooked)	
	Arrowheads, or fresh corms (raw), 3½" diameter	
	Baby corn (canned)*	
	Bamboo shoots	
	Bitter melon or bitter gourd	
	Chayote	
	Chinese celery	
	Chinese eggplant (white or purple)	

Chinese or black mushroom (dried)	2 medium
Hairy melon or hairy cucumber	
Leeks†	
Luffa (angled or smooth)	
Mung bean sprouts	
Mustard greens†	
Peapods or sugar peas†	
Soybean sprouts (cooked or raw)	½ cup
Straw mushrooms	
Turnip†	
Water chestnuts (canned)†	½ cup
Winter melon or wax gourd	
Yard-long beans	

Fruits

Carambola or star fruit (raw)	2 medium
Chinese banana (raw)	1 dwarf
Guava (raw)	1 medium
Kumquats (raw)	5 medium
Litchi or lychee (raw)	10
Litchi or lychee (canned, drained)	½ cup
Longan (raw)	30
Longan (canned, drained)	¾ cup
Mango (raw)†	½ small
Papaya (raw), 3½" diameter, 5⅛" hight	½
Persimmon, Japanese (soft type) (raw)	½
Pummelo (raw)	¾ cup

Milk
Fats

Soybean milk (unsweetened)	1 cup
Coconut milk	1 Tbsp
Sesame paste	1½ tsp
Sesame seeds (whole, dried)	1 Tbsp

TABLE A-23C. CONTINUED

FOOD EXCHANGE GROUP	FOOD	PORTION
Free Foods	Amaranth or Chinese spinach	
	Bok choy	
	Chili pepper (raw)†	1
	Chinese or Peking cabbage†	
	Choy sum or Chinese flowering cabbage	
	Coriander	
	Garland chrysanthemum	
	Ginger	¼ cup
	Mustard greens (salted and soured)	2 Tbsp
	Oriental radish or daikon	
	Watercress	
Combination	Mock duck or wheat gluten (canned)	½ cup (equals ½ starch/ bread, 1 lean meat)

*400 mg or more of sodium per serving.

†Foods are included in *Exchange Lists for Meal Planning*, 1986. © American Diabetes Association and The American Dietetic Association.

‡Probably 400 mg or more of sodium per serving, based on author's estimate.

§Limit high-fat meat choices to 3 times per week.

(From The American Dietetic Association and The American Diabetes Association, Inc.: Ethnic and Regional Food Practices: A Series. Chinese Food Practices, Customs and Holidays. 1990. With permission.)

TABLE A–23D. SUPPLEMENTARY EXCHANGE LISTS FOR HMONG-AMERICAN FOODS

FOOD EXCHANGE GROUP	FOOD	PORTION
Starch/Bread	Cellophane or mung bean noodles (cooked)	¾ cup
	Rice vermicelli or noodles (cooked)	½ cup
	Rice soup	¾ cup
Meat and Meat Substitutes		
Lean Meat	Pheasant†	1 oz
	Squirrel†	1 oz
	Venison†	1 oz
Medium-fat Meat and Substitutes	Pig's feet	2½ oz (equals 2 exchanges)
	Tofu or soybean curd, 2½" × 2¾" × 1"	4 oz or ½ cup
High-fat Meat	Ground pork†‡	1 oz
Vegetables	Bamboo shoots	
(½ cup cooked or	Bitter melon or bitter gourd	
1 cup raw unless	Chinese onion (leeks†)	
indicated otherwise)	Cucuzzi squash (spaghetti squash)	
	Luffa gourd/squash	
	Mustard greens†	
	Mung bean sprouts	
	Pumpkin	
	Sugar peas, snow peas, sweet peas, peapods†	
	Yard-long beans, pod and seeds	½ cup

(Continued)

TABLE A–23D. (CONTINUED)

FOOD EXCHANGE GROUP	FOOD	PORTION
Fruits	Apple pear, Asian pear (raw), 2¼" high, 2½" diameter	1
	Guava (raw)	1½ medium
	Jackfruit (raw)	½ cup
	Mango (raw)†	½ small
	Papaya (raw), 5⅛" high, 3½" diameter†	½ or 1 cup
Fats	Beef fat	1 tsp
	Chicken fat	1 tsp
	Coconut cream or milk	1 Tbsp
	Coconut (raw)†	2 Tbsp
	Pork lard	1 tsp
	Pork intestine, chitterlings†	½ oz
Free Foods	Fish sauce*	
	Pumpkin or squash blossom	
	Soy sauce*†	
	Tender vines and leaves of pumpkin, squash, luffa gourd, and pea plants	
Occasional Foods	Condensed milk, sweetened	1 oz (equals 1½ starch/bread)

*400 mg or more of sodium per serving.
†Foods are included in *Exchange Lists for Meal Planning,* 1986. © American Diabetes Association and The American Dietetic Association.
‡Limit high-fat meat choice to 3 times per week.
(From The American Dietetic Association and The American Diabetes Association, Inc.: Ethnic and Regional Food Practices, a Series. Hmong Food Practices, Customs and Holidays. 1992. With permission.)

TABLE A-23E. DIABETIC EXCHANGES FOR AN INDIAN DIET

FOOD EXCHANGE GROUP	FOOD	PORTION
Starch/Bread	Arrowroot flour (uncooked)	2 Tbsp
	Barley (uncooked)	1½ Tbsp
	Colacassia (cooked)	¼ cup
	Indian breads*	
	Chapati, 5"–6" diameter	1 medium
	Dosa, 5"–6" diameter	1 medium
	Idli, 2½"–3" diameter	1 medium
	Puri, 5" diameter	1 large (omit 2½ fat)
	Phulka, 5" to 6" diameter	1 medium
	Phoa (rice flakes, Indian style) (uncooked)	3 Tbsp
	Plantain (raw)	½ medium
	Rice flour (uncooked)	2 Tbsp
	Sago (uncooked)	1¼ Tbsp
	Suji (cream of wheat) (uncooked)	2 Tbsp
	Upma (plain without vegetable) (cooked)	½ cup
	Vermicelli (thinner than very thin spaghetti) (uncooked)	½ cup
	Whole-wheat flour	2½ Tbsp
Meat and Meat Substitutes		
Lean Meat and Substitutes		
(omit 1 starch/bread for each)	Bengal gram dhal (Chana, whole, split) (uncooked)	2 Tbsp
	Bengal gram dhal (roasted) (uncooked)	3 Tbsp
	Black gram dhal (Urad dhal) (uncooked)	2 Tbsp
	Green gram dhal (Mung dhal) (uncooked)	2 Tbsp
	Masur dhal (uncooked)	2 Tbsp
	Toordhal (uncooked)	2 Tbsp
	Besan (chick pea flour) (uncooked)	3 Tbsp

(Continued)

FOOD EXCHANGE GROUP	FOOD	PORTION
High-Fat Meat and Substitute	Pannir (cheese) made with whole milk	¼ cup
Vegetables	Ashgourd (cooked)	1⅓ cup
(½ cup cooked or 1 cup raw	Bitter gourd (cooked)	
unless indicated otherwise)	Bottle gourd (cooked)	
	Chow-chow (cooked)	
	Cluster beans (cooked)	
	Drumstick (cooked)	
	Fenugreek leaves (cooked)	
	Ladies fingers (cooked) (okra)	
	Ridge gourd (cooked)	
	White radish (cooked)	
Fruits	Guava (fresh)	½ cup
Milk	Curds (yogurt) made from skim milk (plain)	1 cup
Fats	Coconut (grated) (unsweetened)	2 Tbsp
	Coconut chutney	2 Tbsp
	Coconut oil	1 tsp
	Ghee (clarified butter)	1 tsp
	Mustard oil	1 tsp
	Sesame oil	1 tsp

*Exchange values for Indian breads from *Diabetic Diet*, Dietetic Department, Christian Medical College and Hospital, Vellore, India. (Adapted with permission from The American Diabetes Association, Washington, D.C. Area Affiliate, Inc.: Supplement to Exchange Lists for Meal Planning: Indian Cookery.)

TABLE A–23F. SUPPLEMENTARY EXCHANGE LISTS FOR EASTERN EUROPEAN (JEWISH) FOODS*

FOOD EXCHANGE GROUP	FOOD	PORTION
Starch/Bread	Bagel† or bialy	½ small, 1 oz
	Bulgur (cooked)†	½ cup
	Bulke	½ medium
	Farfel (dry)	½ cup
	Hallah	1 slice, 1 oz
	Kasha (cooked)	½ cup
	Kasha (raw)	2 Tbsp
	Lentils†	⅓ cup
	Matzoh†	¾ oz
	Matzoh meal	2½ Tbsp
	Potato starch (flour)	2 Tbsp
	Pumpernickel bread†	1 slice, 1 oz
	Rye bread†	1 slice, 1 oz
	Split peas†	⅓ cup
Starch/Bread Prepared with Fat	Matzoh ball‡	3 balls, 1½ oz (equals 1 starch/bread + 1 fat)
	Potato pancake	½ pancake (equals 1 starch/bread + 1 fat)
Meat		
Lean meat	Flanken†	1 oz
	Gefilte fish	2 oz
	Herring† (smoked, uncreamed)	1 oz
	Lox†	1 oz
	Sardines† (canned, drained)	2 medium
	Smelts	1 oz

(Continued)

TABLE A–23F. (CONTINUED)

FOOD EXCHANGE GROUP	FOOD	PORTION
Medium-fat meat	Beef tongue	1 oz
	Brisket	1 oz
	Chopped liver§	¼ cup
	Corned beef†	1 oz
	Sablefish (smoked)	1 oz
High-fat meat	Salmont (canned)	¼ cup
	Pastrami	1 oz
Vegetables	Borscht (no sugar or sour cream)	½ cup
	Sorrel	½ cup
Fats	Cream cheese†	1 Tbsp
	Nondairy creamer† (liquid)	2 Tbsp
	Nondairy creamer† (powder)	4 tsp
	Schmaltz	1 tsp
	Sour cream†	2 Tbsp
Free Foods	Horseradish†	
(in reasonable amounts)	Pickles, dill†	
Occasional Foods	Sweet kosher wine	½ cup (equals 2 fat)

*Unless otherwise specified, all foods are 1 exchange.
†Foods are included on the American Diabetes Association and American Dietetic Association *Exchange Lists for Meal Planning.* 1986. © American Diabetes Association and The American Dietetic Association.
‡High in sodium.
§No additional salt in recipe.
(From The American Dietetic Association and The American Diabetes Association, Inc. Ethnic and Regional Food Practices, a Series. Jewish Food Practices, Customs and Holidays, 1989. With permission.)

TABLE A–23G. SUPPLEMENTARY EXCHANGE LISTS FOR MEXICAN-AMERICAN FOODS*

FOOD EXCHANGE GROUP	FOOD	PORTION
Starch/Bread	Bolillo (French roll), 4½" to 5" long	¼
	Frijoles cocidos† (cooked beans)	⅓ cup
	Frijoles cocidos	1 cup (equals 2 starch/bread + 1 lean meat)
	Frijoles refritos (refried beans) (no fat added)	⅓ cup
	Tortilla, corn, 7½" across (ready to bake)‡	1
	Tortilla, flour, 7" across (ready to bake)‡	1 (equals 1½ starch/bread)
	Tortilla, flour, 9" across (ready to bake)‡	⅓
Starch/Bread	Frijoles refritos (fat added)	⅓ cup (equals 1 starch/bread + 1 fat)
Prepared with Fat	Taco shell, 5" across (ready to use)	2 (equals 1 starch/bread + 1 fat)
	Tortilla, flour, 7" across (fried with added fat)	1 (equals 1½ starch/bread + 1 fat)
	Tortilla, corn, 7½" across (fried with added fat)	1 (equals 1 starch/bread + 1 fat)
	Tortilla, flour, 9" across (fried with added fat)	1 (equals 3 starch/bread + 2 fat)
Meat		
Lean meat	Menudo (tripe soup)	½ cup
Medium-fat meat	Queso fresco (cheese made with skim milk)	¼ cup (2 oz)
High-fat meat	Chorizo (Mexican sausage)	1 oz (equals 1 high-fat meat + 1 fat)
Vegetables	Chayote (squash) (cooked)	½ cup
	Jícama (yambean root) (raw)	½ cup
	Nopales (cactus) (raw)	½ cup
Fruits	Mango†	½ small
	Papaya†	1 cup
Fats	Avocado†	⅛ medium
Free Foods	Jalapeño chilis	
	Salsa de chile (chili/taco sauce)	
	Verdolagas (purslane)	
Occasional Foods	Pan dulce (sweet bread), 4½" across	1 (equals 4 starch/bread + 1 fat)

*Unless otherwise specified, all foods are 1 exchange.
†Food and amount are same as in 1986 *Exchange Lists for Meal Planning.* © American Diabetes Association, Inc., The American Dietetic Association.
‡Food, amount, or both differ from 1986 *Exchange Lists for Meal Planning* because of new information.
(From The American Dietetic Association and The American Diabetes Association, Inc. Ethnic and Regional Food Practices, a Series. Mexican Food Practices, Customs and Holidays, 1989. With permission.)

TABLE A–23H. SUPPLEMENTARY EXCHANGE LISTS FOR TRADITIONAL NAVAJO FOODS*

FOOD EXCHANGE GROUP	FOOD	PORTION
Starch/Bread	Blue corn mush	¾ cup
	Flour tortilla, 8" diameter	¼
	Steamed corn hominy (cooked)	½ cup
Meat		
Lean meat	Mutton, flesh (lean only) (cooked without added fat)	1 oz
High-fat meat	Mutton, flesh (lean and fat) (cooked without added fat)	1 oz
Fats	Piñon nuts	1 Tbsp (about 25 nuts)

*Nutrition practitioners who work with Navajo clients with noninsulin-dependent diabetes mellitus do not often use the Exchange system in client education sessions. This listing is presented for the few occasions when supplementary Exchange values may be needed.

(From The American Dietetic Association and The American Diabetes Association, Inc. Ethnic and Regional Food Practices, a Series. Navajo Food Practices, Customs and Holidays, 1991. With permission.)

TABLE A-23I. DIABETIC EXCHANGES FOR A GENERAL ASIAN-AMERICAN DIET

FOOD EXCHANGE GROUP	FOOD	PORTION
Starch/Bread		
	Arrowroot	3 small
	Arrowroot starch	2 Tbsp
	Cellophane noodles (cooked)	½ cup
	Chestnuts (shelled)	¼ cup
	Chowmein noodles	½ cup (omit 1 fat)
	Congee (rice soup)*	1 cup
	Cornstarch*	2 Tbsp
	Fungi (woodears) (dried)	1 oz (omit 1 Fruit)
	Gingko seeds (dried)	1½ oz
	Glutinous rice, (cooked)*	¼ cup
	Glutinous rice flour*	1 Tbsp
	Lanka (jackfruit)	⅓ cup
	Lotus root	⅔ segment
	Lotus seeds (dried)	1 oz
	Millet	1 oz (omit ½ Bread)
	Mung bean noodles	½ cup
	Rice noodles (sticks)	
	Cooked	½ cup
	Dry	1 oz
	Tamarind	1 oz
	Tapioca pearles (dry)	1 Tbsp
	Taro (dasheen)	¼ cup

(Continued)

TABLE A–23I. (CONTINUED)

FOOD EXCHANGE GROUP	FOOD	PORTION
Meat and Meat Substitutes		
Lean Meat and Substitutes	Dried beans and peas (cooked)	½ cup (omit 1 Bread)
	Black-eyed peas	
	Broad beans (horse beans)	
	Garbanzo	
	Kidney	
	Lentils	
	Lima	
	Mung	
	Navy	
	Pinto	
	Abalone	1 oz
	Chicken wings	1 wing
	Dried duck feet	½ oz
	Gefilte fish	1 oz
	Octopus	1¾ oz
	Shrimp (dried)	½ oz
	Squid (calamares)	1¾ oz
Medium-Fat Meat and Substitutes	Bean curd cheese	2 oz
	Fishmaw (fish stomach)	2 oz
	Oxtail	1 oz
	Soybeans (cooked)	⅓ cup
	Tofu (soybean curd) 2½″ × 2¾″ × 1″	1 portion
High-Fat Meat and Substitutes	Anchovies	10
	Chinese sausage	1 oz
	Eel	1 oz
	Pork feet (fresh)	2 oz (omit 1 Fat)
	Preserved duck egg	⅔ egg

Vegetables

Bok choy (cooked)	1 cup
Bamboo shoots (canned, drained)	¾ cup
Banana flower	½ cup
Bitter melon (balsam pear)	½ cup
Chinese radish (daikon)	1 cup
Dried Chinese mushrooms (soaked)	½ cup
Green beans (Chinese)	½ cup
Hairy cucumber	½ cup
Kohlrabi	¾ cup
Leek (Chinese onion)	½ cup
Lotus seeds	1 oz
Mung bean sprouts	1 cup
Mustard green root	½ cup
Pear squash (chayote)	½ medium
Salted celery cabbage	Free
Salted Chinese cabbage	½ cup
Scallions, 5" × ½"	3
Seaweed (dried, soaked, drained)	½ cup
Snow peas	½ cup
Straw mushrooms	½ cup
Water chestnuts	4
White eggplant (Chinese)	½ cup
Winter melon (Wax gourd)	1 cup

Fruit

Carambola (star fruit)	1
Dried red dates	4
Guava (fresh)	½ cup
Kumquats (fresh)	3
Litchis (dried or fresh)	6
Longans (dried)	5
Pomegranate	½

Milk

Coconut milk*	1 cup (omit 12 fats)
Soymilk	1 cup (add ½ starch/bread)

(Continued)

TABLE A–23I. (CONTINUED)

FOOD EXCHANGE GROUP	FOOD	PORTION
Fats	Chicken fat or pork fat	1 tsp
	Nuts	
	Cashew	7 large (omit 1 Vegetable)
	Macadamia	6
	Pine	⅓ oz
	Pistachio (shelled)	⅓ oz
	Oils	1 tsp
	Peanut	
	Safflower	
	Sesame	
	Soy (tou yo)	
	Seeds (dried)	
	Pumpkin	1 Tbsp
	Sesame	1 Tbsp
	Watermelon	½ oz
	Sesame seed paste	1 tsp
Miscellaneous Foods		
YES! YES! YES!	Anise, curry powder, flower spice, ground ginger, mustard sauce, oyster sauce, parsley, soy sauce, tangerine peel, tea, vinegar, 5-spices powder.	
NO! NO! NO!	Brown sugar, hoisin sauce, molasses, moon cake, plum sauce, red preserved ginger, rock sugar, sweet buns, sweet coconut tarts, sweet mung bean soup.	

*See Professional Guidelines, *In* American Diabetes Association, Washington, D.C. Area Affiliate, Inc.: Supplement to Exchange Lists for Meal Planning Oriental Cookery, 1979, p. 18.
(Adapted with permission from The American Diabetes Association, Washington, D.C. Area Affiliate, Inc.: Supplement to Exchange Lists for Meal Planning Oriental Cookery. 1979.)

TABLE A—23J. DIET EXCHANGES FOR A VEGETARIAN DIET*

FOOD EXCHANGE GROUP	FOOD	PORTION
Starch/Bread	Brown rice (cooked)	⅓ cup
	Buckwheat flour (dark)	3 Tbsp
	Bulgur wheat	2 Tbsp
	Millet (cooked)	½ cup
	Miso	3 Tbsp
	Oats (dry)	¼ cup
	Pita (Syrian) bread	½ of a 2½-oz loaf
	Rye flour	3 Tbsp
	Wheat berries (cooked)	⅓ cup
	Wild rice (cooked)	½ cup
Meat and Meat Substitutes		
Lean Meat and Substitutes	Dried beans and peas (cooked) (omit 1 bread for each listing)	½ cup
	Black-eyed peas	
	Broad beans	
	Garbanzo	
	Kidney	
	Lentils	
	Lima	
	Mung	
	Navy	
	Pinto	
	Soy flour	¼ cup (omit ½ bread)
Medium-fat Meat and Substitutes†	Cheeses	
	Camembert	1 oz
	Edam	1 oz
	Liederkranz	1 oz
	Soybeans	⅓ cup
	Tofu, 2½" × 2¾" × 1"	1 portion
High-fat Meat and Substitutes	Cheeses	
	Blue, Roquefort	1 oz
	Brick	1 oz
	Gorgonzola	1 oz
	Gouda	1 oz
	Gruyère	1 oz
	Limburger	1 oz
	Muenster	1 oz
	Parmesan	1 oz
	Swiss	1 oz
	Hummus	4 Tbsp (omit 1 bread)
	Peanuts‡	4 Tbsp (omit ½ bread and 2 fat)
	Pignolia nuts‡	6 Tbsp (omit ½ vegetable and 1 fat)
	Pumpkin seeds‡	4 Tbsp (omit ½ bread and 1½ fat)
	Sesame seeds‡	4 Tbsp (omit ½ bread and 2 fat)
	Sunflower seeds‡	4 Tbsp (omit ½ bread and 2 fat)
Vegetables	Bamboo shoots	¾ cup
	Bean sprouts (raw or cooked)	
	Alfalfa	1 cup
	Mung	1 cup
	Soy	1 cup
	Water chestnuts	4
Fruit	Carrot juice	½ cup
Milk	Kefir	1 cup (omit 2 fats)
	Soy milk (fortified)	1 cup (add ½ bread)
Fats	Tahini	1 tsp

Food containing complementary proteins may be eaten together, thereby increasing protein quality. Examples of foods that may be complemented to yield high-quality protein are listed below.

FOOD	COMPLEMENTARY PROTEIN
Grains	Combine rice with: cheese, legumes, sesame
	Combine wheat with: legumes, peanuts and milk, sesame, and soybean
	Combine corn with: legumes
Legumes	Combine beans with: wheat, corn
	Combine soybeans with: rice and wheat, corn and milk, wheat and sesame, peanuts and sesame, peanuts and wheat and rice
Nuts and seeds	Combined sesame with: beans, peanuts and soybeans, soybeans and wheat
	Combine peanuts with: sunflower seeds

DIET PATTERNS

Lacto-Ovovegetarian	Strict Vegetarian
Calories: 1,500	Calories: 1,500
CH_2O—190 g 50%	CH_2O—190 g 50%
Protein—75 g 20%	Protein—75 g 20%
Fat—47 g 30%	Fat—47 g 30%
Daily Food Allowance	Daily Food Allowance
3 Skim Milk Exchanges	3 Soybean Milk Exchanges (Note: Add ½ bread for each cup)
2 Vegetable Exchanges	
4 Fruit Exchanges	2 Vegetable Exchanges
7 Bread Exchanges	4 Fruit Exchanges
4 Lean Meat Exchanges	7 Bread Exchanges
1 Medium-fat Meat Exchange	4 Lean Meat Exchanges
6 Fat Exchanges	1 Medium-fat Meat Exchange
	6 Fat Exchanges
Meal Pattern	Meal Pattern
Breakfast	*Breakfast*
1 Fruit Exchange	1 Fruit Exchange
2 Bread Exchanges	2 Bread Exchanges
1 Medium-fat Meat Exchange	1 Medium-fat Meat Exchange
2 Fat Exchanges	2 Fat Exchanges
1 Skim Milk Exchange	1 Milk Exchange
Lunch	*Lunch*
2 Lean Meat Exchanges	2 Lean Meat Exchanges
2 Bread Exchanges	2 Bread Exchanges
1 Vegetable Exchange	1 Vegetable Exchange
2 Fruit Exchanges	2 Fruit Exchanges
2 Fat Exchanges	2 Fat Exchanges
Dinner	*Dinner*
2 Lean Meat Exchanges	2 Lean Meat Exchanges
2 Bread Exchanges	2 Bread Exchanges
1 Vegetable Exchange	1 Vegetable Exchange
1 Fruit Exchange	1 Fruit Exchange
2 Fat Exchanges	2 Fat Exchanges
1 Skim Milk Exchange	1 Milk Exchange
Bedtime Snack	*Bedtime Snack*
1 Skim Milk Exchange	1 Milk Exchange
1 Bread Exchange	1 Bread Exchange

TABLE A—23J. CONTINUED

GUIDELINES FOR THE PROFESSIONAL

You may revise the patient's meal plan to allow more calories from carbohydrate (50 to 60%) because of the high consumption of complex carbohydrates by vegetarians.

Many vegetarians use butter instead of margarine because it is considered a natural food.

The commercial meat analogues are very high in sodium, ranging in values from 300 mg to 3,000 mg/100 g edible portion. Nutritional analyses of these products are available upon request from Loma Linda Foods, Riverside, California 92505, and Worthington Foods, Miles Laboratories, Worthington, Ohio 43085.

Some vegetarians use diet supplements, such as wheat germ and brewer's yeast. Include these in the diet as follows:

Brewer's yeast, powder: 1 level Tbsp = ½ Lean Meat Exchange
Wheat germ: ¼ cup = 1 Bread Exchange

Vegetarian diets, unless fortified, could be deficient in iron. Iron absorption is enhanced by the inclusion of a vitamin C—rich food at each meal.

Vegetarian diets excluding dairy products may be inadequate in riboflavin and calcium. Two cups daily of fortified soybean milk or appropriate supplements should prevent deficiency.

For the strict vegetarian, vitamin B_{12} is also required as a vitamin supplement if 2 cups of fortified soybean milk are not consumed daily.

SUGGESTED READING FOR VEGETARIANS

1. Position of the American Dietetic Association: Vegetarian Diets, J. Am. Diet. Assoc., *88*:3, 351—355, 1988.
2. Lappe, F.M.: Diet for a Small Planet. New York, Ballantine Books, 1991.
3. Robertson, L., Flinders, C., Ruppenthal, B.: The New Laurel's Kitchen. Berkeley, CA, Ten Speed Press, 1986.
4. Hodgkin, G., Maloney, S.: Diet Manual Utilizing a Vegetarian Diet Plan. 7th Ed. Loma Linda, CA, The Seventh Day Adventist Dietetic Association, 1990.
5. Hinman, B., Snyder, N.: Lean and Luscious and Meatless. Prima Publications, Rocklin, CA, 1992.
6. Mangum, K.: Life's Simple Pleasures: Fine Vegetarian Cooking for Sharing and Celebration. Pacific Press Publications, Boise, ID, 1990.
7. Baird, P.: Quick Harvest: A Vegetarian's Guide to Microwave Cooking. New York, Prentice-Hall, 1991.

*Supplement to Exchange Lists for Meal Planning Vegetarian Cookery. American Diabetes Association, Washington, D.C. Area Affiliate, Inc., Food and Nutrition Committee, 1978. See Table A—23a for Standard Exchange lists.

†Meat analogs: Vegetable protein foods that closely duplicate the flavor, texture, and appearance of meat—"meatless" meats. See company information in the Guidelines for the Professional given above.

‡Seeds and nuts can be considered a "High-fat Meat" exchange and a complete protein only when they are complemented.

TABLE A-24A. GLYCEMIC INDEX VALUES OF SOME FOODS ADJUSTED SO THE GLYCEMIC INDEX OF WHITE BREAD IS 100*

FOOD	MEAN	FOOD	MEAN
Breads		**Legumes**	
Rye (crispbread)	95	Baked beans (canned)	70
Rye (wholemeal)	89	Bengal gram dal	12
Rye (whole grain, i.e., pumpernickel)	68	Butter beans	46
Wheat (white)	100	Chick peas (dried)	47
Wheat (wholemeal)	100	Chick peas (canned)	60
Pasta		Green peas (canned)	50
Macaroni (white, boiled 5 min)	64	Green peas (dried)	65
Spaghetti (brown, boiled 15 min)	61	Garden peas (frozen)	65
Spaghetti (white, boiled 15 min)	67	Haricot beans (white, dried)	54
Star pasta (white, boiled 5 min)	54	Kidney beans (dried)	43
Cereal Grains		Kidney beans (canned)	74
Barley (pearled)	36	Lentils (green, dried)	36
Buckwheat	78	Lentils (green, canned)	74
Bulgur	65	Lentils (red, dried)	38
Millet	103	Pinto beans (dried)	60
Rice (brown)	81	Pinto beans (canned)	64
Rice (instant, boiled 1 min)	65	Peanuts	15
Rice (polished, boiled 5 min)	58	Soya beans (dried)	20
Rice (polished, boiled 10-25 min)	81	Soya beans (canned)	22
Rice (parboiled, boiled 5 min)	54	**Fruit**	
Rice (parboiled, boiled 15 min)	68	Apple	52
Rye kernels	47	Apple juice	45

Food	Glycemic Index		Food	Glycemic Index
Sweet corn	80		Banana	84
Wheat kernels	63		Orange	59
Breakfast Cereals			Orange juice	71
"All Bran"	74		Raisins	93
Cornflakes	121		**Sugars**	
Muesli	96		Fructose	26
Porridge oats	89		Glucose	138
Puffed rice	132		Honey	126
Puffed wheat	110		Lactose	57
Shredded wheat	97		Maltose	152
"Weetabix"	109		Sucrose	83
Cookies			**Dairy Products**	
Digestive	82		Custard	59
Oatmeal	78		Ice cream	69
"Rich tea"	80		Skim milk	46
Plain crackers (water biscuits)	100		Whole milk	44
Shortbread cookies	88		Yogurt	52
Root Vegetables			**Snack Foods**	
Potato (instant)	120		Corn chips	99
Potato (mashed)	98		Potato chips	77
Potato (new/white boiled)	80			
Potato (Russett, baked)	116			
Potato (sweet)	70			
Yam	74			

*Glycemic index is defined as the blood glucose repsonse to a 50-g available carbohydrate portion of a food expressed as a percentage of the response to the same amount of carbohydrate from a standard food, in this case white bread (see Chap. 39). (From Wolever, T. M. S.: World Rev. Nutr. Diet., 62:120–185, 1990.)

TABLE A-24B. DIETS FOR WEIGHT REDUCTION AND FOR DIABETIC PERSONS*

NUTRIENT CLASS	TOTAL DAILY INTAKE (kcal)			
	800	1,200	1,800	2,250
Carbohydrate (g)	109 (54%)	154 (51%)	249 (55%)	309 (55%)
Protein	54 (27%)	60 (20%)	84 (19%)	107 (19%)
Fat (g)	17 (19%)	40 (29%)	54 (27%)	65 (26%)
FOOD GROUP	TOTAL EXCHANGES FOR ONE DAY (see Table A-23)			
Skim milk	2	2	2	2
Vegetable	2	2	3	6
Fruit	3	4	5	7
Bread†	2	4	9	10
Meat	4‡	4	5	7
Unsaturated Fat	1	4	4	4
MEAL	SAMPLE MEAL PATTERN (servings based on exchanges)			
Breakfast				
Skim milk	½	1	1	1
Fruit	1	1	1	1 + 1 midmeal
Bread	1	1	2	2 + 1 midmeal
Meat	0	0	0	1
Unsaturated fat	1	1	1	1
Lunch				
Skim milk	1	½	0	0
Vegetable	0	1	1	2 + 2 midmeal
Fruit	1	1	2	1 + 1 midmeal
Bread	½	1	3	2
Meat	1	1	2	2
Unsaturated fat	0	1	1	1
Dinner				
Skim milk	½	0	0	0
Vegetable	2	1	2	2
Fruit	1	1	1	2
Bread	½	1	2	3
Meat	3	3	3	4
Unsaturated fat	0	1	1	1
Evening				
Skim milk	0	½	1	1
Vegetable	0	0	0	0
Fruit	0	1	1	1
Bread	0	1	2	2
Meat	0	0	0	0
Unsaturated fat	0	1	1	1

*This table, prepared by us with assistance from Ms. Lori Cohen, R.D., is based on the dietary recommendations in Nutrition Guide for Professionals: Diabetes Education and Meal Planning, Powers, M. (Ed.), American Diabetes Association, Inc., and The American Dietetic Association, 1988. See Table A-25 for nutrition guidelines.

†In Exchange lists, trace fat is listed for breads. For calculation purposes, 1 g fat can be used when amount of breads contribute significantly to diet (i.e., > 6 servings per day).

‡Lean meat exchanges are used to calculate the 800-kcal meal pattern. All other meal patterns are based on medium-fat meat exchange.

TABLE A-25. NUTRITION GUIDELINES FOR PERSONS WITH NONINSULIN-DEPENDENT DIABETES MELLITUS

	LEAN PERSONS	OBESE PERSONS
Energy	Enough to maintain desirable body weight Men and physically active women require 30 kcal/kg desirable body weight Sedentary persons and persons older than 55 years require 28 kcal/kg desirable body weight	Enough to achieve reasonable body weight* 20 kcal/kg desirable body weight
Carbohydrate Sucrose	Up to 55 to 60% of total energy Can be included with an individualized diet plan†	Same Low nutrient density; limit on low-calorie diets
Fiber	Up to 40 g/day, with emphasis on water-soluble fiber	25 g/1,000 kcal
Protein	Recommended dietary allowance is 0.8 g/kg body weight	Minimum of 60 g when restricted to ≤1,200-kcal diet‡

Editor's Footnote: The information in the above table has been slightly modified in the new 1994 nutrition recommendation for diabetes from the American Diabetes (1, 2) and Dietetic Associations. These recommendations can be found in their entirety in the references cited. The statement of philosophy from the Commentary and translation article states:

"The 1994 reccomendations, the fifth published by the American Diabetes Association since 1950, present two major changes in the philosophy of nutrition care for diabetes. First, an individually developed dietary prescription based on metabolic, nutrition, and lifestyle requirements replaces the calculated caloric prescription tailored to meet individual needs. This change in philosophy is guided by the recognition that diabetes encompasses a variety of metabolic abnormalities and that a single diet formula does not adequately treat all types of diabetes.

The second philosophical change is in the approach to nutrition management of noninsulin-dependent (type II) diabetes. Glucose and lipid goals join weight loss as the focus of therapy for overweight persons. A variety of strategies to achieve these metabolic goals are advocated, only one of which is weight loss. This change indicates that nutrition interventions besides weight loss can be effective in achieving blood glucose and lipid goals in persons with type II diabetes."(3)

We believe that the guidelines in Table A-25 work within the new framework of the 1994 reccomendations. We suggest the current recommendations be reviewed and incorporated into the overall management of persons being treated for diabetes.

1. American Diabetes Association. Nutrition recommendations and principles for people with diabetes mellitus. Diabetes Care. 1994;17:519-522

2. Franz MJ, Horton ES, Bantle JP, Beebe CA, Brunzell JD, Coulston AM, Henry RR, Hoogwerf BF, Stacpoole PW. Nutrition principles for management of diabetes and related complications. Technical review. Diabetes Care. 1994;17:490-518.

3. Diabetes Care and Education, A Practice Group of the American Dietetic Association; Tinker LF, Heins JM, Holler HJ. Commentary and translation: 1994 nutrition recommendations for diabetes. JADA. 1994;94:507-511

(Continued)

TABLE A–25. (CONTINUED)

	LEAN PERSONS	OBESE PERSONS
Fat	Ideally <30% of energy	Same
Polyunsaturated fats	Up to 10% of energy	
Saturated fats	<10% of energy	
Monounsaturated fats	10 to 15% of energy	
Cholesterol	<300 mg/day	
Alternative Sweeteners	Use is acceptable	Same
Sodium	Not to exceed 3,000 mg/day	Same
Alcohol	Occasional or no use; limit to 1 to 2 alcohol equivalents 1 to 2 times per week	Same
Vitamins/Minerals	No evidence that diabetes causes increased need	
Snacks	Individualized on the basis of preferences and glucose patterns; snack should be coordinated with insulin schedule if on insulin	Not necessary; if desired, should be included in total day's meal plan. If on insulin, coordinate with insulin schedule or adjust insulin as needed.

*Reasonable body weight is that which is achievable and maintainable for the patient, although it may not be in the range considered desirable. For example, a reasonable weight goal for a patient weighing 105 kg may be 95 kg, although desirable body weight may actually be closer to 84 kg. Losing 4.5 to 9 kg may dramatically improve a person's glucose intolerance and may be a maintainable weight loss. Individual weight goals should be discussed and set.

†Individualization should be based on nutritional adequacy, promotion of diet adherence, and glucose and lipid control. Postprandial glucose response to a high-sucrose snack or meal should be evaluated; use of food and glucose records is helpful.

‡For example, 12% of a 1,200-kcal diet is only 36 g protein, which is less than the Recommended Dietary Allowance (9) for a 163-cm-tall woman; 20% of a 1,200-kcal diet will provide the recommended 60 g protein.

(From Beebe, C. A., Pastors, J. G., Powers, M. A., et al.: Nutrition management for individuals with noninsulin-dependent diabetes mellitus in the 1990's: A review by the Diabetes Care and Education dietetic practice group. J. Am. Diet. Assoc., *91*:199, 1991. With permission.)

TABLE 1-26A. RENAL DIETS

Purpose: The diet for chronic renal insufficiency (CRI) is designed to slow the progression of kidney disease and possibly delay the need for maintenance dialysis. The diet for chronic renal failure (CRF) is designed to meet nutritional requirements, minimize uremic complications, and maintain acceptable blood chemistries, blood pressure, and fluid status in patients with impaired renal function.

Use: The CRI diet (often called the predialysis diet) is indicated for patients with chronic renal insufficiency who do not yet require dialysis. The CRF diet is used for patients requiring hemodialysis or peritoneal dialysis treatments.

Modifications: The CRI diet is restricted in two major areas—protein and phosphorus. Restrictions of sodium, potassium, fluid, and calories are based on individual needs.[1-5] Generally, the CRF diet reflects controlled intake of protein, potassium, sodium, phosphorus, and fluids. Additional modifications of fat, cholesterol, triglycerides, and fiber may be necessary based on individual requirements.[6,7] Certain underlying conditions may require the adjustment of kilocalories.

SUMMARY OF NUTRIENT RECOMMENDATIONS FOR ADULT PATIENTS WITH CRI, HEMODIALYSIS, AND PERITONEAL DIALYSIS[4-12]

Nutrient	CRI	Hemodialysis	Peritoneal Dialysis
Protein	0.6-0.8 g/kg ideal body weight	1.1-1.4 g/kg ideal body weight; at least 60% high biologic value	1.2-1.5 g/kg ideal body weight 1.2-1.3 maintenance 1.5 repletion 1.2 reduction or with diabetes
Energy	Normal weight: 35 kcal/kg ideal body weight: Obese: 20-30 kcal/kg ideal body weight Underweight or catabolic: 45 kcal/kg ideal body weight	30-35 kcal/kg ideal body weight	20-50 kcal/kg ideal body weight 25-35 maintenance 35-50 repletion 20-25 reduction 35 with diabetes (for CAPD and CCPD, include dialysate calories)*
Phosphorus	5-10 mg/kg ideal body weight (IBW)	< 17 mg/kg IBW or approximately 800-1,200 mg/day	< 17 mg/kg IBW or approximately 1,200 mg/day
Sodium	1,000-3,000 mg/day if necessary; additional sodium may be required with salt-losing nephropathic conditions	1,000-3,000 mg/day	Individualized based on blood pressure and weight; CAPD and CCPD, 3,000-4,000 mg/day; IPD, 2,000-3,000 mg/day*
Potassium	Generally not restricted unless potassium is elevated and urine output is < 1 L/d	40 mg/kg ideal body weight or approximately 50-80 mEq/day	Generally unrestricted with CAPD and CCPD; IPD, 2,000-3,000 mg/day*

(Continued)

TABLE 1–26A. (CONTINUED)

SUMMARY OF NUTRIENT RECOMMENDATIONS FOR ADULT PATIENTS WITH CRI, HEMODIALYSIS, AND PERITONEAL DIALYSIS[4-12]

Nutrient	CRI	Hemodialysis	Peritoneal Dialysis
Fluid	Generally unrestricted; balance fluid intake with urine output in patients with edema or congestive heart failure	500-750 ml/day plus urine output or approximately 750-1,500 ml/day	CAPD and CCPD, approximately 2,000-3,000 ml/day based on daily weight fluctuations and blood pressure; IPD, same as for hemodialysis*
Calcium	1,200-1,600 mg/day	Approximately 1,000-1,800 mg/day supplement as needed to maintain normal serum level	Same as for hemodialysis
Fat	None	Limit cholesterol to < 300 mg/day; emphasize use of polyunsaturated fats	Same as for hemodialysis

Adequacy: The CRI diet is deficient in calcium, iron, vitamin B_{12}, and zinc because of the low-phosphorus, low-protein intake. The need for vitamin and mineral supplementation should be assessed on an individual basis.[10] CRF diets containing less than 60 g of protein may be deficient in niacin, riboflavin, thiamin, and calcium for men and calcium and iron for women, according to the 1989 Recommended Dietary Allowances.

REFERENCES
1. Zeller, K.: N. Engl. J. Med., *324:*78–84, 1991.
2. Ihle, B. V.: N. Engl. J. Med., *321:*1773–1777, 1989.
3. Mitch, W. E.: *In* Nutrition and the Kidney. Edited by W. E. Mitch and S. Klahr. Boston, Little Brown, 1988.
4. Kopple, J. D.: *In* Modern Nutrition in Health and Disease. Edited by M. E. Shils and R. Young. Philadelphia, Lea & Febiger, 1988.
5. Blumen Krantz, M. J.: *In* Handbook of Dialysis. Edited by J. T. Daugirdas and T. S. Ing. Boston, Little Brown, 1988.
6. Alvestrand, A. S.: *In* Nutrition and the Kidney. Edited by W. E. Mitch and S. Klahr. Boston, Little Brown, 1988.
7. Diamond, S. M. Henrich, D. E.: *In* Nutrition and the Kidney. Edited by W. E. Mitch and S. Klahr. Boston, Little Brown, 1986.
8. Bergstrom, J.: Clin. Nephrol., *21:*29–35, 1984.
9. Hruska, A.: *In* Nutrition and the Kidney. Edited by W. E. Mitch and S. Klahr. Boston, Little Brown, 1988.
10. Wolkens, K., Schiro, K. (eds.): Suggested Guidelines for the Nutrition Care of Renal Patients. 2nd Ed. Chicago, The American Dietetic Association, 1992.
11. Renal Dietitians Dietetic Practice Group: National Renal Diet. Chicago, The American Dietetic Association, to be published.
12. Gillit, D., Stover, J., Spinozzi, N.S. (Eds.): A Clinical Guide to Nutrition Care in End-Stage Renal Disease. Chicago, American Dietetic Association, 1987.

*CAPD = continuous ambulatory peritoneal dialysis; CCPD = continuous cyclic peritoneal dialysis; IPD = intermittent peritoneal dialysis.
(Modified from The Manual of Clinical Dietetics. 4th Ed. Chicago, American Dietetic Association, 1992. With permission.)

TABLE A–26B-1. SAMPLE MENU FOR CHRONIC RENAL INSUFFICIENCY (70-kg man; 40 g protein, 2,000 kcal, 600 mg phosphorus)

BREAKFAST	LUNCH	DINNER
Orange juice (½ cup)	Roast beef (1 oz)	Baked chicken thigh (1 oz)
Cinnamon applesauce (½ cup)	Bread (2 slices)	White rice (½ cup)
Cornflakes (1 cup)	Mayonnaise (1 Tbsp)	Green beans (½ cup)
Toast (1 slice)	Lettuce salad (1 cup)	Low-sodium vegetable soup (½ cup)
Margarine (1 tsp)	Vinegar and oil dressing (1 Tbsp)	Dinner roll (1 small)
Jelly or jam (1 tsp)	Sliced canned peaches (1 cup)	Margarine (2 tsp)
Liquid nondairy creamer (½ cup)	Graham crackers (2)	Jelly
Coffee or tea with sugar	Lemon-lime soda (1 cup)	Strawberries (1 cup)
		Tea with sugar
		Lemonade (½ cup)
	SNACK	
	Apple pie (1 slice)	
	Tea with sugar	

APPROXIMATE NUTRIENT ANALYSIS

Energy (kcal)	2,057.2	Sodium (mg)	1,798.4
Protein (g) (7.9% of kcal)	40.6	Zinc (mg)	5.7
Carbohydrate (g) (61.8% of kcal)	317.6	Vitamin A (µg RE)	994.8
Total fat (g) (32.4% of kcal)	74.2	Vitamin C (mg)	180.2
Saturated fatty acids (g)	14.6	Thiamin (mg)	1.6
Monounsaturated fatty acids (g)	28.0	Riboflavin (mg)	1.4
Polyunsaturated fatty acids (g)	26.7	Niacin (mg)	19.1
Cholesterol (mg)	64.7	Folate (µg)	309.0
Calcium (mg)	258.1	Vitamin B$_6$ (mg)	1.3
Iron (mg)	12.5	Vitamin B$_{12}$ (µg)	1.0
Magnesium (mg)	172.9	Dietary fiber (g)	17.7
Phosphorus (mg)	549.3	Water-insoluble fiber (g)	11.4
Potassium (mg)	2,138.0		

(From The Manual of Clinical Dietetics. 4th Ed. Chicago, American Dietetic Association, 1992. With permission.)

TABLE A–26B-2. SAMPLE MENU FOR HEMODIALYSIS (70-kg man; 85 g protein, 2 g sodium, 2 g potassium, 1,000 mg phosphorus, 1,000 ml fluid)

BREAKFAST	LUNCH	DINNER
Cranberry juice (½ cup)	Low-sodium vegetable soup (½ cup)	Broiled chicken (3 oz)
Grapefruit (½)	Unsalted crackers (4)	White rice (½ cup)
Cornflakes (¾ cup)	Lean hamburger patty (3 oz)	Green beans (½ cup)
White toast (2 slices)	Hamburger bun (1)	Hard dinner roll (1)
Margarine (2 tsp)	Unsalted mayonnaise (1 Tbsp)	Margarine (2 tsp)
Jelly (1 tbsp)	Lettuce	Lettuce salad (1 cup)
Hard-boiled egg (1)	Canned pears (½ cup)	Salt-free vinegar and oil dressing (1 Tbsp)
Coffee (½ cup)	Graham crackers (4)	Baked apple with sugar (1)
Sugar (4 tsp)	Lemonade (½ cup)	2% milk (½ cup)
Liquid nondairy creamer (½ cup)		

SNACK THROUGHOUT DAY

Hard candy (6 pieces)
Lollipop (1 small)
Ginger ale (1 cup)

APPROXIMATE NUTRIENT ANALYSIS

Energy (kcal)	2,618.4	Sodium (mg)	1,901.7
Protein (g) (12.6% of kcal)	82.2	Zinc (mg)	9.7
Carbohydrate (g) (58.4% of kcal)	382.3	Vitamin A (μg RE)	860.3
Total fat (g) (30% of kcal)	87.2	Vitamin C (mg)	132.0
Saturated fatty acids (g)	21.8	Thiamin (mg)	1.6
Monounsaturated fatty acids (g)	32.7	Riboflavin (mg)	1.7
Polyunsaturated fatty acids (g)	25.0	Niacin (mg)	26.4
Cholesterol (mg)	347.8	Folate (μg)	235.0
Calcium (mg)	458.0	Vitamin B_6 (mg)	1.8
Iron (mg)	15.4	Vitamin B_{12} (μg)	3.0
Magnesium (mg)	196.5	Dietary fiber (g)	17.9
Phosphorus (mg)	946.4	Water-insoluble fiber (g)	11.9
Potassium (mg)	2,069.4		

(From The Manual of Clinical Dietetics. 4th Ed. Chicago, American Dietetic Association, 1992. With permission.)

TABLE A–26B-3. SAMPLE MENU FOR PERITONEAL DIALYSIS (70-kg man; 105 g protein, 3 g sodium, 1.4 g phosphorus, 3–4 g potassium)

BREAKFAST	LUNCH	DINNER
Cranberry juice (½ cup)	Low-sodium vegetable soup (1 cup)	Green salad (3½ oz)
Cornflakes (¾ cup)	Lean hamburger patty (3 oz)	Vinegar and oil dressing (1 Tbsp)
Banana (½)	Hamburger bun	Broiled chicken breast (4 oz)
White toast (2 slices)	Sliced tomato (2 oz) and lettuce	Herbed white rice (½ cup)
Margarine (2 tsp)	Fresh fruit salad (½ cup)	Broccoli spears (2)
Skim milk (½ cup)	Graham crackers (4)	Hard dinner roll (1)
Coffee/tea	Coffee/tea	Margarine (2 tsp)
		Fresh strawberries (¾ cup)
		Coffee/tea
	SNACK	
	Unsalted crackers (5)	
	Tuna salad (½ cup)	
	Orange (1 medium)	

APPROXIMATE NUTRIENT ANALYSIS

Energy (kcal)	2,125.6	Sodium (mg)	1,964.8
Protein (g) (20.2% of kcal)	107.6	Zinc (mg)	10.2
Carbohydrate (g) (46.8% of kcal)	248.8	Vitamin A (µg RE)	1,077.0
Total fat (g) (33.4% of kcal)	78.8	Vitamin C (mg)	278.4
Saturated fatty acids (g)	19.3	Thiamin (mg)	1.9
Monounsaturated fatty acids (g)	28.2	Riboflavin (mg)	1.9
Polyunsaturated fatty acids (g)	24.3	Niacin (mg)	40.0
Cholesterol (mg)	193.6	Folate (µg)	340.3
Calcium (mg)	549.9	Vitamin B_6 (mg)	2.9
Iron (mg)	16.5	Vitamin B_{12} (µg)	3.9
Magnesium (mg)	280.5	Dietary fiber (g)	18.7
Phosphorus (mg)	1,069.6	Water-insoluble fiber (g)	10.9
Potassium (mg)	3,170.0		

Note: Calories provided may need to be adjusted based on calories absorbed from the dialysate exchanges.
(From The Manual of Clinical Dietetics. 4th Ed. Chicago, American Dietetic Association, 1992. With permission.)

TABLE A–26C. AVERAGE CALCULATION FIGURES FOR PLANNING CRI AND CRF DIETS*

FOOD EXCHANGES	kcal	Pro (g)	Na (mg)	K (mg)	Phos (mg)
Milk	120	4.0	80	185	110
Milk substitutes†	140	0.5	40	80	30
Meat	65	7.0	25	100	65
Starches	90	2.0	80	35	35
Vegetables‡					
Low K	25	1.0	15	70	20
Medium K	25	1.0	15	150	20
High K	25	1.0	15	270	20
Fruits					
Low K	70	0.5	Trace	70	15
Medium K	70	0.5	Trace	150	15
High K	70	0.5	Trace	270	15
Fats	45	Trace	55	10	5
High-calorie choices§	100	Trace	15	20	5
Beverages	Varies	Varies	Varies	Varies	Varies
Salt choices	—	—	250	—	—

*Serving sizes for each food choice are shown in the following renal exchange lists (Table A–26d).

†Milk substitute choices are nondairy products that can be used in lieu of milk and milk products.

‡Average sodium level values do not include canned vegetables. Add 250 mg sodium for canned vegetables with added salt.

§High-calorie choices are foods high in carbohydrates that contain only a trace of protein and minimal electrolytes. These should be used to raise calorie intake to the desired level.

TABLE A–26D. RENAL EXCHANGE LISTS

MILK EXCHANGES FOR CRI AND CRF PATIENTS

(Average per choice: 4 g protein, 120 kcal, 80 mg sodium, 185 mg potassium, 110 mg phosphorus)

Milk (nonfat, low-fat, whole)	½ cup
Alterna	1 cup
Buttermilk, cultured	½ cup
Chocolate milk	½ cup
Light cream or half and half	½ cup
Ice milk or ice cream	½ cup
Yogurt, plain or fruit-flavored	½ cup
Evaporated milk	¼ cup
Cream cheese	3 Tbsp
Sour cream	4 Tbsp
Sherbet	1 cup
Sweetened condensed milk	¼ cup

NONDAIRY MILK SUBSTITUTES FOR CRI AND CRF PATIENTS

(Average per choice: 0.5 g protein, 140 kcal, 40 mg sodium, 80 mg potassium, 30 mg phosphorus)

Dessert, nondairy frozen	½ cup
Dessert topping, nondairy frozen	½ cup
Liquid nondairy creamer, polyunsaturated	½ cup

MEAT EXCHANGES FOR CRI AND CRF PATIENTS

(Average per ounce: 7 g protein, 65 kcal, 25 mg sodium, 100 mg potassium, 65 mg phosphorus)

Prepared without added salt

Beef

Round, sirloin, flank, cubed, T-bone, and porterhouse steak; tenderloin, rib, chuck, and rump roast; ground beef or ground chuck	1 oz

Pork

Fresh ham, tenderloin, chops, loin roast, cutlets	1 oz

(Continued)

Lamb	
Chops, leg, roasts	1 oz
Veal	
Chops, roasts, cutlets	1 oz
Poultry	
Chicken, turkey, Cornish hen, domestic duck, and goose	1 oz
Fish	
All fresh and frozen fish	1 oz
Lobster, scallops, shrimp, clams	1 oz
Crab, oysters	1½ oz
Canned tuna, canned salmon (unsalted)	1 oz
Sardines (unsalted)*	1 oz
Wild game	
Venison, rabbit, squirrel, pheasant, duck, goose	1 oz
Egg	
Whole	1 large
Egg white or yolk	2 large
Low-cholesterol egg product	¼ cup
Chitterlings	2 oz
Organ meats*	1 oz
Prepared with added salt	
Beef	
Deli-style roast beef†	1 oz
Pork	
Boiled or deli-style ham†	1 oz
Poultry	
Deli-style chicken or turkey†	1 oz
Fish	
Canned tuna, canned salmon†	1 oz
Sardines†	1 oz
Cheese	
Cottage†	¼ cup

High in sodium, phosphorus, and/or saturated fat (should be used in limited quantities)

Bacon

Frankfurters, bratwurst, Polish sausage

Lunch meats, including bologna, braunschweiger, liverwurst, picnic loaf, salami, summer sausage

All cheese except cottage cheese

STARCH EXCHANGES FOR CRI AND CRF PATIENTS

(Average per choice: 2 g protein, 90 kcal, 80 mg sodium, 35 mg potassium, 35 mg phosphorus)

Breads and rolls

Bread (French, Italian, raisin, light rye, sourdough white)	1 slice (1 oz)
Bagel	½ small (1 oz)
Bun, hamburger or hot dog	½
Danish pastry or sweet roll, no nuts	½ small
Dinner roll or hard roll	1 small
Doughnut	1 small
English muffin	½
Muffin, no nuts, bran or whole-wheat	1 small (1 oz)
Pancake‡§	1 small
Pita or pocket bread, 6"	½
Tortilla, corn, 6"	2
Tortilla, flour, 6"	1
Waffle‡§	1 small (1 oz)

Cereals and grains

Cereals, ready-to-eat, most brands§	¾ cup
Puffed rice	2 cups
Puffed wheat	1 cup
Cooked cereal	
Cream of rice or wheat, farina, Malt-O-Meal	½ cup
Oat bran or oatmeal, Ralston	⅓ cup
Corn meal, cooked	¾ cup
Grits, cooked	½ cup
Flour, all-purpose	2½ Tbsp
Pasta (noodles, macaroni, spaghetti), cooked	½ cup

(Continued)

TABLE A–26D. CONTINUED

Pasta made with egg (egg noodles), cooked	⅓ cup
Rice, white or brown, cooked	½ cup
Crackers and snacks	
Crackers (saltines, round butter)	4
Graham crackers	3 squares
Melba toast	3 oblong
RyKrisp§	3
Popcorn, plain	1½ cups popped
Tortilla chips	¾ oz (9 chips)
Pretzels, § sticks or rings	¾ oz (10 sticks)
Desserts	
Cake, angelfood	1/20 cake or 1 oz
Cake, 2" × 2"	1 square or 1½ oz
Sandwich cookies‡§	4
Shortbread cookies	4
Sugar cookies	4
Sugar wafers	4
Vanilla wafers	10
Fruit pie (apple, berry, cherry, peach)	⅛ pie
Sweetened gelatin	½ cup
High in poor-quality protein and phosphorus (should be used rarely and in limited quantities)	
Bran cereal or muffins, Grape-Nuts, granola cereal or bars	
Boxed, frozen, or canned meals, entrees, or side dishes	
Pumpernickel, dark rye, whole-wheat or oatmeal breads	
Whole-wheat crackers	
Whole-wheat cereals	
Starchy vegetables for CRI PATIENTS	
Corn	⅓ cup or ½ ear
Green peas	¼ cup
Potatoes, boiled, mashed	½ cup
Potatoes, baked, white or sweet	1 small (3 oz)

Potatoes, french fried — ½ cup or 10 small
Potatoes, hashed brown — ½ cup
Squash, butternut, mashed — ½ cup
Squash, winter, baked (all other varieties), cubed — 1 cup

VEGETABLE EXCHANGES FOR CRI PATIENTS

(Average per choice: 1 g protein, 25 kcal, 15 mg sodium, 20 mg phosphorus. See starch list for other vegetables. Prepared or canned without added salt.‖)

1 cup serving

Alfalfa sprouts
Cabbage
Celery
Cucumber (or ½ whole)
Eggplant
Endive
Escarole
Lettuce, all varieties
Pepper, green, sweet
Radishes, sliced (or 15 small)
Turnips
Watercress

½ cup serving

Artichoke
Bamboo shoots
Bean sprouts
Beans, green or wax
Beets
Carrots (or 1 small)
Cauliflower
Chard
Chinese cabbage
Collard greens
Kale
Kohlrabi
Mushrooms, fresh (or 4 medium)
Onions
Parsnips¶
Pumpkin
Rutabagas¶
Squash, summer
Tomato (or 1 medium)
Tomato juice, unsalted
Tomato juice, regular#
Tomato puree
Turnip greens
Vegetable juice cocktail, unsalted
Vegetable juice cocktail, regular#

¼ serving

Asparagus (or 2 spears)
Avocado (¼ whole)
Beet greens
Mushrooms, cooked
Mustard greens
Okra

(Continued)

Broccoli
Brussels sprouts
Chili pepper

Snow peas
Spinach
Tomato sauce

VEGETABLE EXCHANGES FOR CRF PATIENTS

(Average per choice: 1 g protein, 25 kcal, 15 mg sodium, 20 mg phosphorus. ½ cup per choice unless otherwise indicated. Prepared or canned without added salt.‖)

Low potassium (0–100 mg)

Alfalfa sprouts (1 cup)
Bamboo shoots, canned
Bean sprouts
Beans, green or wax
Cabbage, raw
Chard, raw
Chinese cabbage, raw

Cucumber, peeled
Endive
Lettuce, all varieties (1 cup)
Escarole
Pepper, green, sweet
Watercress
Water chestnuts, canned

Medium potassium (101–200 mg)

Artichoke
Broccoli
Cabbage, cooked
Carrots (1 small raw)
Cauliflower
Celery, raw (1 stalk)
Collards
Corn (or ½ ear)¶
Eggplant
Kale

Mushrooms, canned¶ or fresh
Mustard greens
Onions
Peas, green¶
Radishes
Snow peas¶
Spinach, raw
Squash, summer
Turnip greens
Turnips

High potassium (201–350 mg)

Asparagus¶ (5 spears)
Avocado (¼ whole)
Bamboo shoots,** fresh cooked
Beet greens** (¼ cup)

Potato,** hash browned
Potato chips** (1 oz or 14 chips)
Pumpkin
Rutabagas

Beets
Brussels sprouts¶
Celery, cooked
Chard**
Kohlrabi
Mushrooms,¶ fresh cooked
Okra¶
Parsnips¶
Pepper, chili
Potato,** baked (½ medium)
Potato,¶ boiled or mashed

Spinach, cooked¶**
Sweet potato¶**
Tomato (1 medium)
Tomato juice, unsalted
Tomato juice, regular#
Tomato paste¶ (2 Tbsp)
Winter squash¶ (¼ cup)

FRUIT EXCHANGES FOR CRI PATIENTS

(Average per choice: 0.5 g protein, 70 kcal, 15 mg phosphorus)

1 cup serving
Apple (1 medium)
Apple juice
Applesauce
Cranberries
Cranberry juice cocktail

½ cup serving
Apricot nectar
Banana (½ small)
Blueberries
Figs, canned
Fruit cocktail
Grape juice
Grapefruit (½ medium)
Grapefruit juice
Grapes (15 small)
Gooseberries

Papaya nectar
Peach nectar
Pear nectar
Pear, canned or fresh (1 medium)
Tangerine (1 medium)

Lemon (½ medium)
Lemon juice
Mango (½ medium)
Nectarine (½ medium)
Orange (½ medium)
Peach, canned or fresh (½ medium)
Pineapple
Plums, canned or fresh (1 medium)
Rhubarb
Strawberries

(Continued)

TABLE A-26D. CONTINUED

Kiwifruit (½ medium)

¼ cup serving
Apricots (2 halves)
Apricots, dried (2)
Blackberries
Cantaloupe (⅛ small)
Cherries
Dates (2 Tbsp)
Figs, dried (1 whole)

Watermelon

Honeydew melon (⅛ small)
Orange juice
Papaya (¼ medium)
Prune juice
Prunes, cooked (5)
Raisins (2 Tbsp)
Raspberries

FRUIT EXCHANGES FOR CRF PATIENTS

(Average per choice: 0.5 g protein, 70 kcal, 15 mg phosphorus, ½ cup per choice unless otherwise indicated)

Low potassium (0–100 mg)

Applesauce	Lemon (½)
Blueberries	Papaya nectar
Cranberries (1 cup)	Peach nectar
Cranberry juice cocktail (1 cup)	Pear nectar
Grape juice	Pears, canned

Medium potassium (101–200 mg)

Apple (1 small, 2½" diameter)	Papaya
Apple juice	Peach, canned
Apricot nectar	Peach, fresh (1 small, 2" diameter)
Blackberries	Pineapple, canned or fresh
Cherries, sour or sweet	Plums, canned or fresh (1 medium)
Fruit cocktail	Raisins (2 Tbsp)
Gooseberries	Raspberries
Grapefruit (½ small)	Rhubarb
Grapefruit juice	Strawberries
Grapes (15 small)	Tangerine (2½" diameter)
Lemon juice	Watermelon (1 cup)
Mango	

High potassium (201–350 mg)

Apricots, canned or fresh (2 halves)	Kiwifruit (½ medium)
Apricots, dried (5)	Nectarine (1 small, 2" diameter)
Banana** (½ medium)	Orange (1 small, 2½" diameter)
Cantaloupe (⅛ small)	Orange juice
Dates (¼ cup)	Pear, fresh (1 medium)
Figs, dried (2 whole)	Prune juice**
Honeydew melon (⅛ small)	Prunes,** dried or canned (5)

FAT EXCHANGES FOR CRI AND CRF PATIENTS

(Average per choice: trace protein, 45 kcal, 55 mg sodium, 10 mg potassium, 5 mg phosphorus)

Unsaturated fats

Margarine	1 tsp
Reduced-calorie margarine	1 Tbsp
Mayonnaise	1 tsp
Low-calorie mayonnaise	1 Tbsp
Oil	
Safflower, sunflower, corn, soybean, olive, peanut, canola	1 tsp
Salad dressing, mayonnaise-type	2 tsp
Salad dressing, oil-type	1 Tbsp
Low-calorie salad dressing (mayonnaise-type)††	2 Tbsp
Low-calorie salad dressing†† (oil-type)	2 Tbsp
Tartar sauce	1½ tsp

Saturated fats

Butter	1 tsp
Coconut	2 Tbsp
Powdered coffee whitener	1 Tbsp
Solid shortening	1 tsp

HIGH CALORIE CHOICES FOR CRI AND CRF PATIENTS

(Average per choice: trace protein, 100 kcal, 15 mg sodium, 20 mg potassium, 5 mg phosphorus)

Beverages (count within fluid allowance)

Carbonated beverages	1 cup	
Fruit flavors, root beer, colas,‡‡ or pepper type		
Fruit-flavored drink		1 cup
Kool-Aid		1 cup
Limeade		1 cup

(Continued)

TABLE A-26D. CONTINUED

Cranberry juice cocktail	1 cup	Lemonade	1 cup
Frozen desserts (count within fluid allowance)		Tang	1 cup
Fruit ice	½ cup	Wine§§	½ cup
Juice bar (3 oz)	1 bar		
Candy and sweets		Popsicle (3 oz)	1 bar
Candy corn	20 or 1 oz	Sorbet	½ cup
Gumdrops	15 small		
Hard candy	4 pieces	Butter mints	14
Jellybeans	10	Fruit chews	4
LifeSavers or cough drops	12	Chewy fruit snacks	1 pouch
Marshmallows	5 large	Fruit Roll-Ups	2
Honey	2 Tbsp	Cranberry sauce or relish	¼ cup
Sugar, brown or white	2 Tbsp		
Jam or jelly	2 Tbsp		
Sugar, powdered	3 Tbsp		
Marmalade	2 Tbsp		
Syrup	2 Tbsp		
Special low-protein products for CRI PATIENTS			
Low-protein gelled dessert	½ cup		
Low-protein bread	1 slice		
Low-protein cookies	2		
Low-protein pasta	½ cup		
Low-protein rusk	2 slices		

SALT CHOICES FOR CRI AND CRF PATIENTS

(Average per choice: 250 mg sodium)

Salt	⅛ tsp
Seasoned salts (onion, garlic)	⅛ tsp
Accent	¼ tsp
Barbecue sauce	2 Tbsp
Bouillon	⅓ cup

Catsup	1½ Tbsp
Chili sauce	1½ Tbsp
Dill pickle	⅙ large or ½ oz
Mustard	4 tsp
Olives, green	2 medium or ⅓ oz
Olives, black	3 large or 1 oz
Soy sauce	¾ tsp
Steak sauce	2½ tsp
Sweet pickle relish	2½ Tbsp
Taco sauce	2 Tbsp
Tamari sauce	¾ tsp
Teriyaki sauce	1¼ tsp
Worcestershire sauce	1 Tbsp

BEVERAGE CHOICES FOR CRF PATIENTS

The following beverages may be used as desired within daily fluid allowance.

Carbonated beverages (except Moxie, colas, and pepper-type)
Ice
Lemonade
Limeade
Mineral water
Water

The following beverages contain moderate amounts of potassium and/or phosphorus and should be used in limited quantities.

Beer and wine§§
Coffee, regular or decaffeinated
Coffee substitute (cereal grain beverage)
Fruit-flavored drinks with added vitamin C
Tea
Thirst quencher beverages

(Continued)

TABLE A–26D. (CONTINUED)

The following liquids are very high in sodium and/or potassium and should only be used as advised by a physician or dietitian.
Bouillon
Broth
Consomme
Salt-free broth or bouillon containing potassium chloride (KCl)
Remember: anything that is liquid or melts at room temperature must also be counted in fluid allowance (for example, ice cream, Popsicles, sherbet, gelatin).

*High phosphorus—≥ 100 mg/serving.
†High sodium—each serving counts as 1 meat choice and 1 salt choice.
‡High phosphorus—≥ 70 mg/serving.
§High sodium—each serving counts as 1 starch choice and 1 salt choice.
‖For vegetables canned with salt, add 250 mg sodium and count as 1 vegetable choice and 1 salt choice.
¶High phosphorus—≥ 40 mg/serving.
#Very high sodium—each serving counts as 1 vegetable choice and 2 salt choices.
**Very high potassium—≥ 300 mg/serving.
††High sodium—each serving counts as 1 fat choice and 1 salt choice.
‡‡High phosphorus—≥ 20 mg/serving.
§§Check with physician for recommendation regarding alcohol.
Alterna, Ross Laboratories; Malt-O-Meal, Malt-O-Meal Co; Ralston, RyKrisp, Ralston Purina Co; Grape-Nuts, Kool-Aid, Tang, General Foods Corp; Popsicle, Popsicle Industries Inc; LifeSavers, Nabisco Brands, Inc; Fruit Roll-Ups, General Mills, Inc; Accent, Pet Inc; Moxie, Monarch Co, Atlanta GA 30341.
(Modified from Renal Dietitians Dietetic Practice Group: National Renal Diet. Chicago, The American Dietetic Association. In press. With permission.)

TABLE A–27A. SODIUM-CONTROLLED DIETS

Purpose: The goal of sodium restriction is to manage hypertension in sodium-sensitive individuals and promote the loss of excess fluids in edema and ascites.

General Rules

1. Avoid the use of all salt, baking soda, and/or baking powder in cooking and for table use.
2. Avoid medicines, laxatives, and salt substitutes unless prescribed by a physician.
3. Read labels carefully for sodium or salt content of packaged foods.

Modifications

1. *3,000 mg sodium (130 mEq).* Eliminate high-sodium processed foods and beverages, such as fast foods; salad dressings; smoked, salted, and koshered meats; regular canned food; pickled vegetables; luncheon meats; and commercially softened water. Allow up to 0.25 tsp table salt in cooking or at the table.
2. *2,000 mg sodium (87 mEq).* Eliminate processed and prepared foods and beverages high in sodium. Do not allow any salt in the preparation of foods or at the table. Limit milk and milk products to 16 fl oz daily. Check labels of canned and instant grain products for high-sodium sources.

3. *1,000 mg sodium (45 mEq).* Eliminate processed and prepared foods and beverages high in sodium. Omit regular canned foods, many frozen foods, deli foods, fast foods, cheeses, margarines, and regular salad dressings. Limit regular breads to 2 servings per day. Limit milk and milk products to 16 fl oz daily. Do not allow any salt in food preparation or for table use.
4. *500 mg sodium (22 mEq).* Omit canned or processed foods containing salt. Do not use any salt in food preparation or at the table. Omit vegetables containing high amounts of natural sodium. Limit meat to 6 oz daily, and milk and milk products to 8 fl oz daily. Use low-sodium bread in place of regular, and distilled water for cooking and drinking. This meal plan is used on a short-term basis only.
5. *250 mg sodium (11 mEq).* Use this meal plan for short terms only. Include the same foods as those in the 500-mg sodium diet, but use low-sodium milk in place of regular milk.

Adequacy: Based on the individual's food choices, the diets are adequate in all nutrients according to the 1989 National Research Council's Recommended Dietary Allowances. Unless carefully planned, however, the 250-mg and the 500-mg sodium diets can be inadequate in some nutrients.

(From The Manual of Clinical Dietetics. 4th Ed. Chicago, American Dietetic Association, 1992. With permission.)

TABLE A–27B-1. SAMPLE MENU FOR 3,000-MG SODIUM DIET*

BREAKFAST	LUNCH	DINNER
Orange juice (½ cup)	Low-sodium vegetable soup (1 cup)	Green salad (3½ oz)
Whole-grain cereal (¾ cup)	Unsalted crackers (4)	Vinegar and oil dressing (1 Tbsp)
Banana (½)	Lean beef patty (3 oz)	Broiled skinless chicken breast (3 oz)
Whole-wheat toast (2 slices)	Hamburger bun (1)	Herbed brown rice (½ cup)
Margarine (2 tsp)	Mustard (1 Tbsp)	Steamed broccoli (½ cup)
Jelly or jam (1 Tbsp)	Catsup (1 Tbsp)	Whole-grain roll (1)
2% milk (1 cup)	Sliced tomato (2 oz) and lettuce	Margarine (2 tsp)
Coffee/tea	Fresh fruit salad (½ cup)	Low-fat frozen yogurt (½ cup)
	Graham crackers (4)	Medium apple (1)
	2% milk (1 cup)	Coffee/tea
	Coffee/tea	

APPROXIMATE NUTRIENT ANALYSIS

Energy (kcal)	2,144.7	Sodium (mg)	2,334.8
Protein (g) (19.2% of kcal)	103.1	Zinc (mg)	13.3
Carbohydrate (g) (54.1% of kcal)	290.2	Vitamin A (μg RE)	1,409.2
Total fat (g) (29.2% of kcal)	69.6	Vitamin C (mg)	167.1
Saturated fatty acids (g)	22.6	Thiamin (mg)	1.8
Monounsaturated fatty acids (g)	25.0	Riboflavin (mg)	2.4
Polyunsaturated fatty acids (g)	15.0	Niacin (mg)	31.1
Cholesterol (mg)	186.6	Folate (μg)	400.3
Calcium (mg)	1,147.8	Vitamin B$_6$ (mg)	2.9
Iron (mg)	16.9	Vitamin B$_{12}$ (μg)	4.3
Magnesium (mg)	459.8	Dietary fiber (g)	24.2
Phosphorus (mg)	1,604.3	Water-insoluble fiber (g)	17.2
Potassium (mg)	4,056.5		

*May use up to ¼ tsp salt per day in cooking and at the table.
(From The Manual of Clinical Dietetics. 4th Ed. Chicago, American Dietetic Association, 1992. With permission.)

TABLE A–27B-2. SAMPLE MENU FOR 2,000-MG SODIUM DIET

BREAKFAST	LUNCH	DINNER
Orange juice (½ cup)	Low-sodium vegetable soup (1 cup)	Green salad (3½ oz)
Whole-grain cereal (¾ cup)	Unsalted crackers (4)	Salt-free vinegar and oil dressing (1 Tbsp)
Banana (½)	Lean beef patty (3 oz)	Broiled skinless chicken breast (3 oz)
Whole-wheat toast (2 slices)	Hamburger bun (1)	Herbed brown rice (½ cup)
Margarine (2 tsp)	Mustard (1 Tbsp)	Steamed broccoli (½ cup)
Jelly or jam (1 Tbsp)	Low-sodium mayonnaise (1 Tbsp)	Whole-grain roll (1)
2% milk (1 cup)	Sliced tomato (2 oz) and lettuce	Margarine (2 tsp)
Coffee/tea	Fresh fruit salad (½ cup)	Italian fruit ice (½ cup)
	Graham crackers (4)	Medium apple (1)
	2% milk (1 cup)	Coffee/tea
	Coffee/tea	

APPROXIMATE NUTRIENT ANALYSIS

Energy (kcal)	2,239.7	Sodium (mg)	1,749.0
Protein (g) (17.5% of kcal)	98.1	Zinc (mg)	12.3
Carbohydrate (g) (53.2% of kcal)	297.8	Vitamin A (μg RE)	1,393.9
Total fat (g) (31.5% of kcal)	78.5	Vitamin C (mg)	165.2
Saturated fatty acids (g)	22.9	Thiamin (mg)	1.8
Monounsaturated fatty acids (g)	27.8	Riboflavin (mg)	2.2
Polyunsaturated fatty acids (g)	20.8	Niacin (mg)	30.7
Cholesterol (mg)	190.9	Folate (μg)	388.9
Calcium (mg)	989.5	Vitamin B$_6$ (mg)	2.9
Iron (mg)	16.2	Vitamin B$_{12}$ (μg)	3.9
Magnesium (mg)	422.8	Dietary fiber (g)	23.3
Phosphorus (mg)	1,462.2	Water-insoluble fiber (g)	16.4
Potassium (mg)	3,751.4		

(From The Manual of Clinical Dietetics. 4th Ed. Chicago, American Dietetic Association, 1992. With permission.)

TABLE A–27B-3. SAMPLE MENU FOR 1,000-MG SODIUM DIET

BREAKFAST	LUNCH	DINNER
Orange juice (½ cup)	Low-sodium vegetable soup (1 cup)	Green salad (3½ oz)
Shredded wheat cereal (¾ cup)	Unsalted crackers (4)	Salt-free vinegar and oil dressing (1 Tbsp)
Banana (½)	Lean beef patty (3 oz)	Broiled skinless chicken breast (3 oz)
Low sodium whole-wheat toast (2 slices)	Low-sodium bread (2 slices)	Herbed brown rice (½ cup)
Unsalted margarine (2 tsp)	Low-sodium mayonnaise (1 Tbsp)	Steamed broccoli (½ cup)
Jelly or jam (1 Tbsp)	Sliced tomato (2 oz) and lettuce	Whole-grain roll (1)
2% milk (1 cup)	Fresh fruit salad (½ cup)	Unsalted margarine (2 tsp)
Coffee/tea	Graham crackers (4)	Italian fruit ice (½ cup)
	2% milk (1 cup)	Medium apple (1)
	Coffee/tea	Coffee/tea

APPROXIMATE NUTRIENT ANALYSIS

Energy (kcal)	2,255.1	Sodium (mg)	1,040.7
Protein (g) (17.9% of kcal)	100.9	Zinc (mg)	13.4
Carbohydrate (g) (54% of kcal)	304.2	Vitamin A (µg RE)	1,111.9
Total fat (g) (31.1% of kcal)	78.0	Vitamin C (mg)	153.9
Saturated fatty acids (g)	22.7	Thiamin (mg)	1.5
Monounsaturated fatty acids (g)	27.5	Riboflavin (mg)	1.9
Polyunsaturated fatty acids (g)	20.8	Niacin (mg)	28.2
Cholesterol (mg)	191.1	Folate (µg)	336.4
Calcium (mg)	952.5	Vitamin B_6 (mg)	2.6
Iron (mg)	14.6	Vitamin B_{12} (µg)	3.9
Magnesium (mg)	469.6	Dietary fiber (g)	26.7
Phosphorus (mg)	1,563.6	Water-insoluble fiber (g)	19.7
Potassium (mg)	3,863.0		

(From The Manual of Clinical Dietetics. 4th Ed. Chicago, American Dietetic Association, 1992. With permission.)

TABLE A–27B-4. SAMPLE MENU FOR 500-MG SODIUM DIET

BREAKFAST	LUNCH	DINNER
Orange juice (½ cup)	Low-sodium vegetable soup (1 cup)	Green salad (3½ oz)
Shredded wheat cereal (¾ cup)	Unsalted crackers (4)	Salt-free vinegar and oil dressing (1 Tbsp)
Banana (½)	Lean beef patty (3 oz)	Broiled skinless chicken breast (3 oz)
Low sodium whole-wheat toast (2 slices)	Low-sodium bread (2 sices)	Herbed brown rice (½ cup)
Unsalted margarine (2 tsp)	Low-sodium mayonnaise (1 Tbsp)	Steamed broccoli (½ cup)
Jelly or jam (1 Tbsp)	Sliced tomato (2 oz) and lettuce	Low-sodium bread (1 slice)
2% milk (1 cup)	Unsalted pretzels (1 oz)	Unsalted margarine (2 tsp)
Coffee/tea	Fresh fruit salad (½ cup)	Italian fruit ice (½ cup)
	Fruit juice (1 cup)	Medium apple (1)
	Coffee/tea	Coffee/tea

APPROXIMATE NUTRIENT ANALYSIS

Energy (kcal)	2,220.8	
Protein (g) (17.3% of kcal)	96.0	
Carbohydrate (g) (57.2% of kcal)	317.4	
Total fat (g) (28.5% of kcal)	70.3	
Saturated fatty acids (g)	18.6	
Monounsaturated fatty acids (g)	24.8	
Polyunsaturated fatty acids (g)	20.2	
Cholesterol (mg)	170.3	
Calcium (mg)	652.5	
Iron (mg)	15.3	
Magnesium (mg)	438.1	
Phosphorus (mg)	1,316.2	
Potassium (mg)	3,552.3	
Sodium (mg)	594.7	
Zinc (mg)	12.3	
Vitamin A (μg RE)	1,109.7	
Vitamin C (mg)	232.0	
Thiamin (mg)	1.6	
Riboflavin (mg)	1.6	
Niacin (mg)	28.7	
Folate (μg)	347.2	
Vitamin B_6 (mg)	2.6	
Vitamin B_{12} (μg)	3.0	
Dietary fiber (g)	26.6	
Water-insoluble fiber (g)	19.2	

(From The Manual of Clinical Dietetics. 4th Ed. Chicago, American Dietetic Association, 1992. With permission.)

TABLE A-27C. GUIDELINES FOR FOOD SELECTION

FOOD CATEGORY	FOODS RECOMMENDED	FOODS EXCLUDED FOR 3,000-MG SODIUM DIET	ADDITIONAL FOODS EXCLUDED FOR 2,000-MG SODIUM DIET*	ADDITIONAL FOODS EXCLUDED FOR 1,000-MG SODIUM DIET*
Beverages	Milk Eggnog Buttermilk (limit to 1 cup per week) Low-sodium or salt-free vegetable juices Regular vegetable or tomato juice (limit to ½ cup per day)	Greater than ½ cup regular vegetable or tomato juice Commercially softened water for drinking or cooking	Buttermilk (>½ cup), malted milk, chocolate milk, milkshake Regular milk (>2 cups) Regular vegetable or tomato juice	No additional restrictions
Vegetables (2–4 servings per day)	Fresh and frozen vegetables Low-sodium canned, drained vegetables	Sauerkraut Pickled vegetables and others prepared in brine Vegetables seasoned with bacon, ham, or pork	Regular canned vegetables Frozen vegetables prepared in sauce	Frozen peas, frozen lima beans, frozen mixed vegetables
Fruits (2 or more servings per day)	All fruits and fruit juices	No additional restrictions	Fruits processed with salt or sodium-containing compounds	No additional restrictions
Breads and cereals (4 or more servings per day)	Enriched white, wheat, rye, and pumpernickel Most cereals, hard rolls, and dinner rolls Crackers Unsalted snack crackers Breadsticks Biscuits, muffins, cornbread, pancakes, and waffles	Breads and rolls with salted tops Instant hot cereals	Quick breads Instant hot cereals Cooked dry cereals with added sodium Crackers with salted tops Self-rising flour and biscuit mixes Regular bread crumbs or cracker crumbs Commercial bread stuffing	Sweet rolls, crackers, and other products containing salt, baking powder, or self-rising flour Dry cereals

		Commercially prepared	No additional restrictions	Instant potatoes
Potato or substitute	White or sweet potatoes Squash Enriched rice, barley, noodles, spaghetti, macaroni, and other pastas	Commercially prepared potato, rice, and pasta mixes Commercial stuffing		Instant potatoes
Meat or substitute	Homemade bread stuffing Fresh or fresh-frozen meats (beef, lamb, pork, veal, and game) Fresh or fresh-frozen poultry (chicken, turkey, Cornish hen, and others) Fresh-water or fresh-frozen unbreaded fish Most shellfish Canned tuna, rinsed Canned salmon, rinsed Eggs and egg substitutes Cheese in limited amounts Low-sodium cheese as desired Ricotta cheese and cream cheese (limit 2 oz per day) Cottage cheese, drained Regular yogurt Regular peanut butter (3 times per week) Dried peas and beans Frozen dinners (<600 mg sodium)	Any meat, fish, or poultry that is smoked, cured, salted, koshered, or canned (bacon, chipped beef, coldcuts, ham, hot dogs, and sausages) Sardines, anchovies, marinated herring, and pickled meats Pickled eggs Frozen breaded meats Processed cheese, cheese spreads, and sauces Salted nuts	Crab Lobster Regular hard and processed cheese Regular peanut butter Frozen dinner entrees (<500 mg sodium)	All shellfish Egg substitutes

(Continued)

TABLE A–27C. CONTINUED

FOOD CATEGORY	FOODS RECOMMENDED	FOODS EXCLUDED FOR 3,000-MG SODIUM DIET	ADDITIONAL FOODS EXCLUDED FOR 2,000-MG SODIUM DIET*	ADDITIONAL FOODS EXCLUDED FOR 1,000-MG SODIUM DIET*
Fats	Butter or margarine Vegetable oils Low-sodium salad dressing as desired Regular salad dressing in limited amounts Light, sour, and heavy cream	Salad dressings containing bacon, bacon fat, bacon bits, and salt pork Snack dips made with instant soup mixes and/ or processed cheese	No additional restrictions	Nondairy cream (≤1 fl oz allowed per day) Salted butter or margarine Regular mayonnaise
Soups	Commercial canned and dehydrated soups, broth, and bouillon Homemade soups without added salt, made with allowed vegetables Homemade broth Low-sodium canned soups and broths	Excessive amounts of canned or dehydrated soups (>1 cup per week)	Regular canned or dehydrated commercial soups, broths, or bouillon	No additional restrictions
Sweets and desserts	Any sweets and desserts allowed	No additional restrictions	Desserts and sweets made with milk exceeding allowance	All candies made with sweet chocolate, nuts, or coconut Desserts make with rennin, rennin tablets Sherbets and flavored gelatin (>½ cup per day) Salted bakery foods, homemade or commercial

Miscellaneous		No additional restrictions
Limit added salt to ¼ tsp per day used at the table or in cooking	Any seasoning containing salt (garlic salt, celery salt, onion salt, and seasoned salt)	Regular catsup, chili sauce, mustard, pickles, relishes, olives, and horseradish
Salt substitute with physician's approval	Sea salt, rock salt, and kosher salt	Barbecue, Worcestershire, and steak sauce
Pepper, herbs, and spices	Any other seasoning containing salt and sodium compounds (meat tenderizers, monosodium glutamate [MSG: Accent])	Canned gravies and mixes
Vinegar		
Lemon or lime juice		
Hot pepper sauce	Regular soy sauce	
Low-sodium soy sauce	Teriyaki sauce	
Unsalted tortilla chips, pretzels, potato chips, popcorn	Most flavored vinegars	
	Regular snack chips	

Guidelines for food selection for 500-mg sodium diet. Use the 1000-mg sodium diet guidelines with the following modifications:

- Use low sodium bread only.
- Omit sherbet and flavored gelatin.
- Limit meat to 6 oz per day. One egg may be used per day in place of 1 oz of meat.
- Omit the following vegetables: beets, beet greens, carrots, kale, spinach, celery, white turnips, rutabagas, mustard greens, chard, peas, and dandelion greens.
- Use distilled water.
- Limit milk and milk products to 8 oz per day.

*The foods listed under the 2 "Additional Foods Excluded" categories represent additions to the foods already excluded either in the preceding column (for 2,000-mg diet) or in the preceding 2 columns (for 1,000-mg diet).

(Adapted from The Manual of Clinical Dietetics. 4th ed. Chicago, American Dietetic Association, 1992. With permission.)

TABLE A–28A. RECOMMENDED DIET MODIFICATIONS TO LOWER BLOOD CHOLESTEROL

Purpose: The general aim of dietary therapy is to reduce elevated cholesterol levels while maintaining a nutritionally adequate eating pattern.

Use: Dietary therapy should occur in two steps, the Step-One and Step-Two Diets, that are designed to progressively reduce intakes of saturated fatty acids and cholesterol and to promote weight loss in patients who are overweight by eliminating excess total calories. The Step-One Diet should be prescribed and explained by the physician and his or her staff. This diet involves an intake of total fat less than 30% of calories, saturated fatty acids less than 10% of calories, and cholesterol less than 300 mg/day. The Step-Two Diet, used if the response to the Step-One Diet is insufficient, calls for a further reduction in saturated fatty acid intake to less than 7% of calories and in cholesterol to less than 200 mg/day. The Step-One Diet calls for the reduction of the major and obvious sources of saturated fatty acids and cholesterol in the diet; for many patients this can be achieved without a radical alteration in dietary habits. The Step-Two Diet requires careful attention to the whole diet to reduce intake of saturated fatty acids and cholesterol to a minimal level compatible with an acceptable and nutritious diet. Involvement of a registered dietitian is useful, particularly for intensive dietary therapy, such as the Step-Two Diet.

After starting the Step-One Diet, the total serum cholesterol level should be measured and adherence to the diet assessed at 4 to 6 weeks and at 3 months. If the total cholesterol monitoring goal is met, the LDL-cholesterol level should be measured to confirm that the LDL goal has been achieved. If this is the case, the patient enters a long-term monitoring program and is seen quarterly for the first year and twice yearly thereafter. At these visits total cholesterol level should be measured, and dietary and behavior modifications reinforced.

If the cholesterol goal has not been achieved with the Step-One Diet, the patient should generally be referred to a registered dietitian. With the aid of the dietitian, the patient should progress to the Step-Two Diet, or to another trial on the Step-One Diet (with progression to the Step-Two Diet if the response is still not satisfactory). On the Step-Two Diet, total cholesterol levels should again be measured and adherence to the diet assessed after 4 to 6 weeks and at 3 months of therapy. If the desired goal for total cholesterol (and for LDL-cholesterol) lowering has been attained, long-term monitoring can begin. If not, drug therapy should be considered. A minimum of 6 months of intensive dietary therapy and counseling should usually be carried out before initiating drug therapy; shorter periods can be considered in patients with severe elevations of LDL-cholesterol (> 225 mg/dl) or with definite coronary heart disease. Drug therapy should be added to, and not substituted for, dietary therapy.

Adequacy: Based on the individual's food choices, the diets are adequate in all nutrients according to the National Research Council's Recommended Dietary Allowances.

NATIONAL CHOLESTEROL EDUCATION PROGRAM: STEP-ONE AND STEP-TWO DIETS

NUTRIENT	RECOMMENDED INTAKE	
	Step-One Diet	Step-Two Diet
Total fat	Less than 30% of total calories	
Saturated fatty acids	Less than 10% of total calories	Less than 7% of total calories
Polyunsaturated fatty acids	Up to 10% of total calories	
Monounsaturated fatty acids	10% to 15% of total calories	
Carbohydrates	50% to 60% of total calories	
Protein	10% to 20% of total calories	
Cholesterol	Less than 300 mg/day	Less than 200 mg/day
Total calories	To achieve and maintain desirable weight	

(With permission from The National Cholesterol Education Program, Report of the Expert Panel on Detection, Evaluation, and Treatment of High Blood Cholesterol in Adults. U.S. Department of Health and Human Services, Public Health Service National Institutes of Health Publication No. 89-2925, 1989.)

TABLE A–28B. STEP-ONE DIET

FOOD CATEGORY	CHOOSE	DECREASE
Fish, chicken, turkey, and lean meat	Fish; poultry without skin; lean cuts of beef, lamb, pork or veal; shellfish	Fatty cuts of beef, lamb, pork; spare ribs; organ meats; regular cold cuts; sausage; hot dogs; bacon; sardines; roe
Skim and low-fat milk, cheese, yogurt, and dairy substitutes	Skim or 1% fat milk (liquid, powdered, evaporated); buttermilk	Whole milk (4% fat) (regular, evaporated, condensed); cream; half and half; 2% milk; imitation milk products; most nondairy creamers; whipped toppings
	Nonfat (0% fat) or low-fat yogurt	Whole-milk yogurt
	Low-fat cottage cheese (1% or 2% fat)	Whole-milk cottage cheese (4% fat)
	Low-fat, farmer, or pot cheeses (all of these should be labeled no more than 2 to 6 g fat/oz)	All natural cheeses (e.g., blue, roquefort, camembert, cheddar, swiss)
	Low-fat or "light" cream cheese, low-fat or "light" sour cream	Cream cheeses, sour cream
	Sherbet or sorbet	Ice cream
Eggs	Egg whites (2 whites = 1 whole egg in recipes), cholesterol-free egg substitutes	Egg yolks

Fruits and vegetables	Fresh, frozen, canned, or dried fruits and vegetables	Vegetables prepared in butter, cream, or other sauces
Breads and cereals	Homemade baked goods using unsaturated oils sparingly, angel food cake, low-fat crackers, low-fat cookies	Commercial baked goods: pies, cakes, doughnuts, croissants, pastries, muffins, biscuits, high-fat crackers, high-fat cookies
	Rice, pasta	Egg noodles
	Whole-grain breads and cereals (oatmeal, whole-wheat, rye, bran, multigrain, etc.)	Breads in which eggs are major ingredient
Fats and oils	Baking cocoa	Chocolate
	Unsaturated vegetable oils: corn, olive, rapeseed (canola oil), safflower, sesame, soybean, sunflower	Butter, coconut oil, palm oil, palm kernel oil, lard, bacon fat
	Margarine or shortening made from one of the unsaturated oils listed above	
	Diet margarine	
	Mayonnaise, salad dressings made with unsaturated oils listed above	Dressings made with egg yolk
	Low-fat dressings	
	Seeds and nuts	Coconut

TABLE A–28C-1. SAMPLE MENU FOR STEP-ONE DIET

BREAKFAST	LUNCH	DINNER
Orange juice (½ cup)	Vegetable soup (1 cup)	Green salad (3½ oz)
Whole-grain cereal (¾ cup)	Saltine crackers (4)	Vinegar and oil dressing (1 tbsp)
Banana (½)	Lean beef patty (3 oz)	Broiled skinless chicken breast (3 oz)
Whole-wheat toast (2 slices)	Hamburger bun (1)	Herbed brown rice (½ cup)
Diet margarine (2 tsp)	Mustard (1 tbsp)	Steamed broccoli (½ cup)
Jelly or jam (1 tbsp)	Low-fat mayonnaise (2 tsp)	Whole-grain roll (1)
1% milk (1 cup)	Sliced tomato (2 oz) and lettuce	Diet margarine (2 tsp)
Coffee/tea	Fresh fruit salad (½ cup)	Low-fat frozen yogurt (½ cup)
	Graham crackers (4)	Medium apple (1)
	1% milk (1 cup)	Coffee/tea
	Coffee/tea	

APPROXIMATE NUTRIENT ANALYSIS

Energy (kcal)	2,054.7	Iron (mg)	16.5	Thiamin (mg)	1.8
Protein (g) (19.9% of kcal)	102.1	Magnesium (mg)	456.4	Riboflavin (mg)	2.4
Carbohydrate (g) (55.5% of kcal)	285.3	Phosphorus (mg)	1,610.8	Niacin (mg)	29.0
Total fat (g) (27.1% of kcal)	61.8	Potassium (mg)	3,978.0	Folate (µg)	400.6
Saturated fatty acids (g)	19.4	Sodium (mg)	3,190.1	Vitamin B$_6$ (mg)	2.8
Monounsaturated fatty acids (g)	21.1	Zinc (mg)	14.4	Vitamin B$_{12}$ (µg)	4.4
Polyunsaturated fatty acids (g)	14.8	Vitamin A (µg RE)	1,378.8	Dietary fiber (g)	24.1
Cholesterol (mg)	167.8	Vitamin C (mg)	165.2	Water-insoluble fiber (g)	17.0
Calcium (mg)	1,126.4			

(From The Manual of Clinical Dietetics. Chicago, American Dietetic Association, 1992. With permission.)

TABLE A–28C-2. SAMPLE MENU FOR STEP-TWO DIET

BREAKFAST	LUNCH	DINNER
Orange juice (½ cup)	Vegetable soup (1 cup)	Green salad (3½ oz)
Whole-grain cereal (¾ cup)	Saltine crackers (4)	Vinegar and oil dressing (1 tbsp)
Banana (½)	Sliced turkey (3 oz)	Broiled skinless chicken breast (3 oz)
Whole-wheat toast (2 slices)	Whole-wheat bread (2 slices)	Herbed brown rice (½ cup)
Diet margarine (2 tsp)	Mustard (1 tbsp)	Steamed broccoli (½ cup)
Jelly or jam (1 tbsp)	Low-fat mayonnaise (2 tsp)	Whole-grain roll (1)
Skim milk (1 cup)	Sliced tomato (2 oz) and lettuce	Diet margarine (2 tsp)
Coffee/tea	Fresh fruit salad (½ cup)	Low-fat frozen yogurt (½ cup)
	Graham crackers (4)	Medium apple (1)
	Skim milk (1 cup)	Coffee/tea
	Coffee/tea	

APPROXIMATE NUTRIENT ANALYSIS

Energy (kcal)	1,892.5	Iron (mg)	15.6
Protein (g) (21.6% of kcal)	102.3	Magnesium (mg)	471.0
Carbohydrate (g) (61.2% of kcal)	289.7	Phosphorus (mg)	1,734.4
Total fat (g) (20.4% of kcal)	42.9	Potassium (mg)	4,024.4
Saturated fatty acids (g)	10.6	Sodium (mg)	3,565.7
Monounsaturated fatty acids (g)	13.3	Zinc (mg)	12.4
Polyunsaturated fatty acids (g)	14.7	Vitamin A (µg RE)	1,392.5
Cholesterol (mg)	126.5	Vitamin C (mg)	165.3
Calcium (mg)	1,129.9	Thiamin (mg)	1.7
		Riboflavin (mg)	2.1
		Niacin (mg)	32.6
		Folate (µg)	413.5
		Vitamin B$_6$ (mg)	2.8
		Vitamin B$_{12}$ (µg)	3.1
		Dietary fiber (g)	25.3
		Water-insoluble fiber (g)	18.0

(From The Manual of Clinical Dietetics. Chicago, American Dietetic Association, 1992. With permission.)

TABLE A-29A. GUIDELINES FOR FOOD SELECTION FOR FAT-RESTRICTED DIET (25 g or 50 g of FAT)

FOOD CATEGORY	RECOMMENDED	MAY CAUSE DISTRESS
Beverages	Skim milk; skim buttermilk; powdered and evaporated skim milk; coffee; tea; soda; other nondairy drinks	1%, 2%, whole milks; buttermilk made with whole milk; chocolate milk; evaporated milk; cream
Breads and cereals	Whole-grain breads; enriched breads; saltines; soda crackers; cold and cooked cereals; whole-grain cereal except granola-type; unbuttered popcorn; plain corn or flour tortillas	Biscuits; breads containing egg or cheese; sweet rolls; pancakes; French toast; doughnuts; waffles; fritters; buttered popcorn; muffins; granola-type cereals and breads to which extra fat is added; popovers; snack crackers with added fat; snack chips; stuffing; fried tortillas
Desserts	Sherbet; fruit ice; gelatin; angel food cake; vanilla wafers; graham crackers; meringues; pudding made with skim milk; fat-free commercial baked products; nonfat ice cream and frozen yogurt	All other cakes, cookies, pies, and pastries; puddings made with whole milk or eggs; cream puffs

Fats
Amount listed equals 1 fat equivalent; 3 to 5 equivalents/day allowed for 50-g fat diet. (Unsaturated fats are recommended.)
	Unsaturated
	Margarine (1 tsp)
	Diet margarine (1 Tbsp)
	Mayonnaise
	  reduced-calorie (1 Tbsp)
	  regular (1 tsp)
	Creamy salad dressings
	  reduced-calorie (1 Tbsp)
	  regular (2 tsp)
	Other salad dressings
	  reduced-calorie (2 Tbsp)
	  regular (1 Tbsp)
	Vegetable oils (1 tsp)
	Nuts
	  almonds (6 whole)
	  cashews (1 Tbsp or 2 whole)
		Any in excess of amounts prescribed on diets and all others

peanuts (20 small or 10 large)
peanut butter (2 tsp)
cashew butter (2 tsp)
walnuts (2 whole)
pistachios (18 whole)
other nuts (1 Tbsp)
Seeds
  sesame (1 Tbsp)
  sunflower (1 Tbsp)
  pumpkin (2 tsp)
Olives (10 small or 5 large)

Saturated
Bacon (1 slice)
Bacon fat (1 tsp)
Butter (1 tsp)
Whipped butter (2 tsp)
Chitterlings (½ oz)
Shredded coconut (2 Tbsp)
Cream
  light, coffee, table (2 Tbsp)
  heavy whipping (1 Tbsp)
Sour cream (2 Tbsp)
Cream cheese (1 Tbsp)
Coffee whitener
  liquid (2 Tbsp)
  powder (4 tsp)
Lard (1 tsp)
Oil
  coconut (1 tsp)
  palm (1 tsp)
Shortening (1 tsp)
Sour cream (2 Tbsp)
Salt pork (¼ oz)

(Continued)

TABLE A-29A. CONTINUED

FOOD CATEGORY	RECOMMENDED	MAY CAUSE DISTRESS
Fruits	Fresh, frozen, canned, or dried fruit; fruit juices	Avocado

Meats and meat substitutes
For 50-g fat diet, 6 oz/day
For 25-g fat diet, 5 oz/day
(Recommended preparation methods are broiling, roasting, grilling, or boiling; weigh meat after cooking.)
	Poultry
	  breast meat without skin
	Veal
	  all cuts
	Lean beef
	  USDA good or choice cuts (i.e., round, sirloin, flank steak, tenderloin, and chopped beef); roast (rib, chuck, rump); steak (cube, Porterhouse, T-bone); meatloaf made with ground beef (95% lean)
	Lean pork
	  fresh, canned, cured, or boiled ham; Canadian bacon; tenderloin; chops; loin roast; Boston butt; cutlets
	Lean lamb
	  chops, leg, or roast
	Fish
	  all fresh, frozen, or canned in water: crab, lobster, scallops, shrimp, clams, oysters, tuna; herring (uncreamed or smoked); sardines (canned, drained); salmon (canned in water)
	Luncheon meats
	  95% fat-free; lean ham, turkey, or beef
		Any fried, fatty, or heavily marbled meat, fish, or poultry
		Poultry
		  duck, goose
		Beef
		  most USDA prime cuts of beef, ribs, corned beef
		Pork
		  spareribs; ground pork sausage (patty or link); ham hocks; pigs' feet; chitterlings
		Lamb
		  patties (ground lamb)
		Fish
		  tuna (packed in oil)
		  salmon (packed in oil)
		Luncheon meats
		  most, including bologna, salami, pimento loaf
		Sausage
		  Polish; Italian; knockwurst; smoked bratwurst; frankfurter
		Legumes (cooked with added fat)

	Allowed	Not allowed

	Legumes
	  cooked, canned, without added fat
	Tofu, tempeh, natto
	Cheese
	  skim-milk cheeses; cottage cheese;
	  parmesan cheese
	Low-fat yogurt; non-fat yogurt as desired
	Eggs
	  poached; soft or hard cooked; scrambled,
	  not fried in fat; count 1 egg as 1 oz of
	  meat in daily meat allowance; egg
	  substitutes as desired	

Potatoes and potato substitutes	Potatoes; rice; barley; noodles; spaghetti, macaroni, and other pastas	Fried potatoes; fried rice; potato chips; chow mein noodles
Soups	Fat-free broth; fat-free vegetable soup; cream soup made with skim milk and allowed fat; packaged dehydrated soups	All others
Sweets	Sugar; honey; jelly; jam; marmalade; molasses; maple syrup; sourballs; gumdrops; jelly beans; marshmallows; hard candy; cocoa powder	Butter, coconut, chocolate, and cream candies
Vegetables	All fresh, frozen, or canned vegetables prepared without fats, oil, or fat-containing sauces	Buttered, au gratin, creamed, or fried vegetables unless made with allowed fat allowance
Miscellaneous	Catsup; chili sauce; vinegar; pickles; vanilla; unbuttered popcorn; white sauce made with skim milk and allowed fat; mustard; all herbs and seasonings; apple butter	Olives and nuts in excess of specified portions; cream sauces; gravies; buttered popcorn

(From The Manual of Clinical Dietetics. 4th Ed. Chicago. American Dietetic Association. 1992. With permission.)

TABLE A–29B-1. SAMPLE MENU FOR FAT-RESTRICTED DIET (25 g of FAT)

BREAKFAST	LUNCH	DINNER
Orange juice (1 cup)	Fat-free vegetable soup (1 cup)	Green salad (3½ oz)
Whole-grain cereal (¾ cup)	Saltine crackers (4)	Fat-free dressing (1 Tbsp)
Banana (1)	Sliced turkey (2 oz)	Broiled skinless chicken
Whole-wheat toast (2 slices)	Whole-wheat bread (2 slices)	breast (2 oz)
Jelly or jam (2 Tbsp)	Mustard (1 Tbsp)	Herbed brown rice (½ cup)
Skim milk (1 cup)	Fat-free mayonnaise (1 Tbsp)	Steamed broccoli (½ cup)
Coffee/tea	Sliced tomato (2 oz)	Whole-grain roll (1)
SNACK	and lettuce	Jelly or jam (1 Tbsp)
Canned or fresh fruit (1 cup)	Fresh fruit salad (½ cup)	Fruit ice or sorbet (½ cup)
Skim milk (½ cup)	Graham crackers (4)	Medium apple (1)
	Skim milk (1 cup)	Coffee/tea
	Coffee/tea	

APPROXIMATE NUTRIENT ANALYSIS

Energy (kcal)	2,016.4	Sodium (mg)	3,259.9
Protein (g) (18.8% of kcal)	94.7	Zinc (mg)	11.6
Carbohydrate (g) (75.6% of kcal)	380.9	Vitamin A (μg RE)	1,261.1
Total fat (g) (9.8% of kcal)	22.0	Vitamin C (mg)	271.7
Saturated fatty acids (g)	6.8	Thiamin (mg)	1.8
Monounsaturated fatty acids (g)	6.4	Riboflavin (mg)	2.2
Polyunsaturated fatty acids (g)	5.2	Niacin (mg)	28.7
Cholesterol (mg)	110.7	Folate (μg)	493.2
Calcium (mg)	1,169.7	Vitamin B$_6$ (mg)	3.3
Iron (mg)	16.6	Vitamin B$_{12}$ (μg)	2.9
Magnesium (mg)	512.5	Dietary fiber (g)	29.3
Phosphorus (mg)	1,672.1	Water-insoluble fiber (g)	20.2
Potassium (mg)	4,681.4		

(From The Manual of Clinical Dietetics. 4th Ed. Chicago, American Dietetic Association, 1992. With permission.)

TABLE A–29B-2. SAMPLE MENU FOR FAT-RESTRICTED DIET (50 g of FAT)

BREAKFAST	LUNCH	DINNER
Orange juice (½ cup)	Fat-free vegetable soup (1 cup)	Green salad (3½ oz)
Whole-grain cereal (¾ cup)	Saltine crackers (4)	Fat-free dressing (1 Tbsp)
Banana (½)	Lean beef patty (3 oz)	Broiled skinless chicken breast (3 oz)
Whole-wheat toast (2 slices)	Hamburger bun (1)	Herbed brown rice (½ cup)
Margarine (1 tsp)	Mustard (1 Tbsp)	Steamed broccoli (½ cup)
Jelly or jam (1 Tbsp)	Reduced-calorie mayonnaise (1 Tbsp)	Whole-grain roll (1)
Skim milk (1 cup)	Sliced tomato (2 oz) and lettuce	Margarine (1 tsp)
Coffee/tea	Fresh fruit salad (½ cup)	Fruit ice or sorbet (½ cup)
SNACK	Graham crackers (4)	Medium apple (1)
Canned peaches (½ cup)	Skim milk (1 cup)	Coffee/tea
Skim milk (½ cup)	Coffee/tea	

APPROXIMATE NUTRIENT ANALYSIS

Energy (kcal)	2,053.2	Sodium (mg)	3,016.8
Protein (g) (20.1% of kcal)	103.3	Zinc (mg)	14.2
Carbohydrate (g) (60.7% of kcal)	311.7	Vitamin A (µg RE)	1,373.5
Total fat (g) (21.6% of kcal)	49.3	Vitamin C (mg)	171.7
Saturated fatty acids (g)	15.2	Thiamin (mg)	1.8
Monounsaturated fatty acids (g)	18.6	Riboflavin (mg)	2.3
Polyunsaturated fatty acids (g)	9.4	Niacin (mg)	29.7
Cholesterol (mg)	159.0	Folate (µg)	400.4
Calcium (mg)	1141.8	Vitamin B_6 (mg)	2.9
Iron (mg)	16.3	Vitamin B_{12} (µg)	4.5
Magnesium (mg)	440.4	Dietary fiber (g)	24.4
Phosphorus (mg)	1,642.1	Water-insoluble fiber (g)	16.9
Potassium (mg)	4,170.9		

(From The Manual of Clinical Dietetics. 4th Ed. Chicago, American Dietetic Association, 1992. With permission.)

TABLE A–30A. RESTRICTED-FIBER DIET

Purpose: The fiber- and residue-restricted diet is designed to prevent blockage of a stenosed gastrointestinal tract and to reduce the frequency and volume of fecal output while prolonging intestinal transit time.

Suggested General Guidelines:

1. Limit milk and milk products to 2 cups daily. If lactose intolerant, see lactose-controlled diet.
2. Limit fruits to the following: juices without pulp (excluding prune), canned fruit, and ripe bananas. Most raw fruits should be avoided, such as dates, figs, prunes, apples, blackberries, boysenberries, peaches, grapes, pears, pineapple, rhubarb, and fresh grapefruit and orange sections.
3. Limit vegetables to the following: vegetable juices without pulp, lettuce, and cooked/canned vegetables without seeds, such as asparagus, beets, green beans, seedless tomatoes, spinach, eggplant, and acorn squash.
4. Use only white or refined bread and cereal products, or baked products using refined flour. Cooked white and sweet potatoes without skin, white rice, and refined pasta are allowed.
5. Avoid tough fibrous meats with gristle: Allow ground or well-cooked tender beef, lamb, ham, veal, pork, poultry, fish, and organ meats. Eggs and cheese are acceptable.
6. Avoid peanuts, coconut, nuts, seeds, popcorn, dried beans, peas, legumes, and lentils.

Modifications: A low-fiber diet is not synonymous with a low-residue diet. The term residue refers to both the indigestible content of a food that acts as a laxative and the total postdigestive luminal contents that increase fecal output.[1,2] A low-fiber diet also can be a low-residue diet if milk and products that contain milk are limited to 2 cups or less per day, prune juice is omitted, and meat and shellfish with tough connective tissue are avoided. Milk, prune juice, and connective tissue from meats are low in fiber but may increase colonic residue and stool weight by mechanisms other than dietary fiber.[1]

Adequacy: Based on the individual's food choices, the diet is adequate in all nutrients according to the National Research Council's Recommended Dietary Allowances, 1989. Vitamin and mineral supplementation may be indicated, however, when illness results in suboptimal intakes and increased requirements. The benefit of long-term restriction of dietary fiber remains controversial. Strict reductions in milk products, vegetables, and fruit intake may necessitate calcium, ascorbic acid, and folate supplementation. Individual response, particularly in patients with ulcerative colitis and Crohn's disease, must be monitored to avoid an overly restrictive regimen and to determine continued indication for this diet.

References

1. Kramer, P.: The meaning of high and low residue diets. *Gastroenterology,* 47:649, 1964.
2. Connell, A.M.: The role of fibre in the gastrointestinal tract. *In* The Clinical Role of Fibre. Edited by P.E. Bowen, A.M. Connell, et al. Toronto, Ontario, Canada, Medical Education Services, 1985.

(From The Manual of Clinical Dietetics. 4th Ed. Chicago, American Dietetic Association, 1992. With permission.)

TABLE A–30B. HIGH-FIBER DIET

Purpose: The diet is designed to be high in dietary fiber. It is useful for decreasing intraluminal colonic pressure, increasing gastrointestinal motility and increasing the volume and weight of material that reaches the distal colon. Both soluble and insoluble fibers exert these physiologic effects, whereas only soluble fibers exert metabolic effects, such as delayed glucose absorption, increased sensitivity to insulin, altered intestinal enzyme activity, binding of bile acids, and decrease in serum cholesterol and triglyceride levels.

General Guidelines

1. The reported positive effects of fiber are derived from a diet high in fiber-rich foods. Increased fiber intake should come from a variety of food sources rather than dietary fiber supplements. This approach is more likely to ensure increased intake of minerals and other nutrients.

2. Consumption of adequate amounts of liquids (eight 8-fluid-ounce glasses per day) in conjunction with high-fiber intake is recommended.

3. Prior to recommending a twofold increase in dietary fiber consumption, an assessment of current fiber intake should be made. Estimates of fiber content of household portions of foods are shown in Table A–30c.

4. Advise gradual increase of dietary fiber intake to minimize potential side effects.

Fiber Components and Food Sources

Water-soluble fibers are hydrated, resulting in gel-like or viscous substances, and are fermented by colonic bacteria.

Water-soluble fibers:

Gum

Mucilages   Foods containing water-soluble fibers include:

Pectin   Fruits, vegetables, barley,

Some hemicellulose   legumes, oat, and oat bran

Water-insoluble fibers remain essentially unchanged during digestion.

Water-insoluble fibers: Foods containing water-insoluble fibers include:

Cellulose

Lignin   Fruits, vegetables, cereals,

Some hemicellulose   whole-wheat products, and wheat bran

(Continued)

TABLE A–30B. (CONTINUED)

Adequacy: Depending on individual food selection, the high-fiber diet is adequate in all nutrients according to the National Research Council's Recommended Dietary Allowances, 1989.

The adequacy of the high-fiber diet may be questionable for individuals whose mineral intake is marginal because of poor dietary practices or for "at-risk" groups (children, pregnant or lactating women, elderly or chronically ill persons). Some studies indicate that excessive intakes of some dietary fiber sources may bind and interfere with the absorption of the following minerals: calcium, copper, iron, magnesium, selenium, and zinc.[1] It is hypothesized, however, that long-term high-fiber diet would not by itself cause mineral or nutrient imbalances in the general population.[2,3] Intake of adequate fluids is necessary because of hygroscopic nature of fiber.

The American Dietetic Association recommends a daily dietary fiber intake of 20 to 35 g from a variety of sources combined with a low-fat, high-carbohydrate diet.[4]

References

1. Walter, A.: Mineral metabolism. *In Dietary Fibre, Fibre-Depleted Foods and Disease.* Edited by H. Trowell, D. Burkitt, and K. Heaton. Orlando, Academic Press, 1985.
2. Gordon, D.T.: Total dietary fiber and mineral absorption. *In Dietary Fiber Chemistry, Physiology and Health Effects.* Edited by D. Kritchevsky, C. Bonfield, and J.W. Anderson. New York, Plenum Press, 1990.
3. Slavin, J.L.: Dietary fiber: classification, chemical analyses and food sources. J. Am. Diet. Assoc., 87:1164, 1987.
4. Position of The American Dietetic Association: Health implications of dietary fiber. Technical support paper. J. Am. Diet. Assoc., 88:216, 1988.

Further Reading

Anderson, J.W.: Fiber and health: an overview. *Am. J. Gastroenterol,* 82:892, 1986.

Judd, P., Truswell, S.: Dietary fibre and blood lipids in man. *In Dietary Fibre Perspectives, Reviews and Bibliography.* Edited by A. Leeds. London, John Libbey, 1985.

Klurfeld, D.M.: The role of dietary fiber in gastrointestinal disease. *J. Am. Diet. Assoc.,* 87:1178, 1987.

Lanza, E., and Batrum, R.: A critical review of fiber analysis and data. *J. Am. Diet. Assoc.,* 86:732, 1986.

(Modified from The Manual of Clinical Dietetics. 4th Ed. Chicago, American Dietetic Association, 1992. With permission.)

TABLE A–30C. DIETARY FIBER CONTENT OF FOODS IN COMMONLY SERVED PORTIONS

FOOD GROUP	<1 g	1–1.9 g	2–2.9 g	3–3.9 g	4–4.9 g	5–5.9 g	>6 g
Breads (1 slice)	Bagel White French	Whole-wheat	Bran muffin (1)	NA*	NA	NA	NA
Cereals (1 oz)	Rice Krispies Special K Cornflakes	Oatmeal Nutri-Grain Cheerios	Wheaties Shredded Wheat	Most Honey Bran	Bran Chex 40% Bran Flakes Raisin Bran	Corn Bran	All-Bran Bran Buds 100% Bran
Pasta (1 cup)	NA	Macaroni Spaghetti	NA	Whole-wheat spaghetti	NA	NA	NA
Rice (½ cup)	White	Brown	NA	NA	NA	NA	NA
Legumes (½ cup cooked)	NA	NA	NA	Lentils	Lima beans Dried peas	NA	Kidney beans Baked beans Navy beans NA
Vegetables (½ cup unless otherwise stated)	Cucumber Lettuce (1 cup) Green pepper	Asparagus Green beans Cabbage Cauliflower Potato without skin (1) Celery	Broccoli Brussels sprouts Carrots Corn Potato with skin (1) Spinach	Peas	NA	NA	NA
Fruits (1 medium unless other-wise stated)	Grapes (20) Watermelon (1 cup)	Apricots (3) Grapefruit (½) Peach with skin Pineapple (½ cup)	Apple, without skin Banana Orange	Apple, with skin Pear, with skin Raspberries (½ cup)	NA	NA	NA

*Not applicable.

(Slavin, J.L.: Dietary fiber: Classification, chemical analyses, and food sources. J. Am. Diet. Assoc., 87:1164, 1987. Reprinted with permission.)

TABLE A–30D-1. SAMPLE MENU FOR FIBER- AND RESIDUE-RESTRICTED DIET

BREAKFAST	LUNCH	DINNER
Strained orange juice (½ cup)	Vegetable broth (1 cup)	Strained tomato juice (½ cup)
Puffed rice cereal (¾ cup)	Saltine crackers (4)	Broiled skinless chicken breast (3 oz)
Canned peaches (½ cup)	Lean beef patty (3 oz)	White rice (½ cup)
White bread toast (2 slices)	Hamburger bun without seeds (1)	Cooked spinach (½ cup)
Margarine (2 tsp)	Mustard (1 Tbsp)	White roll (1)
Jelly (1 Tbsp)	Catsup (1 Tbsp)	Margarine (2 tsp)
2% milk (1 cup)	Canned fruit cocktail (½ cup)	Low-fat frozen yogurt (½ cup)
Coffee/tea	Vanilla wafer cookies (2)	Applesauce (½ cup)
	2% milk (1 cup)	Coffee/tea
	Coffee/tea	

APPROXIMATE NUTRIENT ANALYSIS

Energy (kcal)	1,857.2	Sodium (mg)	2,954.5
Protein (g) (20.9% of kcal)	97.0	Zinc (mg)	11.7
Carbohydrate (g) (52.1% of kcal)	241.9	Vitamin A (μg RE)	1,398.2
Total fat (g) (27.6% of kcal)	53.0	Vitamin C (mg)	132.1
Saturated fatty acids (g)	20.3	Thiamin (mg)	1.4
Monounsaturated fatty acids (g)	21.3	Riboflavin (mg)	2.0
Polyunsaturated fatty acids (g)	9.2	Niacin (mg)	25.4
Cholesterol (mg)	181.8	Folate (μg)	274.2
Calcium (mg)	1,138.7	Vitamin B$_6$ (mg)	1.7
Iron (mg)	13.2	Vitamin B$_{12}$ (μg)	4.2
Magnesium (mg)	346.5	Dietary fiber (g)	14.3
Phosphorus (mg)	1,315.6	Water-insoluble fiber (g)	9.0
Potassium (mg)	3,482.6		

(From The Manual of Clinical Dietetics. 4th Ed. Chicago, American Dietetic Association, 1992. With permission.)

TABLE A–30D-2. SAMPLE MENU FOR HIGH-FIBER DIET*

BREAKFAST	LUNCH	DINNER
Orange juice (½ cup)	Split pea soup (1 cup)	Green salad (3½ oz)
Whole-grain cereal (¾ cup)	Whole-wheat crackers (4)	Vinegar and oil dressing (1 Tbsp)
Raisins (2 Tbsp)	Lean beef patty (3 oz)	Broiled skinless chicken breast (3 oz)
Whole wheat toast (2 slices)	Hamburger bun (1)	Herbed brown rice (½ cup)
Margarine (2 tsp)	Mustard (1 Tbsp)	Steamed broccoli (½ cup)
Jelly or jam (1 Tbsp)	Catsup (1 Tbsp)	Whole-grain roll (1)
2% milk (1 cup)	Sliced tomato (2 oz) and lettuce	Margarine (2 tsp)
Coffee/tea	Fresh fruit salad (½ cup)	Low-fat frozen yogurt (½ cup)
	Bran muffin (1)	Medium pear (1)
	2% milk (1 cup)	Coffee/tea
	Coffee/tea	

APPROXIMATE NUTRIENT ANALYSIS

Energy (kcal)	2,195.0	Sodium (mg)	3,175.6
Protein (g) (19.4% of kcal)	106.4	Zinc (mg)	14.4
Carbohydrate (g) (54.0% of kcal)	296.0	Vitamin A (µg RE)	1,381.1
Total fat (g) (29.6% of kcal)	72.1	Vitamin C (mg)	160.4
Saturated fatty acids (g)	23.0	Thiamin (mg)	1.8
Monounsaturated fatty acids (g)	25.7	Riboflavin (mg)	2.4
Polyunsaturated fatty acids (g)	16.0	Niacin (mg)	28.6
Cholesterol (mg)	190.9	Folate (µg)	425.4
Calcium (mg)	1,241.8	Vitamin B₆ (mg)	2.4
Iron (mg)	18.4	Vitamin B₁₂ (µg)	4.3
Magnesium (mg)	511.7	Dietary fiber (g)	30.8
Phosphorus (mg)	1,763.0	Water-insoluble fiber (g)	21.1
Potassium (mg)	4,328.5		

*For further fat restriction, decrease servings of margarine and salad dressing. Use skimmed or 1% milk and milk products. (From The Manual of Clinical Dietetics. 4th Ed. American Dietetic Association, 1992. With permission.)

TABLE A–31A. SOFT DIET

Purpose: The soft diet is designed for patients who are physically or neurologically unable to tolerate a general diet.
Adequacy: Based on the individual's food choice, the diet is adequate in all nutrients according to the National Research Council's Recommended Dietary Allowances, 1989.

TABLE A–31B. GUIDELINES FOR FOOD SELECTION FOR SOFT DIET

FOOD CATEGORY	RECOMMENDED	MAY CAUSE DISTRESS
Beverages	Milk and milk products; all other beverages	Alcoholic beverages
Breads and cereals	White, refined-wheat, or light-rye enriched breads, soft rolls and crackers; cooked or ready-to-eat cereals	Coarse cereals (e.g., bran); whole-grain breads or crackers with seeds; bread or bread products with nuts or dried fruits
Desserts	Cakes, cookies, pies, pudding, custard, ice cream, sherbet, and gelatin made with allowed foods; fruit ice and frozen pops	All sweets and desserts containing nuts, coconut, or dried fruits not allowed; fried pastries (e.g., doughnuts)
Fats	Butter or fortified margarine; salad dressings; all fats and oils	Highly seasoned salad dressings
Fruits	All fruit juices; cooked or canned fruit; avocado, banana, grapefruit, and orange sections without membrane; soft fruits (e.g., melons, strawberries)	Other fresh and dried fruits

248   Nutrition Facts Manual

	Foods allowed	Foods to avoid
Meats and meat substitutes	All lean, tender meats, poultry, fish, and shellfish; crisp bacon; eggs; mild-flavored cheeses; creamy peanut butter; soybean and other meat substitutes; plain or flavored yogurt	Strong-smelling or highly seasoned meats, cheeses, or fish (e.g., luncheon meats, frankfurters, sausage); yogurt with nuts or dried fruits
Potato or substitute	Potatoes; enriched rice, barley, spaghetti, macaroni, and other pasta	Potato chips, fried potatoes
Soups	Soups made with allowed foods	Highly seasoned soups and soups made with gas-producing vegetables
Sweets	Sugar; syrup; honey; jelly and seedless jam; hard candies; plain chocolate candies; molasses; marshmallows	Any with nuts or coconut
Vegetables	All vegetable juices; cooked vegetables and lettuce as tolerated; salads made from allowed foods	Raw and fried vegetables; whole kernel corn; gas-producing vegetables (eg, broccoli, Brussels sprouts, cabbage, onions, leeks, cauliflower, cucumber, green pepper, rutabagas, turnips, sauerkraut, dried peas, dried beans)
Miscellaneous	Iodized salt; flavorings; mildly flavored gravies and sauces; pepper, herbs, spices, catsup, mustard, and vinegar in moderation	Strongly flavored seasonings and condiments (e.g., garlic, chili sauce, chili pepper, horseradish); pickles; popcorn; nuts and coconut

(From The Manual of Clinical Dietetics. 4th Ed. Chicago, American Dietetic Association, 1992. With permission.)

TABLE A-31C. SAMPLE MENU FOR SOFT DIET

BREAKFAST	LUNCH	DINNER
Orange juice (½ cup)	Vegetable soup (1 cup)	Tomato juice (6 oz)
Refined cold cereal (¾ cup)	Saltine crackers (4)	Broiled skinless chicken breast (3 oz)
Banana (½ cup)	Lean beef patty (3 oz)	Enriched rice (½ cup)
White toast (2 slices)	Hamburger bun (1)	Steamed green beans (½ cup)
Margarine (2 tsp)	Mustard (1 Tbsp)	Soft dinner roll (1)
Jelly or jam (1 Tbsp)	Mayonnaise (1 Tbsp)	Margarine (2 tsp)
2% milk (1 cup)	Lettuce leaf	Low-fat frozen yogurt (½ cup)
Coffee/tea	Canned fruit cocktail (½ cup)	Applesauce (½ cup)
	Graham crackers (4)	Coffee/tea
	2% milk (1 cup)	
	Coffee/tea	

APPROXIMATE NUTRIENT ANALYSIS

Energy (kcal)	2,142.6	Sodium (mg)	3,581.9
Protein (g) (17.9% of kcal)	96.0	Zinc (mg)	12.5
Carbohydrate (g) (57.1% of kcal)	305.8	Vitamin A (μg RE)	944.5
Total fat (g) (25.5% of kcal)	60.8	Vitamin C (mg)	118.3
Saturated fatty acids (g)	21.8	Thiamin (mg)	2.0
Monounsaturated fatty acids (g)	23.0	Riboflavin (mg)	2.4
Polyunsaturated fatty acids (g)	9.9	Niacin (mg)	30.9
Cholesterol (mg)	185.9	Folate (μg)	327.2
Calcium (mg)	1,038.7	Vitamin B$_6$ (mg)	2.5
Iron (mg)	15.4	Vitamin B$_{12}$ (μg)	4.4
Magnesium (mg)	308.9	Dietary fiber (g)	16.5
Phosphorus (mg)	1,319.1	Water-insoluble fiber (g)	11.1
Potassium (mg)	3,389.7		

(From The Manual of Clinical Dietetics. 4th Ed. Chicago, American Dietetic Association, 1992. With permission.)

TABLE A—32. DYSPHAGIA DIET

Stage I—Dysphagia puree, no liquids
Stage II—Dysphagia puree plus thick liquids
Stage III—Dysphagia puree plus thin liquids
Stage IV—Dysphagia mechanical soft foods, no liquids
Stage V—Dysphagia mechanical soft foods plus thick liquids
Stage VI—Dysphagia mechanical soft foods plus thin liquids

STAGE I—DYSPHAGIA PUREE, NO LIQUIDS

No liquids are provided unless specified by physician's order. Includes smooth, moist, and pureed foods that require little or no chewing but form a moist, cohesive bolus.

Food Group	Foods Allowed	Foods Avoided
Milk products	Pudding, custard, ice cream, plain or flavored yogurt (without fruit)	All others
Meat, poultry, and eggs	Pureed meat, chicken, fish; soufflés, soft cooked or poached eggs	All others
Vegetables and fruits	Pureed vegetables, fruits; applesauce, frozen fruit juices	All others
Breads and cereals	Thick cooked cereals, mashed potato	All others
Fats	Butter, margarine, sour cream	All others
Miscellaneous	Salt, pepper, ketchup, mustard, jelly, gelatin dessert	None

STAGE II—DYSPHAGIA PUREE PLUS THICK LIQUIDS

Includes all foods allowed in stage I with the addition of the following *thick liquids*.

Food Group	Liquids Allowed	Liquids Avoided
Milk products	Thickened eggnog, Carnation Instant Breakfast, milk shakes	All others
Soups	Thick creamed soups	Broth
Fruits	Thinned pureed fruits, nectar, vegetable juice	All others

STAGE III—DYSPHAGIA PUREE PLUS THIN LIQUIDS

Includes all foods allowed in stage II with the addition of the following *thin liquids*.

Food Group	Liquids Allowed	Liquids Avoided
Milk products	Eggnog, Carnation Instant Breakfast, milk	None
Soup	Thin creamed soups, broth	None
Beverages	Coffee, tea, soda, fruit juices	None

Note: Once a patient has mastered stage III, the diet can be either progressed in consistency (i.e., to stage V) or changed to puree.

STAGE IV—DYSPHAGIA MECHANICAL SOFT FOODS, NO LIQUIDS

No liquids are provided unless specified by physician's order. Includes minced and soft foods that require little or no chewing but form a soft, cohesive bolus.

Food Group	Liquids Allowed	Liquids Avoided
Milk products	Pudding, custard, ice cream, cream pies; plain, flavored, fruited yogurt	All others

(Continued)

Food Group	Foods Allowed	Foods Avoided
Cheeses	Small-curd cottage cheese, ricotta cheese, American cheese, grated cheese	All others
Eggs	Soft scrambled eggs, crustless quiche, soufflés, egg salad	All others
Meat, fish, and poultry	Ground meat or poultry with gravy; chicken or tuna salad (without celery); meat loaf; hamburger; baked or broiled fish; salmon loaf; pasta casseroles	
Vegetables	Cooked and diced carrots, beets, chopped or creamed spinach, butternut or acorn squash	Raw vegetables, other cooked vegetables
Potatoes, rice, and noodles	Mashed or baked (without skin) potatoes, macaroni and cheese, egg noodles, spaghetti with gravy or sauce	Rice, coarse grain (kasha, buckwheat, bran)
Fruit	Mashed banana, canned or cooked fruits cut into small pieces	Fruits with pits, raisins; all others
Breads and cereals	Bread, soft rolls, muffins, soft French toast, pancakes, cooked cereal, dry cereals soaked in milk, cakes without nuts	Dry crackers, breads with seeds, raisins, nuts
Fats	Butter, margarine, sour cream, gravy, mayonnaise	Nuts, seeds

STAGE V—DYSPHAGIA MECHANICAL SOFT FOODS PLUS THICK LIQUIDS

Includes all food from stage IV with the addition of *thick liquids* as outlined in stage II.

STAGE VI—DYSPHAGIA MECHANICAL SOFT FOODS PLUS THIN LIQUIDS

Includes all food from stage IV with the addition of *thin liquids* as outlined in stage III.

Note: Once a patient has mastered stage VI, the diet can be either progressed in consistency (i.e., to regular) or changed to mechanical soft foods.

Patients at stages I and IV need to have fluid status monitored and fluid requirements met by alternate means.

Milk products may not be tolerated by individuals who are susceptible to increased mucus production probably secondary to casein, a milk protein. If this becomes a problem, substitutes should be found.

Suggestions for dietitians:

1. A member of the medical or nursing staff or dysphagia team should be present at the bedside when a patient initially receives a dysphagia diet or advances to a higher stage to evaluate the patient's tolerance of the stage.
2. The dietitian should work closely with medical and nursing staff for continued evaluation of the patient's diet tolerance and progression.
3. Calorie counts are indicated to evaluate adequacy of intake and to justify the need for supplementation or nutrition support.

TABLE A—32. CONTINUED

4. The dietitian should work closely with the dysphagia team for physiologic evaluation of the patient's ability to chew and swallow to select the correct diet stage.

5. The dietitian should encourage small, frequent meals, particularly in the first stages of the diet.

6. As a guide, the following list gives a progression of food consistencies in order of increasing swallowing difficulty:

- stiff jelled consistency
- standard jelled consistency
- thick purees
- applesauce consistency
- thick soup consistency
- nectar consistency
- standard thin liquids
- chunk consistency (ground or diced)

Eating tips:

1. Food should be taken in small portions (½ tsp at a time).

2. The patient should sit upright with hips flexed at a 90° angle.

3. If possible, the neck should be at a 90° angle and flexed slightly forward.

4. The patient should sit up for 15 to 30 minutes both before and after meals.

5. Food should be placed on the unaffected side when possible.

6. Cold or hot foods may be better tolerated than foods at room temperature.

(From Antiaspiration-dysphagia Diet. *In* Diet Manual. New York, Memorial Sloan-Kettering Cancer Center, 1989. Reprinted by permission; and Bloch, A.S.: Nutrition Management of the Cancer Patient. Aspen, Rockville, MD, 1990. With permission.)

TABLE A—33A. ANTIDUMPING (POSTGASTRECTOMY) DIET

Purpose: This diet is designed to provide adequate calories and nutrients to support tissue healing and prevent weight loss and dumping syndrome after gastric surgery.[1-6]

Modifications: The diet limits beverages and liquids at meals, limits the intake of simple carbohydrates, and is high in protein and moderate in fat. Small, frequent feedings should be provided daily.[1,2] If no complications occur, additional foods are added as tolerated. Some patients are able to advance to a general diet within 2 to 3 weeks.[1]

After surgery, the diet generally progresses as follows:[1,2]

1. Ice chips held in mouth or small sips of water. Some people tolerate warm water better than ice chips or cold water.

2. Low-carbohydrate, clear liquids, such as broth, bouillon, unsweetened gelatin, or diluted unsweetened fruit juices, are given next.

3. The postgastrectomy diet then begins, with gradual progression to a general diet as tolerated.

(Continued)

TABLE A—33A. (CONTINUED)

It is important to note that the stated guidelines must be tailored to each patient's surgery, food tolerances, and nutrition problems and deficiencies.

General Guidelines[1,2,4,5,7,8]

1. Liquids should be given 30 to 60 minutes after meals and limited to 0.5-to 1-cup servings. At least 6 cups of fluid, however, should be consumed daily to replace losses resulting from diarrhea. Carbonated beverages and milk are not recommended initially.
2. Small, frequent feedings should be provided. The number of feedings depends on the patient's tolerance to specific portions of food. Foods should be eaten slowly and chewed well.
3. The diet should be low in simple carbohydrates, high in complex carbohydrates and protein, and moderate in fat.
4. All food and drink should be moderate in temperature. Cold drinks tend to cause increased gastric motility.
5. If "dumping" is a problem, the patient should lie down 20 to 30 minutes after meals to retard transit to the small bowel.
6. Introduce small amounts of milk to determine tolerance. If milk intolerance is found to be caused by a lactase deficiency, a lactose-restricted diet may be necessary (see Table A—35).
7. If adequate caloric intake cannot be provided because of steatorrhea, use of medium-chain triglyceride products may be needed.
8. Pectin, a dietary fiber found in fruits and vegetables, may be helpful for treating dumping syndrome. Pectin delays gastric emptying, slows carbohydrate absorption, and reduces the glycemic response.

Adequacy: The adequacy of the diet depends on the extent of surgery, as well as on individual food tolerances. With careful selection, this diet is adequate in all nutrients. After gastric surgery some patients experience malabsorption, which may be specific for macronutrients (e.g., carbohydrates, proteins, and fats) or micronutrients (e.g., folate, vitamin B_{12}, iron, vitamin D, and calcium).[2] Vitamin and mineral supplementation may be necessary depending on the extent of surgery and on whether the symptoms of dumping syndrome persist.[1,2]

References

1. Zeman, F.J.: *Clinical Nutrition and Dietetics.* 2nd Ed. New York, Macmillan, 1991.
2. Desai, M. Jeejeebhoy, K.N. *In* Modern Nutrition in Health and Disease. 7th Ed. Edited by M.E. Shils and V.R. Young. Philadelphia, Lea & Febiger, 1988.
3. Braga, M., Zuliani, L., Foppa, L., et al.: Br. J. Surg., *75*:477, 1988
4. Jordan, P. *In* Hardy's Textbook of Surgery. 2nd Ed. Edited by J. Hardy. Philadelphia, J.B. Lippincott, 1988.
5. Williams, S.R.: Nutrition and Diet Therapy. 6th Ed. St. Louis, Times Mirror/Mosby College Publishing, 1989.
6. Meyer, J.H. *In* Gastrointestinal Disease: Pathophysiology, Diagnosis, and Management. 4th Ed. Edited by M.H. Sleisenger, J.S. Fordtran. Philadelphia, W.B. Saunders, 1989.
7. Sawyers, J.L.: Am. J. Surg., *159*:8–13, 1990.
8. Alpers, D., Crouse, R., Stenson, W.: Manual of Nutritional Therapeutics. 2nd Ed. Boston, Little Brown, 1988.

TABLE A–33B. GUIDELINES FOR FOOD SELECTION FOR ANTIDUMPING (POSTGASTRECTOMY) DIET

FOOD CATEGORY	RECOMMENDED	MAY CAUSE DISTRESS*
Beverages†	Milk as tolerated; coffee; tea; unsweetened or diluted fruit drinks; unsweetened carbonated beverages	Alcohol; chocolate milk drinks; milkshakes; sweetened fruit drinks; sweetened carbonated beverages
Breads and cereals	Whole-grain or enriched breads and cereals; English muffins and bagels; unsweetened, cooked cereals	Breads made with dried fruits, nuts, and seeds; pastries; donuts; muffins
Cereals	Unsweetened dry and cooked cereals	Sugar-coated cereals, coarse cereals (e.g., bran)
Desserts	Plain cakes and cookies; sugar-free pudding, gelatin dessert; custard, yogurt, and frozen yogurt	All sweets and desserts made with chocolate or dried fruits; sweetened gelatin dessert; fried pastries; ice cream; ice milk; regular fruited or frozen yogurt
Fats	Butter; margarine; salad dressings; mayonnaise; vegetable oils; sour cream; cream cheese as tolerated	None
Fruits	Unsweetened canned fruits and fruit juice†; fresh fruits	All dried fruits; sweetened fruit juice; fruits canned in heavy syrup
Meats and meat substitutes	Lean tender meats; fish; poultry; shellfish; eggs; peanut butter; cottage cheese; mild cheeses; highly seasoned and spicy meats	Fried meats or eggs
Potato and potato substitutes	Potatoes; enriched rice; barley; noodles; spaghetti, macaroni, and other pastas	Any to which sugar has been added (e.g., candied sweet potatoes)
Soups	Soups made with allowed foods; spicy soups as tolerated	Soups prepared with heavy cream or high-fat ingredients
Sweets	Sugar substitutes and sweets made with sugar substitutes	Sugar; syrup; honey; jelly; jam; molasses; marshmallows
Vegetables	Cooked (fresh, frozen, canned) vegetables or vegetable juice†; raw vegetables as tolerated	Any to which sugar has been added
Miscellaneous	Iodized salt; pepper; mildly flavored sauces and gravies; strongly flavored seasonings as tolerated	None

*If no adverse symptoms occur, these foods can be added as tolerated.
†All fluids should be consumed 30 to 60 minutes after meals and limited to ½- to 1-cup servings.
(From The Manual of Clinical Dietetics. 4th Ed. Chicago, American Dietetic Association, 1992. With permission.)

TABLE A-33C. SAMPLE MENU FOR ANTIDUMPING (POSTGASTRECTOMY) DIET*

BREAKFAST	LUNCH	DINNER
Grapefruit (½)	Lean hamburger patty (2 oz)	Broiled skinless chicken breast (3 oz)
Oatmeal (½ cup)	Hamburger bun (1)	Herbed brown rice (½ cup)
Whole-wheat toast (1 slice)	Mayonnaise (1 Tbsp)	Steamed broccoli (½ cup)
Margarine (1 tsp)	Sliced tomato (2 oz) and lettuce	Margarine (2 tsp)
2% milk† (½ cup)	Fresh fruit salad (½ cup)	Unsweetened applesauce (½ cup)
Coffee/tea† (½ cup)	2% milk† (½ cup)	2% milk† (½ cup)
	Coffee/tea† (½ cup)	Coffee/tea† (½ cup)
MIDMORNING SNACK	MIDAFTERNOON SNACK	BEDTIME SNACK
Cheese (1 oz)	Roast beef (1 oz)	Peanut butter (2 Tbsp)
Saltine crackers (4)	Bread (1 slice)	Graham crackers (4)
Banana (½)	Mustard (1 tsp)	2% milk† (½ cup)
	Vegetable soup† (1 cup)	

APPROXIMATE NUTRIENT ANALYSIS

Energy (kcal)	2,055.9	Sodium (mg)	3,016.3
Protein (g) (20.9% of kcal)	107.4	Zinc (mg)	14.1
Carbohydrate (g) (41.7% of kcal)	214.1	Vitamin A (μg RE)	823.3
Total fat (g) (39.4% of kcal)	90.0	Vitamin C (mg)	136.2
Saturated fatty acids (g)	29.8	Thiamin (mg)	1.4
Monounsaturated fatty acids (g)	33.5	Riboflavin (mg)	1.9
Polyunsaturated fatty acids (g)	19.3	Niacin (mg)	27.1
Cholesterol (mg)	215.2	Folate (μg)	240.5
Calcium (mg)	1,035.6	Vitamin B₆ (mg)	2.3
Iron (mg)	12.0	Vitamin B₁₂ (μg)	4.3
Magnesium (mg)	409.9	Dietary fiber (g)	21.6
Phosphorus (mg)	1,652.2	Water-insoluble fiber (g)	14.0
Potassium (mg)	3,270.6		

*The sample menu incorporates six (6) meals per day. The number of feedings depends on the patient's tolerance to food portions and therefore should be adjusted accordingly.

†Liquid should be given 30 to 60 minutes after the meal and limited to ½ cup to 1 cup servings.

(From The Manual of Clinical Dietetics. 4th Ed. Chicago, American Dietetic Association, 1992. With permission.)

TABLE A–34. GLUTEN-RESTRICTED AND GLIADIN- AND PROLAMIN-FREE (Wheat-, Rye-, Oat-, and Barley-Free) DIET INSTRUCTION

This menu pattern is designed to provide adequate nutrition while eliminating wheat, rye, oats, and barley from the diet. The fraction of gluten protein in wheat that injures the intestine of susceptible persons is gliadin. The equivalent toxic protein fractions in barley, rye, and oats are prolamins. When all sources of gliadin and prolamin are removed from the diet, the intestine is able to regenerate, and normal function is usually restored.

Gliadin and prolamin may be either present in foods as a basic ingredient (i.e., listed as wheat, rye, oats, or barley) or added as a derivative when a food is processed or prepared. Thus, *reading labels carefully is very important!* A great deal of confusion occurs about the presence of gliadin- and prolamin-containing additives in foods. This table includes lists of both nebulous ingredients and common additives.

Since flour and cereal products are quite often used in the preparation of foods, it is important to be aware of the methods of preparation used as well as the foods themselves. This is especially true when dining out.

FOOD GROUP WITH SUGGESTED DAILY INTAKE

DAILY INTAKE	FOODS ALLOWED	FOODS TO AVOID
Milk (2 or more cups)	Fresh, dry, evaporated, or condensed milk; cream; sour cream;* whipping cream; yogurt*	Malted milk; some commercial chocolate drinks; some nondairy creamers.†
Meat, fish, poultry	All kinds of fresh meats, fish, other seafood, poultry; fish canned in oil, brine, or vegetable broth; some meat products, such as hot dogs and lunch meats†	Prepared meats containing wheat, rye, oats, or barley, such as some sausages,† hot dogs,† bologna†; luncheon meats†; ground beef and pork with oat bran added in the form of "Oatrim" or "LeanMaker"; chili con carne†; bread-containing products, such as swiss steak, meat loaf, and croquettes; tuna canned with hydrolyzed protein†; turkey with hydrolyzed vegetable protein (HVP) injected as part of the basting solution; "imitation Crab" containing wheat starch or other unacceptable filler.

(Continued)

TABLE A–34. CONTINUED

FOOD GROUP WITH SUGGESTED DAILY INTAKE	FOODS ALLOWED	FOODS TO AVOID
Cheeses (Can be used for meat and milk groups)	All aged cheeses, such as cheddar, swiss, edam, parmesan; cottage cheese;* cream cheese;* pasteurized processed cheese*†	Any cheese product containing *oat gum* as an ingredient.
Eggs	Plain or in cooking.	Eggs in sauce made from wheat, rye, oat, or barley. Usually wheat flour is used in white sauce.
Potato or other starch	White and sweet potatoes; yams; hominy; rice; wild rice; special pasta made from rice, soy, or corn‡; some oriental rice and bean thread noodles.	Regular noodles; spaghetti or macaroni (semolina = wheat); most packaged rice mixes and frozen rice side dishes; frozen potato products with wheat starch or wheat flour added.
Vegetables (2 or more servings)	All plain, fresh, frozen, or canned; dried peas, beans, and lentils; some commercially prepared vegetables†	Creamed vegetables†; vegetables canned in sauce†; some canned baked beans†; commercially prepared vegetables and salads†
Fruits	All fresh, frozen, canned, or dried; all fruit juices; some canned pie fillings	Thickened or prepared fruits; some pie fillings†
Breads (3 or more servings)	Specially prepared breads using only allowed flours. Breads may be purchased ready-to-eat or as mixes to prepare at home. Recipes have been developed for home use and for use in automatic bread machines.‡	Those containing wheat, rye, oats, and/or barley flours. Avoid those with buckwheat, millet, amaranth, quinoa, spelt, or teff.§ *Beware: wheat-free* does not always mean gliadin- and prolamin-free! Breads made from "carob-soy flour" may contain 80% wheat flour!

Category	Foods Allowed	Foods to Avoid
Cereals (1 or more servings)	*Hot cereals* Corn meal Cream of Rice Hominy Rice *Cold cereals* Puffed Rice Corn Pops Fruity and Choc. Pebbles Kenmei Sun Flakes (corn & rice) Special cereals made without malt or malt flavoring.	Those containing wheat, rye, oats, barley, graham, wheat germ, malt or malt flavoring, kasha, bulgar, buckwheat,§ millet,§ amaranth,§ quinoa,§ spelt,§ teff.§ New products with "unusual" grains are constantly being introduced. Do not use them until you can clear them with a reliable source.
Crackers and snack foods	Rice wafers; rice crackers; plain corn and potato chips; rice cakes†; pure cornmeal tortillas; popcorn; caramel corn†	Those with wheat, rye, barley, oats, or other questionable (grain-like) ingredients. *Read labels carefully.* Some coating mixes used on chips contain wheat flour! If the product shows "brown rice syrup," contact the manufacturer to check for "barley malt enzymes" used in processing.
Soups	Homemade broth and soup using allowed ingredients; a few canned soups;† specialty dry soup mixes‡	Most canned soups† and soup mixes†; bouillon and bouillon cubes with hydrolyzed vegetable protein (HVP). HVP may appear as "flavoring" or "natural flavoring" ingredient.
Flours and thickening agents	Arrowroot starch (A) Corn bean (B) Corn flour‡ (B, C, D) Corn germ (B) Corn meal (B, C, D) Potato flour (B, C, E)	Wheat starch Wheat germ, bran Wheat flour Rye Oats Barley

(Continued)

	Potato starch flour (B, C, E)
	Rice bran (B)
	Rice flours
	  Plain (B, C, D, E)
	  Brown (B, C, D, E)
	  Sweet (A, B, C, F)
	  Rice polish‡ (B, C, G)
	  Rice starch (A)
	Soy flour‡ (B, C, G)
	Tapioca starch (A)
		Buckwheat§
		Amaranth§
		Quinoa§
		Spelt§
		Teff§
		"Carob-soy" flour containing 80% wheat flour (made by Sterling Foods Co., Seattle)

A = good thickening agent; B = good combined with other flours; C = best combined with milk and eggs in baked products; D = grainy-textured products; E = drier product than with other flours; F = moister product than with other flours; G = adds distinct flavor to product, use with moderation.

Fats	Butter; margarine; vegetable oil; hydrogenated vegetable oil; nuts; peanut butter; some salad dressings†; mayonnaise† (mayonnaise made with cider or wine vinegar is found at Kosher delis)	Some commercial salad dressings†‖
Desserts	Cakes; quick breads; pastries; puddings made with allowed ingredients; Cornstarch; tapioca; rice puddings; gelatin desserts; cook and serve puddings; "expensive" ice cream with a few simple ingredients; sorbet; frozen Yogurt†; sherbet	Commercial cakes, cookies, pies, made with wheat, rye, oats, barley, millet, amaranth, buckwheat, quinoa, spelt, teff; Jello "instant" pudding; products containing brown rice syrup made with barley malt enzyme.
Beverages	Instant and ground coffee; instant tea; carbonated beverages†; pure cocoa powder; wines made in United States; rums; some root beers†; vodka distilled from grapes or potatoes.	Ovaltine; malted milk; ale; beer; gin; whiskeys‖; vodka distilled from grain; flavored coffees†; some herbal teas with barley or barley malt added†

	INCLUDE	AVOID
Sweets	Jelly; jam; honey; brown and white sugar; molasses; most syrups†; some candy†; chocolate; pure cocoa; coconut; marshmallows†	Some commercial candies; foods with malt/malt flavoring or "natural flavoring"†; See's Molasses Chews; chocolate-coated nuts, which may be rolled in wheat flour†; brown rice syrup made with barley malt enzyme†
Miscellaneous	Spices (salt, pure pepper, cloves, ginger, nutmeg, cinnamon, allspice, etc.); herbs (oregano, rosemary, etc.); food coloring; alcohol-free extracts; yeast; baking soda; baking powder; cream of tartar; dry mustard; cider, rice and wine vinegars; olives; monosodium glutamate (MSG) made in United States	Condiments made with wheat-derived distilled white vinegar‖; alcohol-based extracts‖; some curry powders†; some dry seasoning mixes†; some gravy extracts†; some meat sauces†; most soy sauces†; some chewing gum†; communion wafers/bread#

*Check vegetable gum used.
†Consult label and contact manufacturer to clarify questionable ingredients.
‡See Special Products List for availability and ordering information.
§Additional information is needed before this product can be cleared.
‖Distilled white vinegar uses grain as a starting material. Most often the grain mash includes wheat. Whiskies, including "corn whiskey," use wheat, rye, oats, or barley in their mash. According to chemistry professors consulted, in large-scale distillation processes, such as those used in the manufacture of whiskey and vinegar, it is possible that a very small amount of protein may be carried over into the distillate. The presence of such a small amount of gliadin and/or prolamin must be tested via immunoassay. Currently, we are advising gliadin- and prolamin-intolerant individuals to use cider, wine, or rice vinegar in such food preparation as making salad dressings, pickles, and in cooking. To be 100% safe, purchase or make condiments with cider, wine or rice vinegar. These condiments (ketchup, mustard, mayonnaise, pickles) are usually available in kosher delis. Foods with nongrain vinegars are produced for Passover.
#Contact the Gluten Intolerance Group of North America to obtain instructions for making communion wafers from acceptable ingredients. Note: In Catholic communion, host crumbs are often added to the wine before it is served. A workable solution is to arrange to use a goblet of your own.

NEBULOUS INGREDIENT	INCLUDE	AVOID
"Hydrolyzed vegetable protein" or "hydrolyzed protein"	Those from soy, corn, or milk	Mixtures of wheat, corn, and soy*
"Flour" or "cereal products"	Rice flour, corn flour, corn meal, potato flour, soy flour	Wheat, rye, oats, barley, amaranth, quinoa, spelt, teff, millet, buckwheat
"Vegetable protein"	Soy, corn	Wheat, rye, oats, barley
"Vegetable broth"	In the United States, this must contain two or more of the following: beans, cabbage, carrots, celery, garlic, onions, parsley, peas, potatoes, green bell pepper, red bell pepper, spinach, or tomatoes. It cannot contain any other ingredients. *It can be used.*	

(Continued)

"Malt" or "malt flavoring"	Those derived from barley or barley malt syrup.
	Those derived from corn.
	Rice plus barley malt enzyme.
"Brown rice syrup"	Rice only.
"Starch"	In the United States, it must be *cornstarch*.
"Modified starch" or "modified food starch"	Arrowroot, corn, potato waxy maize, maize.
"Vegetable gum"	Carob bean, locust bean, cellulose, guar, gum arabic, gum acacia, gum tragacanth, xanthan gum
	Wheat starch
	Oat gum.
"Soy sauce" or "soy sauce solids"	Those that *do not* contain wheat *(soy only)*
	Those brewed from wheat and soy.
"Mono-" and "diglycerides"	Those using *non*wheat-based carrier.
	Those using a wheat starch carrier.

These questionable ingredients must be cleared with the manufacturer before they are eaten. A sample letter requesting information on starting materials and packaging and processing ingredients is available at the end of this table.

*Hydrolyzed vegetable protein: A combination of wheat, corn, and soy is primarily used as starting material for hydrolyzed vegetable protein (HVP). When wheat protein is "hydrolyzed," its large amino acid chains are broken down into smaller chains. Some protein researchers believe the same sequence of amino acids found in these smaller chains contain the same toxicity as the intact gliadin subfraction of the gluten protein. Thus, HVP made from wheat is not recommended for use on a gliadin-free diet.

ADDITIVES THAT ARE GLIADIN- AND PROLAMIN-FREE*

Adipic acid	Gums: acacia, arabic, carob bean, cellulose, guar, locust bean, tragacanth, xanthan	Riboflvin
Ascorbic acid		
		Sodium acid pyraphosphate
BHA	Invert sugar	Sodium ascorbate
BHT		Sodium benzoate
Beta carotene	Lactic acid	Sodium caseinate
Biotin	Lactose	Sodium citrate
	Lecithin	Sodium hexametaphosphate
		Sodium nitrate
Calcium chloride	Magnesium hydroxide	Sodium silaco aluminate
Calcium pantothenate	Malic acid	Sorbitol—mannitol
Calcium phosphate		

Carboxymethylcellulose
Carrageenan
Citric acid
Corn sweetener
Corn syrup solids

Demineralized whey
Dextrimaltose
Dextrose—dextrins
Dioctyl sodium sulfosuccinate

Folic acid—folacin
Fructose
Fumaric acid
*The above is not an exhaustive list.

Microcrystallin cellulose
Monosodium glutamate (MSG) made in United States

Niacin—niacinamide

Polyglycerol
Polysorbate 60; 80
Potassium citrate
Potassium iodide
Propylene glycol monostearate
Propylgallate
Pyridoxine hydrochloride

Sucrose
Sulfosuccinate

Tartaric acid
Thiamine hydrochloride
Tri-calcium phosphate

Vanillan
Vitamin A (palmitate)
Vitamins and minerals

MEDICATIONS

All medications have fillers/dispersing agents added. These are usually lactose or corn starch. Wheat starch may also be used. *Before you take any medication, take the following precautions.*

Over-the-Counter Drug: Read the list of active and inactive ingredients carefully. Use the list of "Nebulous Ingredients" in this table to spot potential problems. Ask your pharmacist to "translate" the terms you do not know.

Prescription Drug: Inactive ingredients are *not* listed. Even your pharmacist must call the drug company to obtain this information! When the pharmaceutical company is contacted, they will need the lot number of the product so they can check the formulation of the batch you will be taking. A list of drug companies with addresses and phone numbers can be found in the Physicians' Desk Reference.

Liquid Cold and Flu Medications: These medications often contain alcohol. Check source.

SPECIAL PRODUCTS LIST

AlpineAire Foods
P.O. Box 926
Nevada City, CA 95959
916-272-1971

Freeze-dried foods for backpacking. Vacuumed packed. No preservatives, no added sugar, no artificial flavors or colors. Note: The "vegetable pasta" in Pasta Roma and Vegetable Pasta Stew *contains wheat flour.*
Mail orders accepted.

(Continued)

Bickford Laboratories 282 S. Main Street Akron, OH 44308 216-762-4666	Forty-nine varieties of alcohol-free flavorings. Selection ranges from common flavorings, like vanilla and almond, to exotic. Mail orders accepted.
DeBoles Garden City Park, NY 11040	Corn pasta products, including ribbon noodles, macaroni, and spaghetti.
Dietary Specialties P.O. Box 227 Rochester, NY 14601 1-800-544-0099	A wide assortment of mixes, crackers, cookies, and pasta. Many exclusive imported items. Mail orders accepted.
Ener-G Foods, Inc. P.O. Box 84487 Seattle, WA 98124-5787 1-800-331-5222	Excellent assortment of flours and flour mixes. Will ship in bulk (20# boxes). Variety of baked products, dry soup mixes, flavorings. Mail orders accepted.
Lundberg Family Farms Box 369 Richvale, CA 95974 916-882-4551	Interesting variety of combination rices. Brown rice cereals and rice cakes. Note: Sweet Dreams Brown Rice Syrup is made using barley malt enzyme. Products made with this syrup should be avoided. Soups contain wheat-derived soy sauce. Mail orders accepted.
Med-Diet Inc. 3050 Ranchview Lane Plymouth, MN 55447 1-800-med-diet	Carries various brands of breads, crackers, cookies, cake and muffin mixes, and pasta. Note: Their order blank is not designed for those who must eliminate gliadin and prolamin. Request their list of "wheat/gluten-free foods that contain no wheat starch" so you'll know what to order!
Red Mill Farms, Inc. 290 S. 5th Street Brooklyn, NY 11211 718-384-2150	Three suitable products that are also lactose free: Dutch Chocolate Cake, Banana-Nut Cake, and Coconut Macaroons. All vacuumed packed. Mail orders accepted.
Tad Enterprizes 9356 Pleasant Tinley Park, IL 60477 708-429-2101	Carry a variety of flours for gliadin- and prolamin-free baking. Mail orders accepted.
Van Brode's Milling Clinton, MA 01510	Carries some cold breakfast cereals (malt free). Write for complete product information.

WRITING EFFECTIVE LETTERS TO FOOD MANUFACTURERS*

Clarifying questionable ingredients on product labels and in medications is essential for those following this diet. Manufacturers are usually courteous and prompt when answering questions regarding their products. The usefulness of their reply, however, often depends on how the question is posed. Use the following letter format when you need to contact a a manufacturer.

Your Address

Date

Dear Sir/Madam:

I am on a gluten-restricted, gliadin- and prolamin-free diet for the treatment of celiac sprue (dermatitis herpetiformis). I must avoid the protein found in wheat, rye, oats, and barley, since they cause an immune response which damages the lining of my intestine.

Although I would like to use your product, (insert name), your ingredient listing does not give adequate information for me to determine if it would be suitable. Specifically, I need to know examples would be:

the source of your "food starch modified"

whether your "soy sauce solids" are derived from wheat

what "natural flavorings" you use in this product

from what source your "vegetable gum" is derived

the inacive ingredients used in the medication, including those used in the coatings and capsules

Another likely source of gliadin and prolamin contamination is the incidental ingredients which are used in the packaging and processing of your product. Since these incidental ingredients are not listed on the packaging, I am relying on your thoroughness to clarify these substances.

If it would be possible, I would appreciate a copy of your response to be forwarded to: The Gluten Intolerance Group of North America

P.O. Box 23053

Seattle, WA 98102-0353

This will allow your efforts to be shared with others through our national organization which reaches health-care personnel as well as persons with celiac sprue and dermatitis herpetiformis. If you have questions regarding these disorders and the required dietary restrictions, please direct them to our national office.

Thank you for your efforts on my behalf.

Sincerely,

Your Signature

*Additional information on celiac sprue and dermatitis herpetiformis may be obtained from The Gluten Intolerance Group of North America, P.O. Box 23053, Seattle, WA 98102-0353.
(Table A–34 © Elaine I. Hartsook, Ph.D., R.D. All rights reserved. Printed with permission.)

TABLE A–35A. LACTOSE-CONTROLLED DIET

Purpose: The lactose-controlled diet is designed to prevent or reduce bloating, flatulence, cramping, and diarrhea associated with ingesting lactose-containing products.

Modifications: The diet is a general one that restricts or eliminates lactose-containing foods and beverages. Since tolerance of lactose may vary, the diet is usually administered on a trial-and-error basis.[1] Individual tolerance determines the amount of lactose allowed; many patients may be able to tolerate 5 to 8 g of lactose at a given time, especially if they consume it with a meal.[2]

Labels should be read carefully, and foods containing milk, lactose, milk solids, whey, curds, skim milk powder, and skim milk solids should be avoided. In addition to dairy products, the following food categories may contain lactose: breads, candy and cookies; cold cuts, hot dogs, and bologna; commercial sauces and gravies; cream soups; dry cereals; frostings; frozen breaded fish and chicken; prepared and processed foods; salad dressings containing milk or cheese; sugar substitutes; and instant drink mixes. Moreover, some medications and vitamins may contain lactose as a carrier. Lactate, lactalbumin, lactulate, and calcium compounds are salts of lactic acid and do not contain lactose.

Patients should be encouraged to experiment with the lactose-reduced or lactose-free products currently available. In addition, lactase enzyme is available in droplet form for use with lactose-containing beverages and in tablet form for ingestion prior to consuming a lactose-containing meal. Lactobacillus acidophilus milk is not equivalent to lactase-treated milk.

Tolerance to lactose is variable; if a patient is asymptomatic, no restrictions are necessary. If the patient experiences adverse reactions to lactose, cessation of symptoms should occur within 3 to 5 days on a lactose-controlled diet. Further testing may be necessary if symptoms persist.[2] Small amounts of lactose-containing food (approximately 3 g) several times a day may be tolerated better than a large amount of lactose ingested at one time.[3] Studies have shown that yogurt is significantly better tolerated than milk because of its high lactase activity.[3,4] Different brands and processing methods, however, may affect tolerance to yogurt.

Adequacy: Depending on individual food choices, the diet can provide adequate amounts of all essential nutrients. Calcium, vitamin D, and riboflavin may be deficient if all dairy products are avoided. Use of lactose-hydrolyzed milk and milk products could satisfy these nutrient needs; otherwise, supplementation may be necessary.

References

1. Shils, M.E., Young, V.R. (Eds.): Modern Nutrition in Health and Disease. 7th Ed. Philadelphia, Lea & Febiger, 1988.
2. Martini, M. Savaiano, D.: Am. J. Clin. Nutr., 47:57–60, 1988.
3. Onwulata, C.I., Rao, D.R., Vankineni, P.: Am. J. Clin. Nutr., 49:1233–1237, 1989.
4. Wytock, D.H., DiPalma, J.A.: Am. J. Clin. Nutr., 47:454–457, 1988.

Further Reading

Burlant, A.: Lactose-Free Cooking. Wayne, NJ, Lockley Publishing, 1990.
Dobler, M.L.: Lactose Intolerance. Chicago, The American Dietetic Association, 1991, catalog no. 0881.
Martens, R.A., Martens, S.: The Milk Sugar Dilemma. 2nd Ed. Lansing, Medi-Ed Press, 1987.
Zukin, J.: Dairy-Free Cookbook. Rocklin, CA, Prima Publishing and Communications, 1989.

Special Product Information

Lactaid can be purchased in tablets, drops, or as lactase-treated milk and cheese products.

Lactaid Hotline
800-257-8650
9 AM—4 PM Eastern time
Monday through Friday
In Canada: 800-387-5711

Lactaid, Inc.
P.O. Box 111
Pleasantville, NJ 08232

Lactase tablets are produced by:

Kremers-Urban Company
P.O. Box 2038
Milwaukee, WI 53201

Dairy Ease tablets and lactose-treated milk (skim, 1%, and 2% fat) are produced by:

Winthrop Consumer Products
Glenbrook Laboratories
Division of Sterling Drug, Inc.
90 Park Ave.
New York, NY 10016

(From The Manual of Clinical Dietetics. 4th Ed. Chicago, American Dietetic Association, 1992. With permission.)

TABLE A-35B. GUIDELINES FOR FOOD SELECTION FOR LACTOSE-CONTROLLED DIET*

FOOD CATEGORY	RECOMMENDED	MAY CAUSE DISTRESS*
Beverages	All beverages with allowed ingredients; soybean milks; other lactose-free supplements; lactase-hydrolyzed milk	Milk, milk products, or acidophilus milk as tolerance dictates
Breads and cereals	Whole-grain or enriched breads and cereals	Depending on tolerance, some breads and cereals prepared with milk or milk products may need to be avoided
Desserts	Cakes, cookies, pies; flavored gelatin desserts; water ices made with allowed foods	Any prepared with milk or milk products (e.g., sherbet, ice cream, ice milk, custard, pudding, commercial desserts, and mixes)
Fats	Butter or margarine; salad dressings; nondairy creamer; all oils	Any prepared with lactose-containing ingredients
Fruits	All fruits and juices	None
Meats and meat substitutes	All meats, poultry, fish; eggs; peanut butter; dried peas and beans; hard, aged, and processed cheese, if tolerated; yogurt as tolerated	Cold cuts and frankfurters that contain lactose filler; cottage cheese
Potatoes and potato substitutes	Potatoes; enriched rice; barley; noodles, spaghetti, macaroni, and other pastas	Potatoes or substitutes prepared with milk or milk products; mixes prepared with lactose-containing ingredients
Soups	Broth; bouillon; soups made with allowed ingredients	Soups prepared with milk or milk products
Sweets	Sugar; corn syrup; pure maple syrup; honey; jellies; jams; pure sugar candies; marshmallows	Chocolate; caramels; any candies made with lactose-containing ingredients
Vegetables	All	Vegetables prepared with milk or milk products
Miscellaneous	All spices, seasonings, flavorings	Any prepared with milk or milk products

*A lactose-free diet, from which virtually all known sources of lactose are eliminated, may be indicated for patients with severe intolerance or a congenital lactase deficiency.

(From The Manual of Clinical Dietetics. 4th Ed. American Dietetic Association, 1992. With permission.)

TABLE A–35C. SAMPLE MENU FOR LACTOSE-CONTROLLED DIET*

BREAKFAST	LUNCH	DINNER
Orange juice (½ cup)	Vegetable soup (1 cup)	Green salad (3½ oz)
Whole-grain cereal (¾ cup)	Saltine crackers (4)	Oil and vinegar dressing (1 Tbsp)
Banana (½)	Lean beef patty (3 oz)	Broiled skinless chicken breast (3 oz)
Whole-wheat toast (2 slices)	Hamburger bun (1)	Herbed brown rice (½ cup)
Margarine (2 tsp)	Catsup (1 Tbsp)	Steamed broccoli (½ cup)
Jelly or jam (1 Tbsp)	Mustard (1 Tbsp)	Whole-grain roll (1)
Lactose-reduced 2% milk (1 cup)	Sliced tomato (2 oz) and lettuce	Margarine (2 tsp)
Coffee/tea	Fresh fruit salad (½ cup)	Fruit ice (½ cup)
	Graham crackers (4)	Medium apple (1)
	Lactose-reduced 2% milk (1 cup)	Coffee/tea
	Coffee/tea	

APPROXIMATE NUTRIENT ANALYSIS

Energy (kcal)	2,157.2	Sodium (mg)	3,069.8
Protein (g) (15.6% of kcal)	83.9	Zinc (mg)	11.7
Carbohydrate (g) (56.8% of kcal)	306.3	Vitamin A (µg RE)	1,111.5
Total fat (g) (30.1% of kcal)	72.1	Vitamin C (mg)	256.8
Saturated fatty acids (g)	18.3	Thiamin (mg)	1.7
Monounsaturated fatty acids (g)	27.3	Riboflavin (mg)	1.4
Polyunsaturated fatty acids (g)	19.4	Niacin (mg)	29.0
Cholesterol (mg)	144.4	Folate (µg)	471.0
Calcium (mg)	1,413.5	Vitamin B$_6$ (mg)	2.5
Iron (mg)	16.1	Vitamin B$_{12}$ (µg)	2.2
Magnesium (mg)	380.2	Dietary fiber (g)	23.5
Phosphorus (mg)	1,121.7	Water-insoluble fiber (g)	16.4
Potassium (mg)	3,580.2		

*If lactose-reduced milk is not tolerated, substitute ½ cup nondairy creamer at breakfast and fruit juice at lunch. A calcium supplement should also be provided.
(From The Manual of Clinical Dietetics. 4th Ed. Chicago, American Dietetic Association, 1992. With permission.)

TABLE A–35D. LACTOSE CONTENT OF SELECTED MILK, MILK PRODUCTS, AND SUBSTITUTES*

PRODUCT		LACTOSE (APPROX. g/UNIT)
Milk	1 cup—244 g	11
Low-fat milk (2% fat)	1 cup—244 g	9–13
Skim milk	1 cup—244 g	12–14
Chocolate milk	1 cup—244 g	10–12
Sweetened condensed whole milk	1 cup—306 g	35
Dried whole milk	1 cup—128 g	48
Nonfat dry milk, instant	1½ cup—91 g	46
Buttermilk fluid	1 cup—245 g	9–11
Whipped cream topping	1 Tbsp—3 g	0.4
Light Cream	1 Tbsp—15 g	0.6
Half and Half	1 Tbsp—15 g	0.6
Low-fat yogurts†	8 oz—227–258 g	11–15
Cheese:		
Blue, cream, Parmesan, Colby	1 oz—28 g	0.7–0.8
Camembert, Limburger	1 oz—28 g	0.1
Cheddar, Gouda	1 oz—28 g	0.4–0.6
Cheese, pasteurized, processed:		
American	1 oz—28 g	0.5
Pimento	1 oz—28 g	0.5–1.7
Swiss	1 oz—28 g	0.4–0.6
Cottage cheese	1 cup—210 g	5–6
Cottage cheese, low-fat (2% fat)	1 cup—226 g	7–8
Butter	2 pats—10 g	0.1
Oleomargarine	2 pats—10 g	0
Ice cream		
Vanilla, regular	1 cup—133 g	9
French, soft	1 cup—173 g	9
Ice milk, vanilla	1 cup—131 g	10
Sherbet, orange	1 cup—193 g	4
Ice, orange	100 g	0

*Lactaid milk and other dairy products have lactose reduced by 70%. With further treatment, these products can be 100% lactose-free.

†Bacterial lactase in unpasteurized yogurt survives transit through the stomach, thus allowing digestion of the lactose present in yogurt. This process enables lactase-deficient individuals to consume these dairy products in moderate amounts (from ½ to 1 pint) with fewer or no symptoms. Data from Kolars, J.C., Levitt, M.D., Aouji, M., et al.: N. Engl. J. Med., *310*:1–3, 1984.

Lactase-deficient patients have been reported to experience no gastrointestinal distress after consuming pasteurized yogurt (500 g) even though the lactase activity is significantly destroyed by pasteurization. In contrast, cultured milk does result in gastrointestinal distress for lactose-intolerant individuals. Data from Savaiano, D.A., AbouElAnouar, A., Smith, D.E., et al.: Am. J. Clin. Nutr., *40*:1219–1223, 1984.

(From Walsh, J.D.: Am. J. Clin. Nutr., *31*:592–596, 1978. With permission of the author and publisher.)

TABLE A-36. OXALATE CONTENT OF SELECTED FOODS AND FOOD GROUPS

FOODS TO USE: THESE CONTAIN SMALL AMOUNTS OF OXALATE
0–2 mg OXALATE PER SERVING

Vegetables	Fruits	Beverages	Miscellaneous
Broccoli	Avocados	Apple juice	Butter
Brussels sprouts	Bananas	Barley water	Cheese, cheddar
Cabbage	Cherries	Beer, bottled	Chicken noodle soup
Cauliflower	Grapes, Thompson seedless	Cider	Cornflakes
Chives	Mangoes	Coca-Cola	Eggs
Cucumbers	Melons	Grapefruit juice	Egg noodle (chow mein)
Lettuce	Nectarines	Lemon squash drink (lemonade)	Fish (except sardines)
Mushrooms	Peaches, canned	Lucozade, bottled	Jelly with allowed fruit
Onions	Hiley	Milk	Lemon juice
Peas	Stokes	Orange juice	Lime juice
Potatoes, white	Pineapples	Pepsi-Cola	Macaroni
Radishes	Plums, golden gage, green gage	Pineapple juice	Margarine
Rice		Sherry, dry	Meats
Turnips		Wine	Oatmeal, porridge
			Oxtail soup
			Poultry
			Red plum jam
			Sweets, boiled

FOODS TO AVOID: THESE CONTAIN LARGE AMOUNTS OF OXALATE
>15 mg OXALATE PER SERVING

Vegetables	Fruits	Beverages	Miscellaneous
Beans in tomato sauce	Blackberries	Beer, lager	Chocolate
Beets	Blueberries	Tuborg Pilsner	Cocoa
Celery	Currants, red	Ovaltine (24 mg/8 oz)	Grits (white corn)

(Continued)

TABLE A-36. CONTINUED

Chard, Swiss	Gooseberries, green	Tea (132–181.2 mg/8 oz)
Collards	Grapes, Concord	Peanuts
Dandelion greens	Lemon peel	Pecans
Eggplant	Lime peel	Soybean crackers
Escarole	Raspberries, black	Wheat germ
Leeks	Rhubarb	
Okra		
Parsley		
Peppers, green		
Pokeweed		
Potatoes, sweet		
Rutabagas		
Spinach		
Squash, summer		

LOW-OXALATE MEAL PLAN (40–50 mg)

	Little or No Oxalate Content <2 mg Oxalate/Serving Eat as Desired	Moderate Oxalate Content 2–10 mg Oxalate/Serving Limit: 2 (½ cup) Servings/Day	High Oxalate Content >10 mg Oxalate/Serving Avoid Completely
Foods			
Beverages/Juices	Apple juice	Coffee, any kind (8 oz serving)	Beer: draft
	Beer, bottled	Cranberry juice (4 oz)	Stout, Guinness Draft
	Coca-Cola (12 oz limit/day)	Grape juice (4 oz)	Lager, Tuborg Pilsner
	Distilled alcohol	Orange juice (4 oz)	Juices containing berries
	Grapefruit juice	Tomato juice (4 oz)	Ovaltine and other mixed
	Lemonade or limeade without peel	Nescafé powder	beverage mixes
	Wine, red, rosé		Tea, cocoa
	Pepsi-Cola (12 oz limit/day)		
	Pineapple juice		

Milk (2 or more cups)
- Tap water (preferred for extra calcium)
- Buttermilk
- Low-fat milk
- Low-fat yogurt with allowed fruit
- Skim milk

Meat Group
- Eggs
- Cheese, cheddar
- Lean lamb, beef, or pork
- Poultry
- Seafood
- Sardines
- Baked beans canned in tomato sauce
- Peanut butter
- Soybean curd (Tofu)

Vegetables
- Brussels sprouts
- Cauliflower
- Cabbage
- Mushrooms
- Onions
- Peas, green
- Potatoes (Irish)
- Radishes
- Asparagus
- Broccoli
- Carrots
- Corn, sweet white, sweet yellow
- Cucumbers, peeled
- Green peas, canned
- Lettuce, iceberg
- Lima beans
- Parsnips
- Tomato, 1 small
- Turnips
- Beans, green, wax, dried
- Beets, tops, root, greens
- Celery
- Chard, Swiss
- Chives
- Collards
- Dandelion greens
- Eggplant
- Escarole
- Kale
- Leeks
- Mustard greens
- Okra
- Parsley
- Peppers, green
- Pokeweed
- Potatoes, sweet
- Rutabagas
- Spinach
- Squash, summer
- Watercress

(Continued)

Fruits	Avocados	Apples	Blackberries
	Banana	Apricots	Blueberries
	Cherries, Bing	Cherries, edible portion	Currants, red
	Grapefruit	Currants, black	Dewberries
	Grapes, Thompson seedless	Oranges, edible portion	Fruit cocktail
	Mangoes	Peaches, Alberta	Gooseberries
	Melons	Pears	Grapes, Concord
	cantaloupe	Pineapples	Lemon peel
	casaba	Plums, Damson	Lime peel
	honeydew	Prunes, Italian	Orange peel
	watermelon		Raspberries
	Nectarines		Rhubarb
	Peaches, Hiley		Strawberries
	Plums, green or Golden Age		Tangerines
Bread Starches	Cornflakes	Cornbread	Fruit cake
	Macaroni	Sponge cake	Grits, white corn
	Noodles	Spaghetti, canned in tomato sauce	Soybean crackers
	Oatmeal		Wheat germ
	Rice		
	Spaghetti		
	White bread		
Fats and Oils	Bacon		Peanuts
	Mayonnaise		Pecans
	Salad dressing		
	Vegetable oils		
Miscellaneous	Jelly or preserves (made with allowed fruits)	Chicken noodle soup, dehydrated	Chocolate, cocoa
	Lemon, lime juice		Pepper (in excess of 1 tsp/day)
	Salt, pepper (1 tsp/day)		Vegetable soup
	Soups with ingredients allowed		Tomato soup
	Sugar		

(From The Low Oxalate Diet Book, General Clinical Research Center, University of California at San Diego Medical Center and San Diego Chapter of National Foundation for Ileitis and Colitis, 1981. With permission.)

TABLE A—37. COMMERCIAL NUTRITION FORMULATIONS FOR ORAL AND TUBE FEEDING*

The sixth and seventh editions included numerous tables providing detailed nutrient composition of a variety of available commercial formulas. In more recent years, the companies making these formulas have uniformly provided updated information in reprints that are widely distributed. These reprints often contain the composition of formulas produced by other companies as well as their own. Additionally, new and revised commercial preparations appear on the market in increasing numbers, whereas some older formulas have been removed. These commercial reference guides make the continued publication of detailed formulations unnecessary and actually undesirable in this volume. Thus, outdated information can be avoided.

A list is provided below of the companies currently producing and marketing such formulations. Address and telephone numbers are included to help the reader to obtain the most current information on a specific product. Each company also produces an enteral product reference list that provides nutrient analysis on each product, as well as other relevant information needed to make informed choices. They may be contacted for such publications or for other educational materials they provide. In addition, a list is included of the names of current formulations by dietary use characteristics.

COMPANY LISTS WITH IDENTIFICATION CODE

CLINTEC Nutrition Company (C)
Affiliated with Baxter Healthcare Corporation
  and Nestles S.A.
Three Parkway North, Suite 500
P.O. Box 760
Deerfield, IL 60015-0760
1-800-422-2752
KENDALL McGAW (K)
2525 McGaw Avenue
P.O. Box 19791
Irvine, CA 92713
714-660-2000
1-800-854-6851 (Technical Assistance)
MEAD JOHNSON ENTERAL NUTRITIONALS (M)
Mead Johnson Nutrition Group
A Bristol Myers Squibb Company
Evansville, IN 47721
1-800-457-3550
ELAN PHARMA (E)
320 Charles Street
Cambridge, MA 02141
617-868-6400
1-800-237-3535
ROSS LABORATORIES (R)
Division of Abbott Laboratories
625 Cleveland Avenue
Columbus, OH 43215
614-227-3333
1-800-544-7495

(Continued)

TABLE A–37. CONTINUED

SANDOZ NUTRITION (S)
5300 West 23rd Street
Minneapolis, MN 55416
1-800-999-9978
SHERWOOD MEDICAL (SH)
1915 Olive Street
St. Louis, MO 63103-1642
314-621-7788
1-800-428-4400
CURRENT LIST OF FORMULATIONS FOR ORAL AND/OR ENTERAL FEEDING BY
DIETARY USE CHARACTERISTICS

Complete Diet Formulations Containing Some Natural Foods with Varying Residue
  Carnation Instant Breakfast (C)
  Carnation Instant Breakfast, no sugar (C)
  Compleat Regular (S)
  Compleat Modified (S)
  Meritene Powder (S)
  Sustagen (M)
  Vitaneed (SH)
Complete Defined-formula Diets with Intact Purified Protein, Low Residue, and No
Lactose
  Attain (SH)
  CitriSource (S)
  Citrotein (S)
  Comply (SH)
  Ensure (R)
  Ensure HN (R)
  Ensure Plus (R)
  Ensure Plus HN (R)
  Entrition 0.5 (C)
  Entrition HN (C)
  Fortical (SH)
  Fortison (SH)
  Fortison, L.S. (SH)
  Introlan (E)
  Introlite (R)
  Isocal (M)
  Isocal HCN (M)
  Isocal HN (M)
  Isolan (E)
  Isosource (S)
  Isosource HN (S)
  Isotein HN (S)
  Magnacal (SH)
  Nitrolan (E)
  Nutren 1.0 (C)
  Nutren 1.5 (C)
  Nutren 2.0 (C)
  Nutrilan (E)
  Osmolite (R)
  Osmolite HN (R)

*Data as of July, 1994. In the interim, new products have come on the market. Please refer to individual manufacturers to receive updated product lists.

Portagen (M)
Pre-Attain (SH)
Pre-Fortison (SH)
Promote (R)
Replete Oral (C)
Resource Liquid (S)
Resource Plus Liquid (S)
Ross SLD (R)
Susta II (M)
Sustacal (M)
Sustacal HC (M)
Sustacal 8.8 (M)
Travasorb MCT (C)
Two Cal HN (R)
Ultralan (E)

Complete Defined Formula Diets with Intact Purified Protein, No Lactose-Containing Fiber

Ensure with Fiber (R)
Fiberlan (E)
Fibersource (S)
Fibersource HN (S)
Jevity (R)
Nutren with Fiber (C)
Profiber (SH)
Replete with Fiber (C)
Sustacal with Fiber (M)
Ultracal (M)

Defined Formula Diets with Hydrolyzed Protein or Amino Acids, Low Residue, and No Lactose

Accupep HPF (SH)
Alitraq (R)
Criticare HN (M)
Peptamen (C)
Reabilan (E)
Reabilan HN (E)
Tolerex (S)
Travasorb HN (C)
Travasorb (C)
Vital HN (R)
Vivonex T.E.N. (S)

Disease-Specific Formulations

Alterna (R)
Aminess Essential Amino Acid Tablets (C)
Amin-Aid (K)
Glucerna (R)
Hepatic-Aid II (K)
Immun-Aid (K)
Impact (S)
Impact with Fiber (S)
Lipisorb (M)
Nepro (R)

(Continued)

TABLE A—37. CONTINUED

Nutri Hep (C)
Nutrivent (C)
Perative (R)
Protain XL (SH)
Pulmocare (R)
Replena (R)
Replete (C)
Stresstein (S)
Suplena (R)
Traum-Aid HBC (K)
TraumaCal (M)
Travasorb Hepatic (C)
Travasorb Renal (C)

( ) = Company identification, see preceding list.
*O'Brien KMI is now Elan Pharma. The Newtrition product line is now the Elan product line.

TABLE A—38. HUMAN BODY PROPORTIONS FOR ASSESSING AMPUTEES

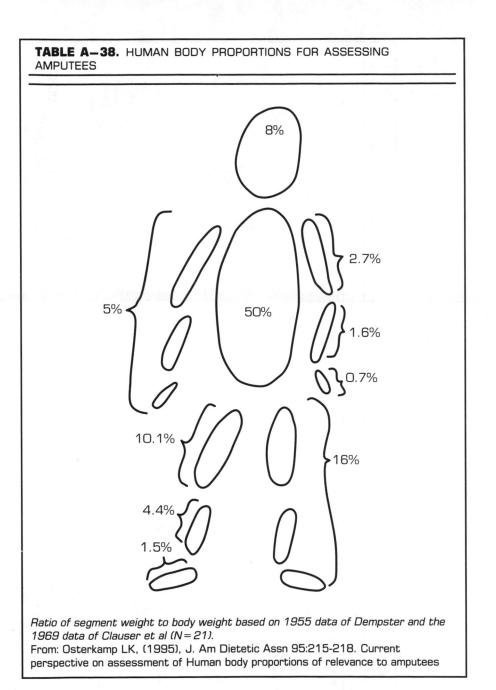

Ratio of segment weight to body weight based on 1955 data of Dempster and the 1969 data of Clauser et al (N = 21).
From: Osterkamp LK, (1995), J. Am Dietetic Assn 95:215-218. Current perspective on assessment of Human body proportions of relevance to amputees

TABLE A–39. NAMES, CODES, AND FORMULAS OF VARIOUS FATTY ACIDS[†]

COMMON NAME	GENEVA NOMENCLATURE	CODE	FORMULA*
Short-chain saturated fatty acids			
butyric acid	butanoic acid	C4:0	$CH_3(CH_2)_2COOH$
Medium-chain saturated fatty acids			
caproic acid	hexanoic acid	C6:0	$CH_3(CH_2)_4COOH$
caprylic acid	octanoic acid	C8:0	$CH_3(CH_2)_6COOH$
capric acid	decanoic acid	C10:0	$CH_3(CH_2)_8COOH$
lauric acid	dodecanoic acid	C12:0	$CH_3(CH_2)_{10}COOH$
Long-chain fatty acids			
myristic acid	tetradecanoic acid	C14:0	$CH_3(CH_2)_{12}COOH$
palmitic acid	hexadecanoic acid	C16:0	$CH_3(CH_2)_{14}COOH$
stearic acid	octadecanoic acid	C18:0	$CH_3(CH_2)_{16}COOH$
palmitoleic acid	9-hexadecaenoic acid	C16:1,n-7 cis	$CH_3(CH_2)_5CH=CH(CH_2)_7COOH$
oleic acid	9-octadecaenoic acid	C18:1,n-9 cis	$CH_3(CH_2)_7CH=CH(CH_2)_7COOH$
elaidic acid	9-octadecaenoic acid	C18:1,n-9 trans	$CH_3(CH_2)_7CH=tCH(CH_2)_7COOH$
linoleic acid	9,12-octadecadienoic acid	C18:2,n-6,9 all cis	$CH_3(CH_2)_4CH=CHCH_2CH=CH(CH_2)_7COOH$
α-linoleic acid	9,12,15-octadecatrienoic acid	C18:3,n-3,6,9 all cis	$CH_3CH_2CH=CHCH_2CH=CHCH_2CH=CH(CH_2)_7COOH$
γ-linoleic acid	6,9,12-octadecatrienoic acid	C18:3,n-6,9,12 all cis	$CH_3(CH_2)_4CH=CHCH_2CH=CHCH_2CH=CH(CH_2)_4COOH$

Common name	Systematic name	Shorthand	Structural formula
columbinic acid	5,9,12-octatrienoic acid	C18: n-6, cis,9 cis, 13 trans	CH₃(CH₂)₄CH=©CHCH₂CH=©CHCH₂CH=tCH(CH₂)₃COOH
Very long-chain fatty acids			
arachidic acid	eicosanoic acid	C20:0	CH₃(CH₂)₁₈COOH
behenic acid	docosanoic acid	C22:0	CH₃(CH₂)₂₀COOH
eicosenoic acid	11-eicosenoic acid	C20:1,n-9 cis	CH₃(CH₂)₇CH=©CH(CH₂)₉COOH
erucic acid	13-docosaenoic acid	C22:1,n-9 cis	CH₃(CH₂)₇CH=©CH(CH₂)₁₁COOH
brassidic acid	13-docosaenoic acid	C22:1,n-9 trans	CH₃(CH₂)₇CH=tCH(CH₂)₁₁COOH
cetoleic acid	11-docosaenoic acid	C22:1,n-11 cis	CH₃(CH₂)₉CH=©CH(CH₂)₉COOH
nervonic acid	15-tetracosaenoic acid	C24:1,n-9 cis	CH₃(CH₂)₇CH=©CH(CH₂)₁₃COOH
"Mead" acid	5,8,11-eicosatrienoic acid	C20:3,n-9,12,15 all cis	CH₃(CH₂)₇CH=©CHCH₂CH=©CHCH₂CH=©CH(CH₂)₃COOH
dihomo-γ-linoleic acid	8,11,14-eicosatrienoic acid	C20:3,n-6,9,12 all cis	CH₃(CH₂)₄CH=©CHCH₂CH=©CHCH₂CH=©CH(CH₂)₆COOH
arachidonic acid	5,8,11,14-eicosatetraenoic acid	C20:4,n-6,9,12, 15 all cis	CH₃(CH₂)₄CH=©CHCH₂CH=©CHCH₂CH=©CHCH₂CH=©CH(CH₂)₃COOH
timnodonic acid	5,8,11,14,17-eicosapentaenoic acid	C20:5,n-3,6,9,12, 15 all cis	CH₃(CH₂CH=©CH)₅(CH₂)₃COOH
clupanodonic acid	7,10,13,16,19-docosapentaenoic acid	C22:5,n-3,6,9,12, 15 all cis	CH₃(CH₂CH=©CH)₅(CH₂)₅COOH
docosahexaenoic acid	4,7,10,13,16,19-docosahexaenoic acid	C22:6,n-3,6,9,12, 15,18 all cis	CH₃(CH₂CH=©CH)₆(CH₂)₂COOH

*t, trans ©, cis

†From Chapter 3 page 72

TABLE A—40. VITAMIN E. ACTIVITIES OF TOCOPHEROL ISOMERS@

COMPOUND	VITAMIN E ACTIVITY
[d]-α-tocopherol (RRR-α-tocopherol)	1.49 IU/mg
[d]-α-tocopheryl acetate (RRR-α-tocopheryl-acetate)	1.36 IU/mg
[dl]-α-tocopherol (all rac-α-tocopherol)	1.1 IU/mg*
[dl]-α-tocopheryl acetate (all rac-α-tocopheryl acetate)	1.0 IU/mg*
"[dl]-α-tocopheryl acetate" ("2-ambo-α-tocopheryl acetate")	1.0 IU/mg
[dl]-β-tocopherol	0.60 IU/mg[†]
[d]-γ-tocopherol	0.15–0.45 IU/mg[†]
[d]-δ-tocopherol	0.015[†]

*The original international standard is no longer available, and the activity of the current replacement compound is being investigated to determine if its specific biologic activity is less than 1 IU/mg.[15,22]

[†]Derived by calculation, since only α vitamers are officially recognized by assigned international units of biologic activity.

(From Bieri, J.G., McKenna, M.C.: Am. J. Clin. Nutr., *34*:289, 1981.)

@From Chapter 18-page 331

TABLE A-41. AVERAGE VITAMIN K CONTENT OF ORDINARY FOODS.[*][†]

FOOD	VITAMIN K µg/100 g	FOOD	VITAMIN K µg/100 g	FOOD	VITAMIN K µg/100 g	FOOD	VITAMIN K µg/100 g
Milk and milk products		**Fats**		**Vegetables**		**Fruits**	
Butter	30	Beef fat	15	Asparagus	57	Applesauce	2
Cheese	35	Corn oil	0	Beans, green	46	Banana	2
Milk (cow)	1	Safflower oil	10	Broccoli	175	Orange	1
Milk (human)	0.2	**Cereal and grain products**		Cabbage	125	Peach	8
Eggs		Bread	4	Kale	729	Raisin	6
Hens (whole)	11	Maize	5	Lettuce	129	Strawberry	10
Meat and meat products		Oats	10	Peas, green	29	**Beverages**	
Bacon	46	Rice	3	Potato	1	Coffee	38
Beef liver	92	Wheat flour	4	Pumpkin	2	Cola	2
Chicken liver	7	Whole flour	17	Spinach	415	Tea, black	—
Ground beef	7			Tomato	6	Tea, green	712
Ham	15			Turnip greens	650	**Tobacco**	
Pork liver	25			Watercress	80	Cigarettes	5000
Pork tenderloin	11			White turnip	1		

(Data from Shearer, M.J., Allan, V., Haroon, Y., et al.: *In* Vitamin K Metabolism and Vitamin K-Dependent Proteins. Edited by J.W. Suttie. Baltimore, University Park Press, 1980, pp. 317–327; Dam, H., Glavind, J.: Biochem. J., *32*:485–490, 1938; Matschiner, J.T., Doisy, E.A. Jr.: J. Nutr., *90*:97–100, 1966; and Doisy, E.A. Jr.: Private communication.)

[*]1 µg vitamin K_1 = 2.2 nmol
[*]From Chapter 19, page 345
[†]An expanded table of the Vitamin K content of foods has been published recently by Booth SL, Sadowski JA, Weihrauch JL, Ferland G in J Food Composition and Analysis 6:109-120, 1993.

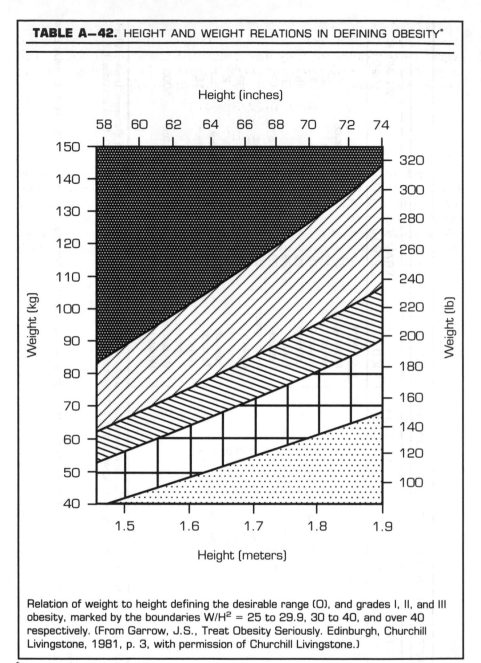

Relation of weight to height defining the desirable range (O), and grades I, II, and III obesity, marked by the boundaries W/H^2 = 25 to 29.9, 30 to 40, and over 40 respectively. (From Garrow, J.S., Treat Obesity Seriously. Edinburgh, Churchill Livingstone, 1981, p. 3, with permission of Churchill Livingstone.)

*From Chapter 59 page 986

As pointed out in Chapter 59 overweight is based on two simple measurements: height without shoes and weight with minimal clothing. The weight/height^2 (W/H^2), called the body mass index (BMI), is then calculated, with weight expressed in kilograms and height in meters. The population, whether male or female, can be divided for degree of obesity as follows:

$$\text{Grade III: W/H}^2 > 40$$
$$\text{II: W/H}^2 \text{ 30 to 40}$$
$$\text{I: W/H}^2 \text{ 25 to 29.9}$$
$$\text{O: W/H}^2 \text{ 20 to 24.9}$$

The BMI range of 20 to 24.9, classified as normal, coincides well with the normal mortality ratio derived from life insurance tables. The mortality ratio begins to increase at BMI levels above 25, and it is here that health professionals should be concerned.

Although the increase in mortality in grade I obesity (W/H^2 = 25 to 29.9) is not great, it is of importance because it is transitional to grades II and III, which truly create health risks for the individual.

TABLE A–43. COMPOUNDS WHOSE ABSORPTION MAY BE REDUCED BY FOOD OR FOOD SUPPLEMENTS[@]

COMPOUND	DOSAGE FORM
Amoxycillin	Capsules
Ampicillin	Capsules
Aspirin	Tablets
Aspirin, calcium	Tablets
Atenolol	Tablets
Captopril	Tablets
Cephalexin	Capsules, suspension
Demeclocycline (demethylchlortetracycline)	Capsules
Doxycycline	Capsules
Ethanol	Solution
Folic acid	Tablets*
Hydrochlorothiazide	Tablets
Iron	Solution, tablets
Isoniazid	Tablets
Ketoconazole	Tablets
Levodopa	Tablets
Lincomycin	Capsules
Methacycline	
Nafcillin	Tablets
Oxytetracycline	
Penicillamine	Tablets
Penicillin G	Tablets, suspension
Penicillin V (K)	Capsules, suspension, tablets
Penicillin V (Ca)	Tablets
Penicillin V (acid)	Tablets
Phenacetin	Suspension
Phenazone (antipyrine)	Syrup
Phenethicillin	Capsules, tablets
Phenylmercaptomethylpenicillin	Capsules
Phenytoin	Capsules[†]
Pivampicillin	Capsules
Propantheline	Tablets
Rifampicin	
Sotalol	Tablets
Tetracycline	Capsules
Theophylline	Capsules, controlled release[‡]

*Absorption reduced by calcium carbonate.

[†]Absorption reduced by folic acid and by enteral formula.

[‡]Absorption reduced by controlled release preparation of theophylline (Theo-Dur Sprinkle, Key Pharmaceuticals).

(Adapted from Welling, P.: Nutrient effects on drug metabolism and action in the elderly. Drug-Nutrient Interac., *4:*183, 1985.)

[@]from Chapter 78-page 1404

TABLE A–44. COMPOUNDS WHOSE ABSORPTION MAY BE INCREASED BY FOOD OR FORMULA@

COMPOUND	DOSAGE FORM
Alafostalin	Capsules
Canrenone	Tablets
Carbamazepine	Tablets
Chlorothiazide	Tablets
Dextropropoxyphene	Capsules
Diazepam	Tablets
Dicoumarol	Tablets
Diftalone	Capsules
Griseofulvin	Tablets or capsule
Hydralazine	Tablets
Hydrocholorothiazide	Tablets
Labetalol	Tablets
Lithium citrate	Tablets
Mebendazole	Tablets
Methoxsalen	Coated tablets
Metoprolol	Tablets
Nitrofurantoin	Capsules, tablets
Phenytoin	Capsules
Pivampicillin	Capsules
Propranolol	Capsules
Riboflavin*	Tablets, solution
Riboflavin-5'-phosphate*	Tablets, solution
Sulfamethoxydiazine	Tablets
α-Tocopherol nicotinate	Capsules

*Absorption is slowed by increased by food by specific dietary fiber sources including bran and by a glucose polymer solution (Polycose.Ross).

(Adapted from Welling, P.: Nutrient effects on drug metabolism and action in the elderly. Drug-Nutrient Interact., 4:193, 1985.)

@from Chapter 78 page 1405

TABLE A—45. WATER FORMED IN THE METABOLISM OF TISSUE AND CALORIC SOURCES*

SOURCE	AMOUNT
Muscle	1 g yields 0.85 ml (0.1 ml from protein + 0.75 ml cellular water)
Mixed tissue	100 kcal yields 10 ml
Fat	1 g yields 1.0 ml
Protein	1 g yields 0.4 ml
Glucose	1 g yields 0.64 ml
Glucose · H_2O	1 g yields 0.60 ml
Mixed diet	100 kcal yields 20 ml
Example: High-glucose TPN solution	
750 ml 10% amino acids	= 300 kcal yields 30 ml H_2O
1175 ml 50% glucose/water	= 2,000 kcal yields 353 ml H_2O
143 ml 10% lipid	= 157 kcal yields 14 ml H_2O
Total: 2068 ml	= 2,457 kcal yields 397 ml H_2O
Example: Glucose-lipid TPN solution	
750 ml 10% amino acids	= 300 kcal yields 30 ml H_2O
750 ml 50% glucose/water	= 1,275 kcal yields 225 ml H_2O
500 ml 20% lipid	= 1,000 kcal yields 100 ml H_2O
Total: 2,000 ml	= 2,575 kcal yields 355 ml H_2O

*from Chapter 80 page 1434